NUTRITION

ASSESSMENT SUPPORT AND MANAGEMENT

Anne Grant, M.S., R.D., C.D.

Susan DeHoog, R.D., C.D.

Fifth Edition, Revised and Expanded

First Edition 1977

Second Edition/Revision 1979

Third Edition/Expanded and Revised 1985

Fourth Edition/Revised/Expanded 1991

Fifth Edition/Revised/Expanded 1999

PUBLISHERS

Anne Grant

Susan DeHoog

    P.O. Box 75057

    Northgate Station

    Seattle, WA 98125

    (206) 362-9323 (MESSAGE)

    (425) 885-2849 (MESSAGE AND/OR FAX)

    (10:00 am - 4:00 pm PST)

AUTHORS

Anne Grant, M.S., R.D., C.D.

    Critical Care Dietitian

    University of Washington Medical Center

    Seattle, WA

Susan DeHoog, R.D., C.D.

    Associate Director Food and Nutrition

    University of Washington Medical Center

    Seattle, WA

CONTRIBUTORS

Joan Zerzan, M.S.,R.D.,C.D.

    NICU Dietitian

    University of Washington Medical Center

    Seattle, WA

    Pediatrics

CONTENTS

Introduction

INTRODUCTION

Nutrition is an integral component of medical disease prevention, treatment and recovery and can have a direct impact on patients/clients health or medical condition. Current interest in nutrition, the recognition of the significance of nutrition care to the maintenance and improvement of health, the rising concern about costs of health care, quality of health care, as well as the issue of health insurance coverage, lends credence to nutrition intervention. Nutrition care is delivered in hospitals, long-term care facilities, nursing homes, congregate feeding sites, patients' homes and physicians offices/clinics. Market forces continue to emphasize decreasing costs and improved services provided.

Nutrition care reflects interdisciplinary treatment. Integrated nutrition care should involve the patient, physician, dietitian, nurse, pharmacist, social worker and other disciplines as appropriate. Patients perceive improved care when a team approach is taken to address their health problems.

Preventative nutrition care decreases the major effect of poor nutrition and poor eating habits on several expensive health problems. Examples include; birth defects, anemia, diabetes, coronary heart disease, hypertension, dental disease and obesity. In some cases, diet is the basic means of managing the disease. Benefits of nutrition support are:

- Improved nutritional status
- Reduced morbidity and mortality
- Potential for decreased length of stay
- Decreased costs to patients and facility
- Reduced liability

Evidence suggests that a significant amount of malnutrition still exists in our hospitals today. Malnutrition in adults occurs in all diagnoses. The likelihood of developing malnutrition (LOM) has been reduced over the past 20 years. High LOMs still are associated with longer hospital stays as shown by recent studies. The nutritional status of hospitalized patients does not decline as much but the importance of nutritional status in the prediction of length of stay and mortality has been confirmed. With the cost of health care increasing and fewer people covered by insurance, patients frequently delay medical exams, which leads to increasing acuity levels in hospitals. The escalation of medical costs has led to legislation aimed at reducing the national health bill. Nutrition is cost-effective as demonstrated by published information:

- Malnutrition is not an acceptable treatment that improves outcome.
- Malnutrition is still a major problem among hospitalized patients.
- Incidence of major infectious and noninfectious complications increase two to six fold in malnourished patients. Death rates increase at least two to four fold.
- Complications significantly increase length of stay and result in increased costs.
- Technology exists to detect, prevent and treat most instances of malnutrition.
- Research shows nutrition intervention and/or support can correct malnutrition and prevent costly complications.

Malnutrition is a hidden cost. Components of the cost are: direct costs (hospital, physician, drug payments); morbidity costs (lost work, earnings and productivity); and mortality costs (future value of earnings lost). Malnourished patients have longer hospital stays, experience slower healing and more complications.

Undesirable medical practices that continue to affect medical and surgical patients hospitalized for seven days or more include:

- Failure to record height and weight routinely
- Prolonged use of glucose and saline intravenous fluid
- Failing to adequately observe all food intake
- Withholding meals for diagnostic tests
- Maintaining NPO status for prolonged periods
- Failure to recognize increased metabolic needs due to stress, illness, and injury
- Undue reliance on antibiotics and lack of knowledge of the importance of nutrition to the immune system
- Inadequate monitoring of nutrition status
- Failure to give adequate nutrition support after surgery
- Delay of nutrition support until depletion is advanced

All who have acute or chronic illness are at nutrition risk and should be evaluated. Other population groups where malnutrition is not uncommon include those who are:

- Obese
- Cachexic
- Elderly
- Adolescent
- Pregnant and adolescent
- Traumatized

Malnutrition has far reaching consequences if allowed to develop or if left untreated. Consequences include:

- Loss of protein and fat store
- Decreased immune competence
- Increased incidence of infection
- Decreased enzyme function
- Decreased ventilatory response
- Fluid and electrolyte imbalance
- Endocrine imbalance
- Increased morbidity and mortality
- Family stress and delayed return to work

Physical and biochemical findings in malnutrition vary with the severity of malnutrition. The table below compares the characteristics of several malnourished states found in adults. The severity of malnutrition is related to the magnitude and duration of nutritional deprivation.

Comparison of Adult Malnourished States

Cause	Anthropometric Measures	Biochemistry Signs	Other clinical Support	Nutritional
Adult Kwashiorkor Protein deficient diet plus catabolic stress in previously well nourished. Rapid onset.	Tend to be maintained due to rapid onset.	Serum proteins depressed.	Edema, altered electrolyte metabolism.	Supplement with fluids, electrolytes, vitamins, protein and minerals.
Adult Marasmus Prolonged and gradual wasting of muscle mass and subcutaneous fat. Poor calorie and protein intake.	Depressed.	Serum proteins normal.	No edema.	Oral feeding of calories and protein. Weight loss more than 20 to 30% requires aggressive support.
Marasmic Kwashiorkor Advanced stage of marasmus. Calorie and protein reserves depressed.	Depressed.	Serum proteins depressed.	Edema. Deterioration of multiple organ systems.	Feeding (oral, parenteral, or both) needed promptly to avoid mortality.

Poor nutritional status is prevalent in nursing homes. More than 50 percent of residents may be malnourished and up to 35% of the residents may suffer dehydration. The most common problems include:

- Under/over weight
- Hypoalbuminemia
- Loss of appetite secondary to depression or drugs
- Hydration and electrolyte imbalance
- Pressure sores
- Chewing and swallowing problems
- Uncontrolled blood sugars or blood pressure

Economic Benefits of Nutrition

Health promotion and disease prevention nutrition programs are necessary, cost-effective, and humanitarian measures for the prevention of and delay in the progression toward disease. Nutrition, the cornerstone of treatment, can prevent, postpone, or mitigate the onset or progression of some diseases, thus saving health care dollars.

In preventative care the goals are to keep people healthy in their communities, reduce the incidence and severity of preventable diseases, improve health and quality of life, and reduce total medical costs, particularly costs for medication, hospitalization, and extended care. The advances of science continue to bring an increasing complexity to health care reform and the aging of America.

In acute care nutrition services play a vital role in the recovery of patients. Evidence indicates that nutrition intervention corrects malnutrition, prevents disease complications, and speeds recovery. To be cost-effective, emphasis should be placed on minimizing iatrogenic malnutrition and unnecessarily prolonged hospitalization.

Medical nutrition therapy provides a cost-effective way to keep people healthy in ambulatory care. Nutrition in outpatient care is a cost-effective way to keep patients/clients healthy and save health care dollars.

In home care, excessive costs can be reduced if the care plan includes nutrition treatment and if patients on enteral and parenteral nutrition therapy are assessed and treated with a sound outcome-based nutrition care plan.

In long-term care, nutrition services should be provided to improve the quality of life, slow the rate of physical deterioration, and prevent further costly hospitalization or the need for a higher level of care. The elderly in nursing homes are prone to suffer from protein-calorie malnutrition as well as from certain micronutrient deficiencies.

Quality nutrition care is essential to decreasing morbidity, mortality, and attendant health care costs for the older American. The elderly make up almost 12 percent of the population but account for 36 percent of health care costs and 30% or more of all hospital stays and drug prescriptions. Eighty-five percent of the older population has a chronic disease such as diabetes, hypertension or cancer. Provision of nutrition decreases costs of medical and institutional care, surgery, and drug therapy. The advances of science continues to bring an increasing complexity to health care along with the aging of America.

The following flow-chart demonstrates the potential economic benefits of nutrition intervention.

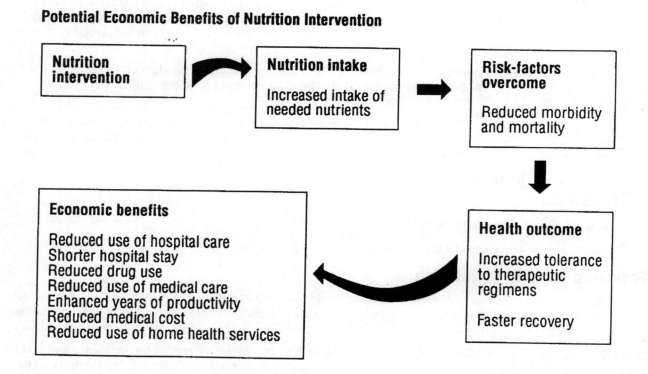

Potential Economic Benefits of Nutrition Intervention

Nutrition intervention

Nutrition intake

Increased intake of needed nutrients

Risk-factors overcome

Reduced morbidity and mortality

Health outcome

Increased tolerance to therapeutic regimens

Faster recovery

Economic benefits

Reduced use of hospital care
Shorter hospital stay
Reduced drug use
Reduced use of medical care
Enhanced years of productivity
Reduced medical cost
Reduced use of home health services

MEDICAL NUTRITION THERAPY PLANNING AND MANAGEMENT

Medical nutrition therapy is an integral part of medical therapy and must be implemented if patients are to receive maximum benefits from their medical therapy. It is well recognized that all patients should receive nutrition support within a few days, if not hours, following hospital admission. Early intervention is the key to minimizing the adverse effects of malnutrition. Also, it has been documented in the literature patients who are not severely compromised may not benefit from aggressive nutrition support. Therefore, a process for assessing who is at nutritional risk is important.

Nursing home populations are increasing. By the year 2000, the nursing home population is expected to be 2.1 million. The elderly are a rapidly growing group with approximately five percent of the elderly population residing in nursing homes.

Multiple risk factors are common among residents of long-term care facilities: 88 percent are elderly; 63 percent are immobile and 47 percent are incontinent. Malnutrition is a major risk factor for the development of pressure ulcers. Immobile patients are at the greatest risk for malnutrition followed by those who are incontinent with fecal matter being the most destructive to tissue. Provision of quality nutrition care over extended time periods presents a challenge.

MEDICAL NUTRITION THERAPY PROCESS

Medical nutrition therapy or the nutrition care process is a system for identifying, planning and meeting the nutrition needs of individuals. The process is not restricted to the hospitalized patient and can be applied in all settings. The components consist of screening, assessment, implementation, documentation, evaluation and/or monitor, and education.

SCREENING

Screening is the first step in determining who is at nutritional risk. The process identifies the appropriate degree of nutrition intervention required in a timely outcome-based, cost-effective manner. Screening identifies patients at risk for malnutrition or those suspected of becoming at risk due to disease and/or treatment modalities. Screening can occur in multiple settings: the home (home health care), the clinic/physician office, congregate feeding sites, long term care facilities, and the hospital. Screening can be done by individuals, such as the dietitian and dietetic technician, or it can be a multidisciplinary process.

The goals of screening are to determine who needs priority nutrition care and who needs further assessment. The screening process involves two steps:

- **Chart Review:** Includes height and weight, physical exam, problem list, labs, indication of constant fever, blood pressure, diet order or lack of, and the diagnosis.

- **Patient Interview:** Addresses estimated height and usual weight, weight patterns, past diet modifications, allergies, food intolerances, chronic medication use (to identify drug/nutrient interactions for appropriate counseling), diet history, and nutrition supplements.

Nutrition intervention may be based on diagnosis alone. A detailed screen (**Figure 1**) of every patient may be unnecessary and impractical.

Figure 1: Nutrition Screen

DATE	TIME

S:

WEIGHT CHANGE	N	V	D	APPETITE CHANGE	DYSPHAGIA/CHEWING DIFFICULTY
☐ Yes ☐ No ☐ N/A				☐ Yes ☐ No ☐ N/A	☐ Yes ☐ No ☐ N/A

VITAMIN/MINERAL SUPPLEMENT	FOOD ALLERGIES
☐ Yes ☐ No Specify:	

SPECIAL DIET

OTHER

O:

AGE	HEIGHT	WEIGHT	USUAL WEIGHT	USUAL WEIGHT %	IDEAL WEIGHT	IDEAL WEIGHT %	SERUM ALBUMIN
							gm/dl ☐ WNL ☐ Depletion

DIAGNOSIS

DIET ORDER

A:

NUTRITIONAL STATUS

☐ High Risk ☐ Moderate Risk ☐ Not Compromised   Further R.D./D.T. Intervention Needed   ☐ Yes ☐ No

COMMENTS

P:

☐ Provide Basic Nutrition Services. Re-evaluate In   5   7   10   Days (Circle One).

☐ Screening Data Not Available. Please Order: _____

☐ Nutritional Assessment _____

☐ Nutrient Intake Analysis (NIA) _____

☐ Nutrition Counseling/Diet Instruction: _____

Drug Nutrient Interaction Identified ☐ Yes ☐ No   OTHER

Action Taken:
☐ Patient At Nutritional Risk/Referal To Dietitian
☐ Information Sheet Given To Patient

A short simple screen (**Figure 2**) may be used for patient populations historically known not at nutritional risk. It also meets the Joint Commission on Accreditation of Hospitals Organization recommendations for nutrition care being multidisciplinary (**Figure 3**). This information can be incorporated into the nursing assessment form, thus meeting the recommendations of assessing within 24 hours of admission.

Figure 2: Short Screen

Nutrition Screen

O: Diagnosis: _____

Height: _____ Weight: _____ UBW: _____ IBW: _____

A: Nutritional Status:

Per review of medical record, patient is not nutritionally compromised at this time.

Drug/Nutrient Interaction Identified: Yes _____ No _____

☐ Previously instructed

P: 1. Provide basic nutrition services.

    2. Will re-evaluate in 6 days or per consult.

Signature _____

Figure 3: Multidisciplinary Screen

Date: _____

S: ☐ Nausea ☐ Diarrhea ☐ Swallowing Problems

☐ Vomiting ☐ Constipation ☐ Chewing Problems

Appetite change ☐ Yes ☐ No

O: Diagnosis: _____ PMH: _____

Diet Order: _____ Pertinent Drugs: _____

Food Allergies: _____ Vit/Min Supp: _____

Height: _____ Admitting Weight: _____ Current Weight: _____

UBW: _____ % UBW _____ IBW: _____ % IBW: _____

A. Chart reviewed and patient interviewed

☐ Nutrition screen indicates potential for compromised nutrition status.

☐ Patient determined not to be nutritionally compromised at this time.

P: ☐ Basic nutrition care to be provided

☐ Nutrition Assessment requested

☐ Re-evaluate if medical conditions changes or in six days

Signature: _____

The screening method will depend upon the facility's policies and procedures. All facilities should have screening policies (see examples).

Examples:

The clinical nutrition staff and/or multidisciplinary staff should identify all patients who need nutrition care (moderate and high nutritional risk) through an established screening process within 24 hours of admission.

All patients with an anticipated LOS > 3 days will be screened for nutritional risk within 24 hours of admission.

Procedure:

All patients* will be screened within 24 hours of admission and assigned the proper level of nutrition care.

*Exceptions may be neurosurgery, orthopedics (foot/ankle, shoulder, hand, hips, knee if less than 65 years of age), sports medicine, ophthalmology, kidney stones, kidney infection, gynecology-oncology nontumor, vaginal hysterectomy, UTIs,**, general psych, general OB, ante/postpartum, limited stay and those readmitted within 3 days of discharge, and those assessed during the screening process.

**These patients are screened and/or assessed under the following conditions: consultation requested, NPO/Cl liq > 3 days and hospital stay exceeding seven days. If a non-compromised patient and/or excepted patient exceeds the length of expected stay, the patient should be reevaluated for nutritional status. Documentation in the medical record stating the patients nutritional status should follow the reevaluation.

If staff is limited, the screening process must be simple, efficient and applicable to the patient population. The criteria used for the process must be specific. **Table 1** demonstrates screening criteria that can be used for major medical centers and acute care hospitals. Risk factors are **diagnosis/treatment**: high probable effect on nutrition status, nutrition requirements, on ingestion, digestion, absorption and/or utilization of food; **age** of < 18 and > 65 captures children and the elderly; **labs**: may reflect abnormal nutrition status and/or require dietary modification; **drugs:** may seriously affect the ability to ingest, absorb or utilize nutrients and require monitoring of lab indices to determine efficacy of, or need for, dietary modification; and **weight:** indicating poor intake and loss of lean body mass.

Table 1: Screening Indicators for Nutritional Risk

	High Risk	Moderate Risk
Age	> 75	65 - 74
	1 Point	**1 Point**
System Cardiovascular	Congestive heart failure Cardiac Transplant Cardiac Cachexia Cardiomypathy	Uncomplicated CABG Mitral valve Replacement Coronary Artery Disease Myocardial Infarct Cardiovascular Accident Hypertension Hyperlipidemia
Endocrine	DKA HHND IDDM - Pregnancy Nephrogenic Diabetes Insipidus Newly Diagnosed Diabetic	Gestational Diabetic Controlled Diabetes
Cancer Leukemia Neoplastic Gastric Cancer	ALL AML BMT Head and Neck Pancreatic/Liver Breast - Stage III Ovarian - Stage III Multiple Myleoma Osteosarcoma Radiation/Chemo Treatment	Non Hodgkin's Lymphoma Oral Hodgkin's Disease Breast - Stage II Ovarian - Stage II Lung w/o surgery Prostate w/o surgery
Gastrointestinal Esophagus Stomach Large Colon Small Intestine	Varices Gastric Surgery, Ileostomy GI Fistulas Acute Crohn's Gastric Outlet Obstruction Acute Gastroenteritis Gastrectomy, Billroth I,II Whipple Celiac Disease	Short Bowel Syndrome Irritable Bowel - Chronic Ulcerative Colitis - Chronic Colostomy Vagotomy
Hepatic	End Stage Liver Disease Liver Transplant Cirrhosis Encephalopathy Zollinger-Ellison Syndrome	Alcoholism Substance Abuse

	High Risk	**Moderate Risk**
Immune Deficiency	AIDS Multi Organ Failure Sepsis, Septicemia Multiple Trauma, Burns	HIV Epstein-Barr Bacterial Endocarditis
Neurological	ALS Acute Spinal Cord Injury	Chronic Spinal Cord Injury Guillain-Barre Syndrome Multiple Sclerosis Myasthenia Gravis Huntington's Chorea Parkinson's Alzheimers
Pancreatic	Acute Pancreatitis Pancreatic Insufficiency Pancreas Transplant Biliary Cirrhosis	Chronic Pancreatitis
Psychiatric	Anorexia Nervosa	Bulimia
Pulmonary	Cystic Fibrosis COPD Respiratory Failure Acute Respiratory Distress Lung-Heart Transplant	Stable Home Dialysis
Renal	Acute Renal Failure Chronic Renal Failure Kidney Transplant End Stage Renal Disease Nephrotic Syndrome	
	2 Point/Diagnosis	**1 Point**
Weight	75 - 80% - UBW 75% - IBW	80 - 90% - UBW
Unintentional Weight loss	> 10% loss - 6 months > 5% loss - 1 month 7.5% loss - 3 months Elderly - BMI < 24 or > 27	< 10% - 6 months
Obesity	Severe > 150% IBW > 40 BM I	> 130% IBW Moderate - BMI > 30 Mild - BMI > 27.5
	2 Points	**1 Point**
Labs	Albumin 2.8 gm/dL or < Prealbumin 10 mg/dL or <	Albumin 2.8 - 3.5 gm/dL Prealbumin 10 - 15 mg/dL
	2 Points	**1 Point**
Feeding Modalities	Impaired ability to ingest or absorb Parenteral Nutrition Enteral (tube) Feeding NPO/Cl Liq > 5 days	NPO/Cl Liq > 3 days

	High Risk	**Moderate Risk**
	2 Points	**1 Point**
Drug/Nutrient Interactions	Chronic use Drugs identified per protocol impacting nutritional status and/or have drug/nutrient implications	Multiple medications (> 5)
	1 Point	**1 Point**
Subjective Nutritional Factors	PO intake < 25% x 3 days Vomiting 2 - 5x past 24 hrs Aspiration Risk Diarrhea 2 - 3 stools per day Nausea no significant po intake Swallowing Problems Procedures: major surgery, long term chemo	PO intake < 50% x 3 days Chewing Problems Procedures: rehabilitation short stay chemo
	1 Point	**1 Point**

Nutritional status should be determined from the following major categories:

- Diagnosis
- Weight/weight patterns
- Age
- Labs
- Feeding modality

Points are totaled to determine the nutritional risk classification. Nutritional risk includes:

- Documented malnutrition
- PN/PPN/TF
- > 6 points = high nutritional risk
- 4 - 6 points = moderate nutritional risk
- 0 - 3 points = not compromised

Nutritional status can quickly be determined by using disease state, weight loss and a prealbumin, if available. With patients entering the hospital at a higher acuity level, attention to the patient's nutritional needs and status is imperative.

Screening in nursing homes follows a process defined by Health Care Finance Association (HCFA). The process is as follows:

Minimum Data Set (MDS)
↓
Resident Assessment Protocols (RAPS)
↓
Interdisciplinary Care Plan (ICP)

MDS is a basic screening tools that identifies risk factors associated with possible functional decline. Factors affecting nutritional status are: disease/diagnosis-health conditions such as constipation, fecal impaction, diarrhea, edema, pain, SOB, vomiting; oral status – chewing problems, swallowing, mouth pain/sores, ill fitting dentures, no dentures, missing teeth, dry mouth, taste changes, oral abscesses and inflamed gums; skin conditions - pressure ulcers; medications; and special treatments such as chemotherapy, radiation, dialysis, tube feeding and parenteral nutrition.

RAPS that specifically address nutrition concerns are: nutrition status, feeding tubes, dehydration/fluid maintenance, dental and pressure ulcers

ICP has three major elements: 1) problem identification; 2) measurable, time-limited goals that seek to maximize strengths, treat weaknesses, rehabilitate and prevent deterioration; and 3) plan of action, including follow-up.

The results of the assessment and RAPs are used to develop a comprehensive nutrition care plan.

Figure 4 is a screening form that can be used in the admitting office. It must be verified when the patient is admitted on the nursing unit.

Figure 4: Admission Screening Nutrition Questionnaire

1. Height: _____ Usual Weight: _____ Actual Weight: _____

2. Have you had a recent weight loss greater than 10 pounds within 30 days?
   ☐ Yes ☐ No

3. Have you been on a weight reduction diet? ☐ Yes ☐ No

4. Have you had a recent change in appetite? ☐ Yes ☐ No

5. Do you have any problems with:
   - Swallowing ☐ Yes ☐ No
   - Chewing ☐ Yes ☐ No
   - Nausea ☐ Yes ☐ No
   - Diarrhea ☐ Yes ☐ No
   - Vomiting ☐ Yes ☐ No
   - Constipation ☐ Yes ☐ No

6. Do you follow any special diet? ☐ Yes ☐ No
   If yes, What? _____

7. What foods are you allergic to?

8. Do you take any vitamin/mineral supplement? ☐ Yes ☐ No
   If yes, please list. _____

9. Do you take any medications? ☐ Yes ☐ No
   If yes, please list: Prescription _____
                        Over-the-counter _____

Figure 5 is a screen for healthy populations. It can be used at health fairs or other gatherings.

Figure 5: Screen Form for the Healthy Population

Name: _____ Age: _____ Sex: _____

Ht: _____ Current Wt: _____ Usual Wt: _____ % Usual Wt: _____

IBW: _____ % IBW: _____

Weight History:

Have you gained or lost weight in the past:

Month	☐ Gained	☐ Lost	Amount _____
6 Months	☐ Gained	☐ Lost	Amount _____
Year	☐ Gained	☐ Lost	Amount _____
2 Years	☐ Gained	☐ Lost	Amount _____

Have you had a change in appetite? ☐ Yes ☐ No

Explain:

Do you take any vitamin/mineral supplements? ☐ Yes ☐ No

List:

Do you follow a special diet at home? ☐ Yes ☐ No

What Kind?

For the elderly in congregate feeding situations **Figure 6** can be used.

Figure 6: Nutrition Questionnaire for the Elderly/Congregate Feeding

1. Age: _____ Height: _____ Weight: _____ BMI: _____

2. Have you had a recent weight loss over the past 6 months?

    ☐ Yes ☐ No How much? _____

3. Have you had a recent change in appetite? ☐ Yes ☐ No

4. Do you have any problems with:

    Swallowing   ☐ Yes ☐ No

    Chewing   ☐ Yes ☐ No

    Nausea   ☐ Yes ☐ No

    Diarrhea   ☐ Yes ☐ No

    Vomiting   ☐ Yes ☐ No

    Constipation ☐ Yes ☐ No

    Pain in the:

        Mouth ☐ Yes ☐ No

        Teeth ☐ Yes ☐ No

        Gums ☐ Yes ☐ No

5. Dietary: _____ number of meals per day _____ meets the RDA

    _____ eats alone _____ allergies

    _____ vit/min supplements

    If yes, please list.

6. Do you take any medications?   ☐ Yes ☐ No

    If yes, please list: Prescription: _____

                            Over-the-counter _____

7. Living conditions: ☐ Lives alone ☐ Poverty level

8. Functional Status:

    ☐ Difficulty shopping ☐ Difficulty preparing food ☐ Difficulty dressing

ASSESSMENT

The first phase of medical nutrition therapy is the nutrition assessment process. Assessment of nutritional status is ideal for everyone during the life cycle and during illness. This process analyzes medical, social, dietary and drug histories; clinical/functional status; anthropometry; biochemical; and nutrient needs and intakes. All patients with known or suspected malnutrition should be assessed. Assessment should occur no later than one day after identification or it during the screening process. Information gathered is used to design an outcome-based, cost-effective nutrition care plan, whether the setting is in the hospital, ambulatory care, or long term care. A comprehensive nutrition assessment determines nutritional status by analyzing the following:

Histories

Collection of medical, social, and dietary intake information on an individual or a population routinely has been part of nutritional status surveys. Frequently histories give clues as to the type of nutritional problems which may be encountered. Significant incidence of malnutrition still occurs in U.S. hospitals. The following is merely a screening tool for identifiying factors which may place a patient at risk of developing medical complications unless attention is given to meeting nutritional needs. It is by no means complete. No positive findings probably indicates that a patient is not compromised. The degree of risk increases with the number of positive findings.

Medical   Medical history is reviewed from a nutritional viewpoint, which helps evaluate factors that can affect nutritional status negatively.

- Usual body weight 20% over or under ideal

- Recent recorded height or weight

- Pregnancy: deviation from normal weight gain

- Elderly:
  Mental deterioration
  Constipation or incontinence
  Poor eye sight or hearing
  Physical disability (e.g., stroke, arthritis)
  Slowed reactions (vision, holding utensils, chewing, swallowing)
  Ill-fitting or missing dentures

- Increased metabolic needs:
  Fever
  Infection
  Trauma
  Pregnancy
  Frequent past pregnancies
  Hyperthyroidism
  Infancy
  Burns

- Increased losses:
  Draining fistula
  Open wounds
  Draining abscesses
  Effusions (escape of body fluids into body organs or tissue, e.g., pleural effusion)
  Chronic blood loss
  Chronic renal dialysis
  Exudative enteropathies (excess loss of protein into GI tract)
  Burns

- Chronic diseases:
  Diabetes mellitus
  Hypertension
  Hyperlipidemia
  Coronary heart disease
  Chronic lung disease
  Chronic renal disease
  Chronic liver disease
  Circulatory problems or heart failure
  Carcinoma
  Mental retardation
  Psychosis
  Epilepsy
  Rheumatoid arthritis
  Peptic ulcer disease

- Recent major surgery or illness

- Prolonged comatose state

- Diseases of GI tract:
  Congenital malformations
  Pancreatic insufficiency
  Malabsorption states (e.g., celiac disease, Crohn's disease, parasites, blind loop syndrome, pernicious anemia)
  Severe diarrhea
  GI fistula

- Surgery of GI tract:
  Resection of stomach or small bowel
  Intestinal bypass

- Head and neck trauma or surgery

Social   Social history identifies factors that may impact nutrition status.

- Inadequate income
- Unable to buy food
- Lives alone
- Eats meals alone
- Handicapped
- Drug addiction
- Alcoholism
- Inadequate refrigeration or cooking facilities
- Smokes
- Elderly:
  Confusion due to environment change
  Poor housing
  Unsuitable housing
  Lacks socialization at mealtime
  Psychological problems
  Poverty

Dietary   Diet history refers to a review of the usual pattern of food intake and food selection variables and usually focuses on nutrient intake. Factors that may impact nutritional status are:

- Meals are not adequate for needs
- Poor appetite
- Excess alcohol intake
- Poor fitting dentures
- Limited, fad or monotonous diet
- Lost taste for food
- Dysgeusia (perverted sense of taste)
- Anorexia nervosa
- Chewing or swallowing problems
- Cultural or religious dietary limitations
- Frequent meals away from home
- Unable to eat for more than 10 days
- Maintained on IV fluids for more than 10 days
- Antibiotics superimposed on poor food intake and prolonged use of IV fluids
- Adverse food and drug interactions
- Elderly
  Long-established poor food habits
  Inadequate knowledge of nutrition
  Follows food fads

A diet history provides an understanding of a patient's baseline nutritional status. The aim is to detect subclinical deficiencies. Accuracy of memory of foods consumed does not decline over time necessarily. Nutrition history implies the incorporation of information from laboratory and clinical data as well as from the diet history.

For individuals, food records and recall are the most common methods for estimating dietary intake. Intake is either done by summarizing prospective intake data or by collecting retrospective intake data. The appropriate method selected depends on the purpose for and the setting in which it is done. The goal is to determine the nutrient content of food and appropriate intake for a particular individual. Calcium, iron, sodium and potassium are the minerals most frequently cited for reasons of dietary intervention. Dietary needs are based on age, sex, activity level, nutrient needs, health status, and dietary modifications.

Prospective methods record data at the time the food is consumed or shortly thereafter. The following are prospective methods:

Seven Day Food Record: This documents dietary intake as it occurs. One week is considered the shortest time feasible to ensure validity. The food record is usually more accurate if the food eaten is recorded the day and time it is consumed. The record is calculated and averaged at the end of the seven day period and then compared to the Recommended Dietary Allowances or the Food Guide Pyramid. In a group setting, the patient/client may record all food taken but not what was actually consumed. When used cautiously, an estimated food diary is a valid method for assessing current intake.

Nutrient Intake Analysis (NIA): NIA (calorie count) is used in hospitals or long-term care facilities to monitor intakes to identify nutritional inadequacies, before deficiencies develop. Other risk factors without the NIA may be invalid. For example, weight can be altered by fluid balance and laboratory values change relatively slow compared to timely nutrient intake documentation. The term Nutrient Intake Analysis is more comprehensive than just a calorie count. All NIAs should include and account for a desired outcome.

Ideally, the NIA is recorded for three consecutive days. Complete records accurately reflect average intake. If the record is incomplete, it may be necessary to extend the duration until a intake trend is established.

Reasons for NIAs are inadequate po (to document need for an alternative feeding modality such as TF or PN) and transition from TF or PN. Reasons for discontinuing NIAs are no change in eating is likely to occur, meeting > 50 - 75 percent of estimated needs, no change in nutrition support is indicated, intake based on trends is likely to meet nutrition needs soon and intake is negligible.

NIA results can be interpreted and documented daily or at the end of the three day period. The patient can participate in their nutrition care by recording intake on the menu or on a special form in their room. A graph can be kept in the patients' room or outside the door to record all intakes, which may include enteral, parenteral nutrition and nourishments.

Retrospective: Data includes information from recollection. The following are types of retrospective data:

Food Frequency: The food frequency (FF) is a retrospective review of intake frequency, i.e., food per day, per week and per month. For ease of evaluation, the food frequency organizes food into groups that have common nutrients. Since the food frequency interview is concerned with the frequency of food group usage, rather than specific nutrients, it is helpful to focus on the diet in general rather than specific nutrients. Foods consumed once a week or more are recalled better than foods eaten less often. Foods eaten infrequently are recalled with the least accuracy. FFs have limited accuracy if a wide variety of foods are consumed secondary to decrease in recall. 5 - 15 percent of foods are omitted from food diaries.

FF can provide a relative measure of food consumption and is reproducible and valid for most foods. FF is appropriate for use in examining relationships between diet and risk of disease.

During illness, various food items can change with the stage of illness. It is helpful if the food frequency can be completed for the period immediately prior to hospitalization. If the intake has been poor, as demonstrated by significant weight loss, it is helpful to get a frequency prior to the illness to arrive at an accurate history.

24 Hour Recall: A 24 Hour recall asks the person to list specific foods consumed in the last 24 hours. Problems encountered include the inability to recall accurately the kinds and amount of food eaten; atypical intakes and a tendency toward over-reporting low intakes and under-reporting high intakes. Foods omitted from recall range from 10 - 40 percent. When both food frequency and a 24 hour recall are used, a more accurate estimation of intake can be made. This is termed cross-check.

Reliability and Validity: Validity is the degree to which the method actually assesses the usual intake. Whenever attention is given to an individual's dietary intake, the person may consciously or unconsciously alter their intake to simplify recording or to impress the person seeking the information. This decreases the validity of the intake.

For example, the obese often under-report their intake, whereas, subjects with anorexic nervosa over-report their intake. Poor reporting by the elderly, the very sick, children, alcohol and drug abusers, the confused and those whose food habits are chaotic impair validity. Validity also can be impaired when symptoms or treatment of a medical condition affect the diet. Also, people just simply forget what they consumed. Some reports from years ago are at least as good as more recent memories. Attention should be paid to both the quality and quantity of diet records to ensure the validity of the record. The food diary is used as the criterion for assessing the validity of other methods of collecting food data.

Reliability refers to the consistency of data obtained. Dietary intake should reflect typical food patterns of the individual to have any significance. Some people actually do not have a dietary pattern, which makes it difficult to assess intake. For patterns, memory lapses, lack of knowledge of portion sizes, over and under estimating consumption all jeopardize reliability of the method used.

Drug: A drug history should be part of the diet history. Information should include drug names, dosages, frequencies, reasons for the drugs, how long they have been taken, and how they are taken. This history includes both prescription and over the counter drugs. Factors that may affect nutritional status include:

- Large number of prescription drugs
- Multiple drugs for the same problem
- High drug dosages
- Drugs taken for extended periods
- Drugs taken with nutritional supplements
- Drugs taken with alcohol
- Use of megavitamins
- Use of over-the-counter drugs
- Laxative abuse
- Antacid abuse
- Poor nutritional status
- Marginal diet
- Pregnancy
- Altered renal function

Food and drugs interact in many ways to affect nutritional status and drug therapy effectiveness. Drug monitoring of will identify any effects the drug may have on the ability to ingest, digest, absorb, or use nutrients. Those most susceptible to drug/nutrient interactions are individuals receiving multi-medications, the chronically ill and the elderly.

In recognition of increased pharmalogic therapeutic complexity , patients need to be instructed on the possibility of any food/drug interactions. The goal is to prevent adverse effects and to promote compliance and maximize medication effectiveness.

For more detail, see the section Drug and Nutrient Interactions.

Anthropometry

Assessment of height, weight, and growth is an important part of the nutrition assessment. Anthropometric data is most valuable when accurately measured and recorded over a period of time. The common failure to measure weight and, more often, height hampers nutrition assessment of change and growth.

Measurements such as height, head circumference, weight, and skinfold thickness, reflect present nutritional status. Ethnic, familial, birth weight and environmental factors affect growth and should be taken into consideration.

Height, weight (usual, ideal) and weight patterns are simple measurements to obtain and evaluate. Degree of weight loss is an extremely important index of change in nutritional status because it usually reflects caloric inadequacy, which mandates an increased loss of protein from the body cell mass. An adult can be deemed at nutritional risk if there has been a five percent weight loss in less than one month or a 10 percent loss in less than six months. An individual measurement shows how a person stands relative to the total population, not to an absolute standard, when comparing the information to reference standards.

Height and weight measurements in children are recorded as a percentile, which reflects the percentage of the total population of children of the same sex or below the height or weight at that age. This allows the child's growth at each age, or growth "curve" to be evaluated.

Height and particularly weight are useful in determining nutritional status in adults. Both should be measured because there is a tendency to overestimate height and underestimate weight. Weight loss reflects the recent ability to meet nutritional requirements and thus may indicate nutritional risk. Determination of weight loss percent is highly reflective of the extent of illness.

The following are useful parameters in assessing a hospitalized patient's nutritional status based on weight:
- Height
- Weight: admission, current and normal (usual)
- Weight patterns (percent of weight change over a period of time)
- Percent above/below usual body weight and /or ideal
- Body weight

For more detail, see the section Anthropometric Assessment

Clinical Assessment

During the medical work-up, the medical plan/treatment is addressed. Consideration should be given to the diagnosis or treatment of potential effects on nutrient status or requirements. Also, metabolic or mechanical problems that affect food ingestion, digestion or absorption must be evaluated.

The clinical assessment includes information from the physical examination and medical history. Significant findings may include temporal wasting, proximal muscle weakness, depleted muscle bulk, or tongue atrophy. The appearance of the skin should be noted for pallor, scaly dermatitis, wounds, quality of wound healing, bruising, and hydration status. Membranes (conjunctiva, orpharynx) should be examined for integrity, hydration, pallor, and bleeding.

Muscosal changes of the gastrointestinal tract are reflected in problems such as diarrhea and anorexia. Symptoms of nutrient deficiencies may or may not be apparent in the physical exam.

Functional status should be included in the physical exam. The focus should be on the mechanics and process needed for good nutritional status:
- Dentition – Presence and condition of teeth/ill fitting dentures.
- Coordination – Ability to handle utensils, hand to mouth coordination, and any need for assistive devices.
- Mental status – Alertness and orientation.
- Respiratory status – Shortness of breath, which may impair eating.
- Swallowing – Observe for normal swallowing, including time the food is held in the mouth.
- Positioning – The ability to sit upright while eating.
- Level of assistance – Need for assistance with food preparation, shopping, eating.

Special attention should be paid to loss of mobility, jaundice, depletion of subcutenous fat, muscle wasting, ascites, and edema. Subjective evaluation can include the change in energy level, lethargy, inability to work, inability to perform activities of daily living (ADLs), and the need for custodial care.

Functional status scales are the Karnofsky and ECOG.

Grade ECOG	Scale Karnofsky	Description
0	90 - 100%	Fully active; able to carry on normal activity.
1	80%	Ambulatory and able to carry out light or sedentary work.
1	70%	Cares for self; unable to carry on normal activity and work.
2	60%	Ambulatory and capable of self care; unable to work.
2	50%	Requires considerable assistance and frequent medical care; < 50% of waking hours spent in bed.
3	40%	Disabled; requires special care and assistance.
3	30%	Severely disabled; confined to bed or chair > 50% of waking hours.
4	10-20%	Completely disabled. Cannot carry on any self care. Totally confined to wheelchair or bed (bedridden).

For more detail, see the section Clinical Assessment

Biochemical Assessment

Some biochemical tests can be the most objective measures of nutritional status. Lab tests can help assess protein status, organ function, and hydration status.

Often the following is used in the medical record to denote lab values. This allows for a quick review of some of the pertinent labs.

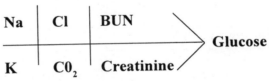

Further information /explanation of nutrition labs can be found in the section Biochemical Assessment.

Assessment parameters for the older population are:
- Weight loss of five percent within one month; 10 percent in six months.
- Clinical observations: peripheral edema, cachexia, pale skin, dull eyes, swollen lips, swollen gums, swollen and/or dry tongue, dry mucous membranes, poor skin turgor and muscle wasting.
- Labs: abnormal values for albumin, Hb, HCT, BUN, creatinine, sodium, potassium and magnesium. If these problems are not corrected, they can lead to confusion, weakness, reduced quality of life and poor rehabilitative progress.

INTERVENTION/IMPLEMENTATION

This process is the formulation of the nutrition care plan. It includes all activities that will enable the patient to meet their nutrition needs.

Formulation of the nutrition care plan consists of:
- Implementing decisions following medical goals for the patient.
- Implementing decisions from the assessment data.
- Specifying/recommending the modality of feeding.
- Recommending macro/micro nutrients plus electrolytes.
- Establishing goal(s) of therapy and/or desired outcome(s).
- Recommending baseline nutrition labs.
- Interdisciplinary planning for nutrition therapy.
- Educational needs and/or a plan for continuum of care.
- Discharge planning needs.

Figure 7 is an example of a discharge summary.

Figure 7: Discharge Summary

Name _____ Discharge Date _____

Hospital Number _____ Admission Date _____

Age _____ Sex _____ Diagnosis _____

Anthropometrics: Ht. _____ Wt.: _____ Admit Wt.: _____ DC Wt: _____

Usual Wt. _____ Activity Level _____

Laboratory Albumin: _____ Prealbumin: _____

Other _____

Estimated Needs: _____ Kcal   _____ gm pro

_____ Kcal/kg   _____ gm/kg

Current Diet: _____ Nutritional Supplements: _____

Major Nutritional Problems:

Ongoing: _____ Follow-up recommendations: _____

Resolved: _____

After the medical nutrition therapy goals are decided, the nutrition care plan can guide the selection of appropriate nutrition support system. Full implementation should occur no later than hospital day two (during the first phase of the nutrition care process).

A nutrition support system is simply a method of meeting an individual's nutrition needs. The system chosen will depend on the patient's disease (whether present or potential), his/her stage of growth and development (e.g., adolescence, pregnancy, aging), and his/her environment (i.e. poverty, drug addiction).

Figure 8 displays the decision process for nutrition support intervention in both adults and children.

Figure 8: Nutrition Support Process

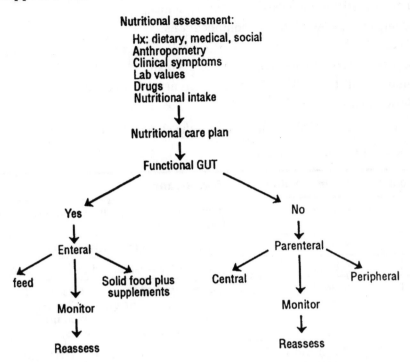

Discharge planning is the process by which a plan is developed for a continuum of care. This allows for a smooth transition from the acute care facility to home or other health care settings. Discharge planning should begin at the time the patient is found at nutritional risk. The planning process is as follows:

Case Finding: High nutrition risk patient may need nutrition care discharge planning.

Assessment: Determine if patient needs nutrition support accompanied by appropriate documentation at discharge.

Planning: Develop a discharge plan that meets the needs of and is acceptable to the patient and provides a provision of continuity of nutritional care.

Implementation: A discharge plan can be implemented after the identification of a nutrition problem and is a potential resource for solving/following the problem.

Evaluation: Need to establish a method for continuous feedback.

MONITORING/EVALUATION

The monitoring function is the follow-up process that demonstrates whether the goal(s) and/or desired outcome(s) of medical nutrition therapy are being met. Monitoring should include evaluation of the patient's clinical status, lab parameters, weight, nutrient intake and route of administration. Frequency is determined by the patient's medical condition and stability, tolerance of nutrition therapy and achievement of goals. Frequent modification of the feeding regimen may be necessary, particularly for clinically unstable patients. Monitoring of the high nutrition risk patient should occur at least every two to three days until discharge or until the patients' medical condition and/or nutritional status changes. Monitoring of the moderate risk patient should occur every three to four days until discharge or the medical condition and/or nutritional status changes.

Parameters of Monitoring Include:
- Monitoring the effectiveness of the care plan/status of goals.
- Monitoring lab tests pertinent to nutrition/hydration status.
- Monitoring feeding modalities/routes for complications.
- Monitoring intake.
- Monitoring the patient's compliance/adherence to the plan.
- Evaluation of nutritional status secondary to the current medical condition.
- Review of anthropometrics.

The following tests can be used to evaluate and monitor the status of various systems:

Tests to Evaluate Gastrointestinal Function

Test	Specimen	Normal Nalue	Significance
D-xylose	Urine	> 20%	Detects diseases of intestinal mucosa resulting in malabsorption.
pH	Stool	< 6	Indicates CHO malabsorption.
Fat	Stool	< 5 gm	Diagnostic of steatorrhea if elevated.
Guaiac	Stool	Negative	Determines the presence of blood in stool. Bleeding from lower colon is bright red. Bleeding from stomach or small intestines is not recognized until guaiac is added to the stool and blue color results.
Schilling	Urine	7% or more of ingested radio-cyanocobalamin	Decreased: Indicates B_{12} deficiency.
Lactase	Blood		Deficiency indicates lactose intolerance. There is no rise in blood glucose or galactose with a lactose load.

Tests to Evaluate Liver Function

Test	Specimen	Normal Value	Significance
Ammonia	Serum	30 - 70 mcg	Elevated with cirrhosis, liver failure and/or porta caval shunt.
Alkaline Phosphatase	Serum	25 - 105 U/L	Increased with hepatic disease, phosphatase malignancy and in chronic obstruction of biliary duct. Is non-specific.
SGGT	Serum	35 U/L or less	Elevated value highly indicative of hepatocellular injury secondary to ethanol abuse.
SGOT	Serum	25 U/L	Elevated levels detects hepatocellular injury secondary to exacerbation of infectious hepatitis.
Bilirubin Direct	Serum	0.2 - 0.4 mg%	Reflects ability of liver to conjugate and excrete bilirubin. Elevated with liver and biliary disease.
Indirect		0.1 - 0.5 mg%	Abnormalities in direct bilirubin indicate biliary obstruction.
Total		0.2 - 0.9 mg%	Abnormalities in indirect bilirubin indicate RBC hemolysis or liver disease.
Bile	Urine	Negative	Liver function test. Indicates biliary tract obstruction if positive.

Tests to Evaluate Pancreatic Function

Test	Specimen	Normal Value	Significance
Amylase	Serum	3.0 U/ml or less 60 - 180 Somogyi U	Elevated with pancreatic dysfunction due to liberation of digestive enzymes from pancreas.
Bilirubin	Serum	0.2 - 0.9 mg%	Elevated values may be due to compression of the distal common duct within the pancreas, biliary stones, inflammation of the liver and bile ducts.
Carotene	Serum	90 - 280 mcg% 100 - 300 IU%	Decreased secondary to fat Malabsorption associated with steatorrhea.
Fecal Fat	Stool	> 6 grams	Elevated with fat malabsorption secondary to impaired digestion of fat due to impaired secretion of pancreatic lipase.
Lipase	Serum	< 1.5 IU/ml	Elevated with liberation of lipase from the pancreas into the blood stream.
Fasting Blood Sugar	Serum	80 - 120 mg%	Elevated with impaired secretion of insulin in response to glucose load because of inflammatory destruction of islets of Langerhans.
Calcium	Serum	9 - 11 mg%	Decreased due to soap formation between interstitial calcium and fatty acids.
Hematocrit	Serum	M: 40 - 54% F: 37 - 47%	Elevated due to hemoconcentration when serum exudes into abdomen. Decreased in severe hemorrhagic pancreatitis.

Tests to Evaluate Renal Function

Test	Specimen	Normal Value	Significance
Specific Gravity	Urine	1.003 - 1.030	Reflects urine osmolarity. The high specific gravity associated with high osmolarity indicates failure to concentrate urine; this may indicate renal failure.
pH	Urine	4.6 - 8.0	Metabolic acidosis due to renal failure.
Protein	Urine	0	Trace levels associated with glomerular involvement. Nephrotic syndrome associated w/ levels of 3.5 - 4.0 gms.
Sugars	Urine	0	Renal threshold refers to the level which glucose is reabsorbed by the kidneys. Glycosuria results when threshold is exceeded.
Creatinine	Serum	90 - 130 ml/min	Used to measure glomerular clearance filtration rate (GFR).

Miscellaneous Tests

Test	Specimen	Normal Value	Significance
Acetone	Urine	Negative	Positive in diabetes, ketosis, fasting, high fat diet or CHO free diet.
Coombs	Serum	Negative	Positive in certain acquired anemias.
Protein-Bound Iodine	Serum	3.5 - 8.5 mg%	Evaluation of thyroid function. Elevated with hyperthyroidism, thyroiditis, and pregnancy. Decreased with hypothyroidism and myxedema.
Glucose Tolerance Test (GTT)	Serum	FBS: 110mg/ml PostPrandial: 1 hour: 170 mg 2 hour: 150 mg	Levels greater than 150 mg indicate Diabetes Mellitus.

The care plan requires revision as the medical condition of the patient changes. If the nutrition care plan needs revision, a statement and rational for any changes in therapy must be documented.

DOCUMENTATION/CHARTING

When the screening criteria identifies a patient at nutritional risk, the patient should be assessed and have a timely documented outcome-based nutrition care plan. Documentation should contain the specifics of what, where, when and how.

Medical records constitute the legally recognized healthcare record of a patient. From a legal perspective, documentation serves a dual function; 1) provides pertinent and useful data about a patients' condition, together with the medical and nutrition regimen(s) employed, and 2) a record of adherence to accepted standards of care. The nutrition information documented should provide a concise record of the patient's nutrition intervention and the outcomes. Benefits of documentation are:

- Demonstration of the continuity of care and proof of ongoing evaluation.
- Provision of legal protection for patient, practitioners and facility.
- Provision of evidence of proof for third party reimbursement of services rendered.
- Provides evidence of accountability in meeting regulatory and professional standards. Legal problems still can occur when an intervention is documented and the plan is not carried out or the clinical response not recorded.

The essence of effective documentation is a systematic written account of the nutrition care process. The documentation should validate the process. Charting should reflect the outcome of the process through nutrition decision making which includes identification of the problem(s), gathering of data, development of the care plan, analysis of the data, and evaluation of measurable outcomes.

There is a need for documentation standards to provide direction and guidance for outcome-based nutrition care plans. Documentation should show a reprocessing of information and continuity of thought. **Figure 9** can be used as an evaluation tool for a chart review of nutrition care and documentation.

Figure 9: Clinical Nutrition Performance Evaluation Tool

Chart Review

Date _____ Dietitian _____

Patient _____ Diagnosis _____

Admit Date _____ Screen Date _____

Initial Assessment Date _____

Evaluation of Nutritional Status: **Evaluation of:**

Weight/wt Patterns	yes	no	Nutritional Needs	yes	no
Lab Values	yes	no			
Diet History	yes	no	Feeding Modality	yes	no
Drug History	yes	no			
Goals/outcomes	yes	no	Functional Status	yes	no
Interdisciplinary Care	yes	no	Discharge Planning	yes	no

Reassessment:	F/u date		F/u date		F/u date		F/u date	
Review of wts	yes	no	yes	no	yes	no	yes	no
Review of labs	yes	no	yes	no	yes	no	yes	no
Review of intake	yes	no	yes	no	yes	no	yes	no
Eval of feeding modality	yes	no	yes	no	yes	no	yes	no
Status of needs	yes	no	yes	no	yes	no	yes	no
Status of goals/progress	yes	no	yes	no	yes	no	yes	no
Discharge plans	yes	no	yes	no	yes	no	yes	no

Discharge Summary includes:

Current nutrition support
Summary of nutrition therapies
Outcome of nutrition therapies
Pertinent information on wts, labs
Statement of expected progress
Recommendations for follow-up

Education includes:

What
Who
Comprehension
Adherence
Goals/learning outcomes
Drug/nutrient education

Comments:

The documented care plan should include an evaluation of nutritional status secondary to the medical condition; estimated nutrition needs; an evaluation of labs pertinent to nutritional status; an evaluation of anthropometric measures; an evaluation of drug/nutrient interactions; an evaluation of diet history; and evaluation of diet order and/or feeding modality. The documentation should demonstrate interdisciplinary nutrition care, goal(s) of therapy and/or desired outcome(s), evaluation of any patient education needs and discharge planning.

There are various styles for documentation.

Source Oriented and Narrative Format

Narrative: Narrative charting has been used since the institution of written health care records. The source or originator can be any member of the health care team who has responsibility to provide information. Each originator describes their own unique observations, activities and evaluations. Department policies dictate who records what, how it is recorded and where and when the information is documented. Disadvantages of narrative documentation are: 1) a potential for a fragmented collection of disjointed, overused, virtually meaningless entries; 2) sometimes difficult to retrieve information without reviewing the entire record; 3) perpetuates a record of "buried messages"; 4) requires a review of each source to determine an overall clinical picture of the patient; 5) potentially time consuming; the open-ended format requires careful consideration when personalizing information about each patient; and 6) tracking the patient's progress and outcomes may be time consuming. This style could be used in any clinical setting.

Narrative, Outcome: The focus of this charting system is on desired patient outcomes rather than on problems. Progress notes are recorded in the narrative style. Major components include: data base (subjective/objective information); problem identification (usual and unusual); nutrition care plan that includes desired outcomes (the focus of care is directed toward patient outcome rather than toward a problem); implementation; and evaluation. Outcome documentation can be adapted to virtually any clinical setting.

Other process-oriented documentation include:

SOAP style (most widely practiced) **Figure 10**

Figure 10: Nutrition Assessment Form

DATE	TIME

DIAGNOSTIC NUTRITIONAL ANALYSIS (_____)

S: _____

_____

_____

_____

_____

_____

_____

O:

AGE	HEIGHT	ADMIT WEIGHT	CURRENT WEIGHT	USUAL WEIGHT	USUAL WEIGHT %	IDEAL WEIGHT	IDEAL WEIGHT %

LAB VALUES:

ALBUMIN	TRANSTHYRETIN (PREALBUMIN)	OTHER

NUTRITIONALLY PERTINENT MEDICATIONS

DIET ORDER

A: NUTRITION SUPPORT

ESTIMATED BASAL ENERGY EXPENDITURE

ESTIMATED NEEDS

kcals	kcals/kg	gms protein	gms protein/kg IBW

_____

_____

_____

_____

_____

_____

_____

P: RECOMMEND _____

_____

_____

_____

_____

SOAP meaning:

Subjective: Patient Interview
- Information provided by patient, family or caretaker.
- Significant nutrition history.
- Perceived appetite change, chewing and swallowing problems.
- Weight patterns, allergies/intolerances.
- Pertinent socioeconomic, cultural information.
- Level of physical activity/functional status.
- Current dietary intake (in terms of nutrients).

Objective: Chart Review
- Factual, reproducible observations (e.g., age, anthropometric and lab data).
- Physical exam: nausea, vomiting, diarrhea.
- Clinical status/functional status.
- Current diet order.
- Nutritionally pertinent medications.
- Diagnosis.
- Goals of medical therapy.

Assessment
- Interpretation of patient's status based on subjective and objective data.
- Evaluation of nutrition history as it pertains to the medical condition, if available.
- Estimation of nutritional requirements.
- Assessment of diet order and/or feeding modality as to appropriateness.
- Assessment of laboratory data as it applies to nutrition/hydration status.
- Assessment of comprehension and motivation and compliance with past dietary modifications, if appropriate.
- Anticipated problems and/or difficulties with patient compliance/adherence.
- Assessment of medications as they pertain to nutritional status.

Plans
- Diagnostic
  1) Suggestions for gaining further useful subjective or objective data.
  2) Further workup, data gathering, consultations.

- Therapeutic
  1) Goal of nutrition therapy.
  2) Recommendations for nutrition care.
  3) Reassessment/follow-up.
  4) Discharge planning.

- Patient Education
  1) Description of specific written or verbal instruction provided.
  2) Description of specific recommendations.

SOAPE (subjective, objective, analysis/assesment, plan, and education).

SOAPIER (subjective, objective, analysis/assessment, plan, interventions, evaluations and revisions): Charted with data organized according to patient problems. Contains initial assessment and discharge information.

Derivations from the SOAP OR SOAPIER include:

APIO (assessment, plan, intervention, outcomes).

HOAPO (history, observation, assessment, plan, outcomes).

POAPO (problem, objectives, assessment, plan, outcomes).

SAP (screen, assess, plan).

PIE (problem, intervention, evaluation) This oriented approach process does away with redundancy. It fosters development of a realistic care plan and decreases the time needed for documentation. It does not, however, lend itself to multidisciplinary or integrated charting. The initial entry can be a diagnostic (problem) statement. A variation is PIO - O being outcome expected or achieved by the intervention (nutrition care plan).

FOCUS/DAR charting is process oriented and patient centered. It uses the nutrition care process to organize documentation of care. It is a positive perspective instead of a negative (problem). It is flexible and can be adapted to virtually any clinical setting. The focus for nutrition care could be nausea, vomiting, malnutrition, or intolerance to tube feeding. When writing in the progress notes, **DAR** construct is used: Data, Action, and Response. **Data** include subjective/objective information that supports observations made at the time of a significant event. **Action** refers to immediate or future nutrition interventions based on the assessment/evaluation of the patient's condition. **Response** provides a description of patient response/outcome to any part of the medical or nutrition care plan.

Diagnostic charting is a clinical judgment about an individual that describes an actual or potential nutrition problem requiring actual/suggested nutrition intervention. For example, nutrition assessment demonstrates a patient is at high risk of malnutrition; elevated blood sugar shows marked glucose intolerance; rising creatinine/BUN, and PO4 suggests worsening renal function; elevated ammonia and LFTs are consistent with worsening liver function. It does not diagnose a disease. Other nutrition diagnosis include: altered nutrition (↑↓), diarrhea, excess fluid volume, impaired skin integrity, impaired swallowing or potential for aspiration. When using a nutrition diagnosis, three components are needed: problem statement, the etiology and signs and symptoms. Written diagnostic statement contains two parts: 1) statement of the problem; and 2) its probable cause. The following demonstrates the process.

Introductory phrase "at risk of, potential for or possibility of," **second part** should have a connective phrase such as "related to or secondary to," and the **closing phrase** might contain the comment "resulting from, induced by or manifested by." For example, "at risk for malnutrition secondary to poor intake with a weight loss of greater than 10% during the past 4 months, and severe, frothy diarrhea, induced by exacerbation of Crohns disease."

Charting By Exception: The focus is on abnormal or exceptional facts or observations. System review and repetitive parameters are predefined and are automatically assumed to have been performed according to standards unless specifically stated otherwise. This type of charting follows the clinical pathways and only the variances are documented in the progress notes.

The style and format of the documentation are secondary considerations. The important issue is the content as it pertains to the issues of nutritional status and nutrition needs.

Each facility should have standards for documentation style and time frame. The following example is a policy for documentation.

Example

Policy: No later than one day after identifying a patient at nutritional risk, an outcome-based medical nutrition care plan will be documented in the medical record. Plan may include:

1. Objective data
   - Age
   - Height (include growth standard for age if less than 18)
   - IBW; % of IBW
   - Usual weight (or pre-illness weight); % of usual weight
   - Current weight
   - Diet history
   - Pertinent medications
   - Current diet prescription

2. Evaluation of pertinent clinical laboratory data

3. Assessment of functioning/nonfunctional GI tract

   Indicating evidence of maldigestion and/or malabsorption (nausea, vomiting, diarrhea, fistula obstruction, severe protein-calorie malnutrition)

4. Evaluation of factors that may affect nutrient intake, digestion, absorption
   - Medications
   - Previous surgeries
   - On-going treatment modalities
   - Chronic disease processes

5. Statement of goal of nutrition therapy and/or outcome, for example to:
   - Stop weight loss
   - Increase anabolism
   - Prevent negative nitrogen balance
   - Promote wound healing and weight maintenance
   - Minimize nitrogen wasting
   - Maintain body weight and protein stores

6. Statement of evaluation of appropriateness of current diet order, if applicable

7. Documentation of nutrition needs:
   - Estimated energy needs; Kcal/kg: round to nearest 50
   - Estimated protein needs; gm/kg IBW: round to nearest 5
   - Vitamin/mineral supplement, if appropriate
   - Estimated fluid needs: round to nearest 50

8. Development/documentation of a nutrition care plan

   Indicating type of nutrition support and its implementation (dietary modifications/delivery system oral, enteral or parenteral)

9. Follow-up documentation should occur within one to two days of the original note and any subsequent notes. The documentation should address the review of weights; labs pertinent to the nutrition/hydration status; review of NIA, if appropriate; evaluation of current feeding modality; status of the goals and/or desired outcomes; statement and rationale for any changes in nutrition therapy; revision of the nutrition care plan if the medical condition necessitates it; and a statement on the education process and status of/progress toward discharge planning. Follow-up documentation

should quickly identify the nutrition progress. These chart notes can use the **IER** format: **I** for intervention, **E** for evaluation and **R** for response. **IER** is outcome oriented linking nutrition intervention with clinical response and/or changes in medical therapy.

10. Statement of patient education, if appropriate, to include:
    - Patient and/or significant other has been instructed
    - Statement on type of instruction given
    - Statement of comprehension
    - Cultural diversity and lifestyle recognition, if appropriate
    - Statement of expected adherence to prescribed diet
    - Patient discharged on medications with food/drug interactions
    - Statement of an expected outcome/goal (for reimbursement purposes)
    - Statement for continuum of care

11. Discharge documentation to include:
    - Current nutrition therapy
    - Summary of nutrition therapies
    - Outcome of nutrition therapies
    - Pertinent information on weights, labs, intake
    - Statement on expected progress
    - Statement for continuum of care

General Guidelines for Documentation

1. Medical records are permanent legal documents; therefore all entries should be written in black pen or typewritten; no soft felt pens, multicolored pens or pencils should be used.
2. Documentation should be complete, clear and concise.
3. Documentation must be legible. Printing is preferred. If an entry cannot be read, it can be argued the services did not occur.
4. Documentation must be accurate.
5. Entries should be documented by service, date and time. Each medical record page should be identified by the patient's stamp or written name and hospital number.
6. Entries should be in chronological order and on consecutive lines.
7. No entry should be made in advance of the procedure performed.
8. The first word of every statement should be capitalized. Periods should be used at the completion of each thought. Complete sentences are not necessary. Grammar and spelling must be correct.
9. All entries should be consistent and noncontradictory.
10. Only institution-approved and authorized abbreviations should be used. Abbreviations with duplicate meanings should be avoided. Each institution should have a document for abbreviations.
11. All entries must be signed at the end of the chart note. The signature should include the first name initial, complete surname and status (e.g., R. Brown, MS,RD).
12. No one should ever document or sign the medical record for another individual.
13. All student notes must be co-signed either by the clinical staff or the clinical instructor. Never countersign an entry without reading or confirming the entry for accuracy. A counter-signature attests to the authenticity and shares equal responsibility.
14. Documentation must be objective and void of conclusions. Words should be carefully chosen, so there is not room for conjecture, doubt or misunderstanding.

15. Documentation must be specific. Many words have different meanings.

16. Personal positions or points should never be argued in the chart. Criticism or doubts about the professionalism of others should not appear in the documentation.

17. Time gaps must be avoided. Documentation must occur as soon as the actual procedure/service is rendered. The frequency depends upon the patient's degree of illness, therapies administered and standards of nutrition care.

18. Late entries should be identified as such, reflecting the date and time of the actual entry followed by the date and time the entry should have been recorded.

19. Medical record entries should never be made non-legible.

Guidelines for Correcting Errors

A. When making a correction NEVER:

    1. Use white out, correction tape or self adhesive labels

    2. Obliterate an entry

    3. Add notes after the fact without accurately authenticating, dating and referencing the original entry

    4. Remove original and replace with a copy

B. Corrections performed at the time an entry is in progress:

    1. Minor error in transcription, spelling, one word, etc

        a. Errors should be corrected by the person who made the initial entry

        b. Line only through an error. Enter the correction

    2. Other errors, for example, an entry in wrong chart:

        a. One line should be drawn through the entry, or an X made through the paragraph or page in error.

        b. Note "error" plus the date and time. Initial the correction.

> ***Example:***
> The patient denies any self-induced vomiting.
> error 04/24/98 0950 S.D.

> The patient would not respond to questions regarding self-induced vomiting.
> (continue entry and sign)

    3. Omitted Information:

        a. Beside the original entry, note an addendum: "See Addendum," enter date and initial.

        b. Write addendum in chart sequence. Identify it as an addendum and reference the original entry.

> ***Example:***
> "4/29/98 0900 Addendum to (progress) note
> of 4/28/98 (continue entry and sign.)

C. Corrections performed after any interval of time since original entry (interval of time: when a chart has been out of the possession of the person).

    1. Minor error in transcription, spelling, one word:

        a. Errors should be corrected by the person who made the error

        b. Line once through the error. Enter the correction, date, time and sign

2. Other errors, test results, misquoted orders, entry in wrong chart:

   a. Errors should be corrected by the person who made the error.

   b. One line should be drawn through the entry or an X should be made through the page.

   c. Note "error" plus date and time. Sign the correction.

Effective documentation has multidimensional characteristics that are applicable to any documentation format or system. These characteristics reflect:

- Current, complete and concise descriptions of patient status, with minimum duplication of data.
- Current problem-solving and decision-making efforts; includes conclusive statements.
- Information clear and presented in a manner useful to the health care team.
- Chronology of care and decision making logic.

In formulating an effective nutrition chart note, the following information must be gathered and evaluated for impact on nutritional status:

- Admit diagnosis
- Medical problems list/medical condition(s) affecting nutritional status
- Anthropometry
- Baseline nutrition labs
- Pertinent diagnostic procedures
- Medical therapy/treatment goals

Example:

For Assessment and Plan

A: 37 year old male with Crohns disease who presents with severe frothy diarrhea x 2 weeks, pain and a 10% weight loss. Prealbumin of 7.3 mg/dL may indicate loss of lean body mass. In accordance with the medical plan, will provide nutrition support to minimize nitrogen loss/loss of lean body mass and to stop/control further weight loss. Recommend 2800 kcal and ~110 gm protein to meet needs.

P: Discuss alternative feeding modalities with the physician, i.e., efficacy of PN. Discuss the nutrition care plan with the patient. Suggest repeating prealbumin once full nutrition support is implemented and needs are being met. Plans for discharge being formulated.

EDUCATION

Today's environment dictates that patient education should be provided wherever it is the most cost and care-effective. Basic education should be provided in the hospital unless the process was implemented prior to admission. Effective education planning begins with day of admission. The patient needs to be counseled on the merits of the care plan and their continued nutrition needs. This provides for the continuum of care after discharge.

Patient education takes place every time an attempt is made to change knowledge, attitudes or behaviors and not just when a planned or scheduled session takes place. The patient's ability to learn, sociocultural background, and development status are some of the many factors that influence the nutrition education approach. Planned education includes notations of identified, specific patient-learning needs; detailed learning objectives; discharge planning; promotion of continuity of care between health care agency and home. The correct behavioral terms must be used to document patient learning outcomes. The emphasis on education is outcome learning. Progress notes usually are the primary location used by providers to document patient learning. A brief description of the education includes:

WHO:

What was taught and **Why**

How the teaching was provided

Outcome(s)

	The patient can
Knowledge	Define, describe, identify, name, select, state
Comprehension	Estimate, explain, generalize, give example, paraphrase, summarize
Adhere	Comply with, stick to

Figure 11 is an example of a nutrition education form.

Figure 11: Nutrition Education Form

Persons Present: ☐ Patient ☐ Partner ☐ Family ☐ Friend ☐ Other

Primary learner (if other than patient): _____ ☐ Interpreter Present

Evidence of Teaching Based on Patient's Needs and Concerns

What Was Taught (summarize)

How It Was Taught

☐ Verbal information provided

☐ Written information provided

☐ Class/group session

Evidence of Learning

Outcome Met

☐ Describes/able to restate information

If Outcome Not Met

☐ Unable to understand:

Barriers:

☐ Education   ☐ Cognitive

☐ Language   ☐ Emotional

☐ Culture   ☐ Physical

☐ Indicates understanding of topic

☐ Refuses information

☐ Needs further instruction

Follow-Up Plan and Needs (if applicable)

☐ Follow-up/referral

☐ Additional topics to be covered

If the patient is referred to an outside agency, a discharge summary must be submitted.

ETHICAL/LEGAL ISSUES

ETHICAL

Comfort and quality of life are the main goals for all patients but especially for the terminally ill. Terminal illness is defined as the end of a specific, progressive, normally irreversible disease when the physician has determined, through objective medical validations, that medical treatment is futile and the disease will cause the patient's death in the foreseeable future. Terminally ill adults have the right to choose the level of treatment and care they receive. The health care professional has an ethical responsibility to respect the sanctity of life and the dignity and rights of all persons and to provide relief from suffering. In nutrition, issues in feeding the terminally ill adult identifies some of the ethical and legal issues that need to be considered when deciding to provide or withhold nutrition support. The most powerful ethical principle to consider is the patient's right of self determination.

Palliative care encourages the alleviation of physical symptoms, anxiety and fear. The patient wishes are known through advance directives. The Do Not Attempt Rescuitation (DNAR) can include the termination of nutrition support. With a DNAR that includes nutrition support, the goal is to maintain current nutrition status. Dietary restrictions are usually inappropriate unless the situation (for example, ESRD) deems it necessary. Mentally competent patients have the right to refuse treatment (e.g., eating, tube feeding or parenteral nutrition). The refusal should be well documented.

LEGAL

The number of medical malpractice suits has increased considerably in recent years. The nutrition professional is not immune to malpractice suits, even when she/he hides behind the veil of legal principle of "respondent superior" (when a physician's and facility's liability ends and the nutrition professionals begins).

The law expects health care professionals to provide safe and reasonable care in accordance with professional standards and to document that care. It is the responsibility of the nutrition health care professional to provide reasonable care and skill in providing quality nutrition care. The question is; what standard of nutrition care in a hospital would the courts deem reasonable? How does the hospital meet its duty to ensure that such a standard of nutrition care is provided?

Nutrition malpractice occurs when a practitioner fails to meet the accepted/stated standards of care. Law of negligence states each person is liable for damage if they fail to meet the standard of care and that failure causes harm. Medical nutrition therapy is a medically proven standard of patient care. Malnutrition is not a medically accepted state for even the most seriously ill patient. The modern standards of nutrition care includes enteral and parenteral nutrition. Failure of the medical profession/community to stay current in the technological advancement can result in malpractice.

Negligence is a failure to do what the reasonable health care practitioner would do under same or similar circumstances. To protect themselves and fulfill their responsibilities, nutrition professionals should always provide and document quality nutrition intervention to those who have been identified at nutritional risk. Nutrition professionals should know the facilities policies and procedures, be familiar with the standard of care and ensure proper care is being provided. If the standard of care in not being met, the nutrition professional has a duty to report it to a higher authority (e.g., risk management and/or the medical director). The court will want to know what measures were taken to ensure information was communicated to the physician.

Written policies and procedures for nutrition care are mandatory. Any discrepancies between the policy and actual practice may be used as evidence of professional malpractice. To ensure policies meet legal and clinical requirements the following must be considered: 1) all policies should be consistent with the facilities philosophy of care and should be processed through the appropriate committee(s) for approval; 2) all policies should reflect accepted standards of care and should be written within the competency levels and legally recognized scopes of practice; 3) any deviations from accepted standards of care should be acknowledged in the policy and the rationale for the deviation substantiated; 4) all policies should be reviewed periodically to ensure compliance with current standards of nutrition care; and 5) all policies that are not followed should be eliminated and replaced with ones reflecting the current nutrition care practices.

Long term care nutrition professionals have a further responsibility to report and document any deficiencies noted. This responsibility includes providing input regarding Medicare/Medicaid guidelines and state rules and regulations governing health care facilities.

Terminology:

Negligence: The failure to exercise that degree of care that a reasonable person would exercise under the same circumstances

Malpractice: A professional's improper conduct in the performance of duties, done either intentionally or through carelessness or ignorance.

Standard of care: How a prudent person would perform in the same or similar manner.

MANAGED CARE

Managed care is a comprehensive system of delivering quality, cost-effective medical care through a contracted network of providers. The basic concept of managed care is all medical care is provided in exchange for a set monthly premium. The overall goals of managed care organizations (MCOs) include increasing enrollment, decreasing utilization of high-cost services, and the referral of routine services to the primary care physician. The primary care physician is either employed by or contracts with the health plan provider. The health care provider needs to deliver care in the most cost-effective manner possible. Nutrition is an essential part of the overall picture. Poor nutritional status is a hidden cost in health care. Improved status can make a difference, not only for the patient but also for the health care providers' financial position.

Managed care plans have varying degrees of requirements to provide health care through the use of case management, practice guidelines and utilization management. Some aspects of managed care are; 1) emphasis on containing costs while maximizing quality; 2) patients utilization of services within a provider network to obtain maximum benefits; 3) coordinates utilization through primary care provider; and 4) capitated plans share risk with providers. The goals MCOs are to provide a full range of health care services and to raise the quality of care while reducing costs. How payment is made and care is provided can differ significantly by the type of managed care organization (MCO). Models of managed care system include: Health Maintenance Organizations (HMOs), Preferred Provider Organizations (PPOs) and Exclusive Provider Organizations.

HMOs:	**Staff**	Hires own salaried medical staff
	Contract	Has a contractual agreement with one or more multispeciality group practice
	Individual	Contracts directly with solo practice practitioners
	Network	Contracts two or more group practices
PPOs:	**Network**	Physicians and hospitals that have agreed to give a sponsoring organization discounts from usual charges
Exclusive:		Similar to PPOs except the beneficiary cannot go outside the network

Nutrition is an integral component of any effective health plan and should be provided as part of the plan, but services may not be part of the plan. The HMO concept, to provide comprehensive and defined medical services, emphasizes comprehensive health care, including treatment and prevention.

The managed care concept provides continuity of care because it covers care wherever it is delivered. The emphasis is on health promotion, early identification and treatment of acute problems and management of chronic conditions to minimize hospitalization. The environmental trends of healthcare are indicated below.

Environmental trends with emphasis on:
- Cost containment
- Influence of government in healthcare
- Changing demographics
- Increasing awareness of diet and health relationship
- Increasing demand for quality and outcome
- Changing technology
- Increasing demand for nutrition education and diverse channel of communication

A glossary of managed care terms is located at the end of this section.

CASE MANAGEMENT

Case management is a system that provides continuity of care for patients who receive care from multiple clinical areas, institutions and/or agencies. Case management is an approach to the clinical and financial management of care of patients and treatment outcomes. It is a systematic process of care planning, monitoring and evaluation and reassessment targeted at individuals who are likely to need more intensive, costly and dependent levels of care. Not all patients need case management. Three essential concepts to case management are:

1. **Comprehensive** for overseeing a patient's entire episode of illness, regardless of the payer system or location of the service provided.
2. **Organized** around a system of interdisciplinary care and resources needed to provide cost-effective high-quality care.
3. **Coordinated** via clinical and financial management of care by coordinators who have financial incentive to manage risk and maximize the quality of care.

Case management is directed toward patients whose cases are complex (with complexity being defined as health, economic, social, emotional and psychological factors). The focus of case management is improving the patient experience, ensuring clinical outcomes are met, assuring accountability, effectively managing resources, and integrating and coordinating the activities of the health care team.

Case managers are generally registered nurses or social workers. All case managers perform five essential functions: assessment, planning, intervention, monitoring, and evaluation.

FINANCIAL MANAGEMENT

The health care sector is growing rapidly in size and complexity. Understanding the financial and economic implications of decision making has become one of the most critical areas encountered by nutrition professionals. Successful decision making skills contribute to a viable operation capable of providing needed nutrition services cost-effectively.

In any business, effective financial management is the product of many factors, such as environmental conditions, personnel capabilities and information quality. A major portion of the total financial management task is the provision of accurate, timely, and relevant information.

When formulating an effective financial policy, it is important to relate to the strategic plan of the facility. The financial plan should not be developed in isolation from the strategic plan, nor should the strategic plan be developed separately from the financial plan.

Strategic planning can be defined as a decision making process analyzing challenges and opportunities that impact a facility and individual departments within that facility. The information is used to set goals and design strategies. Strategic planning is concerned with two basic decision outcomes: first, a statement of mission and/or goals and second, a set of programs or activities to which the organization will commit resources. Strategic plans and goals usually span one year. The clinical nutrition services mission statement is to provide quality nutrition care, thereby enhancing patient outcomes. In ambulatory care the mission statement may be to promote optimal nutritional health and well-being.

On a departmental level, three points concerning the integration of strategic and financial planning should be emphasized. First, strategic and financial planning are the primary responsibility of management (which would incorporate financial plans with the facility's strategic plans). This would not exclude staff members from the process. Second, strategic planning should precede financial planning. Third, administration plays an active role in the financial planning process and has the final approval.

Budget development must be integrated into the management control process, which consists of programming, budgeting, accounting and analysis and reporting.

Programming In this phase an organization determines the nature and size of programs it will use to accomplish its stated goals of objectives. Programming deals with new and existing programs.

Budgeting is the next phase of management control. A budget is defined as a quantitative expression of a plan of action. Another definition is a process by which managers assure resources are obtained and used effectively and efficiently in the accomplishment of an organization's objective. A budget is an integral part of overall management control process of an organization. Budgeting may change programs. A careful and accurate estimate of revenues and costs may prompt action to reevaluate prior program decisions as financially unfeasible.

The budget usually is stated in monetary terms, covers a one year period and allocates resources (people and dollars). In many cases, no review of existing programs is undertaken; the budgeting phase then may be based on a prior year's budget or on the actual results of existing programs. The budgeting process translates program decisions into terms that are meaningful for responsibility centers.

There are several types of budgets. The type of budget used depends on the needs and the policies of the organization.

Forecast/Fixed Budget:

The forecast/fixed budget lists labor, supply, equipment and other anticipated costs and the estimated dollar amount for each. Justification for each cost/item should relate to the mission and vision statement of the department.

A forecast/fixed budget is developed for a specific, predetermined level of annual volume (patient days, consults, acuity level). This budget compares current budget with projected estimates for the next fiscal year.

Flexible Budget:

A flexible budget adjusts targeted levels of costs for change in volume. For example, the budget for a food service operating at 95 percent occupancy would be different from the budget operating at 80 percent occupancy. Forecast budget would make no formal differentiation in the allowed budget between these two levels. In clinical nutrition, forecast budgeting may be used in staffing whereas in food service, flexible budgeting may apply.

Zero-Base Budget:

The goal of a zero-base budget (ZBB) is to ensure fiscal responsibility in allocating resources and controlling costs. ZBB is a process of periodically reevaluating all existing programs, their associated levels of expenditure, and determining the efficacy of the entire expenditure. ZBB assumes that no existing program is entitled to automatic approval. ZBB requires that a budget be prepared for each department activity and that each activity be justified. It encourages evaluation of the current state of the operation and justifies the costs and benefits of existing as well as new programs.

Budget process steps consist of:
1. Reviewing the mission statement of the facility.
2. Reviewing the mission statement of the department.
3. Reviewing the goals and objectives (vision statement).
4. Collecting statistical data to use in making budget decisions.
5. Preparation of any revenue budget.
6. Preparation of expenses.

All professionals need to understand their facility's budget process. To get an adequate budget approved, a realistic budget must be developed based on the objectives of the facility and the nutrition department. A successful process requires that each staff member must participate in the following:

- Development of the budget in relation to the organization's overall goals and objectives.
- Justification of how each expenditure contributes to the achievement of the goals and objectives of the operation.
- Identification of the impact of carrying budget levels on the level and quality of service.
- Projection of the payback time for expenditures, if appropriate.
- Projection of the revenue generated by the expenses incurred, if appropriate.

Cost is a major concern of the health care industry. Clinical nutrition is caught between an increase in the demand for services and a decrease in available resources. Every task/function should be cost-effective and maintain quality care. Nutrition care can be cost effective by identifying patients at nutritional risk, providing appropriate care, providing economical care and monitoring for outcomes.

Types of Cost: **Direct and Indirect**

Direct Costs include all resources expended directly in providing nutrition care. Operating expenses include personnel (salaries and wages, benefits), equipment (computers and pagers), supplies, education materials, education/travel, professional fees, and subscriptions, plus depreciation and amortization if appropriate.

Personnel is the biggest part of direct cost. Personnel costs are usually 60 percent of the total expenditures. The cost is calculated by full time equivalent (FTE). An FTE is based on one employee who works on a full-time basis either by the day, week, month or year. The FTE is based on a number of hours not on an actual employee. **Table 2** shows the FTEs needed for RDs.

Table 2: Daily FTE Determination

1. Daily FTEs = Labor hours per day/8 hours per FTE per day.
   Example: Daily FTEs = 60 hours/8 hours = 7.5 FTEs
2. Weekly FTEs = Labor hours per week/40 hours per FTE per wk.
   Example: Weekly FTEs = 300/40 hours = 7.5 FTEs
3. Monthly FTEs = Labor hours per month/173.3 hours per FTE.
   Example: Monthly FTEs = 1299.75/173.3 = 7.5 FTEs
3. Yearly FTEs = Labor hours per year/2080 per FTE per year.
   Example: Yearly FTEs = 15600/2080 hours = 7.5 FTEs

Sick leave and vacation must be factored into the FTE equation. For example, a two - three week vacation per FTE would equate to .43 FTE vacation relief needed per year (7.5 x 3 = 22.5 weeks x 40 hours = 900/2080). Sick leave can be cross-covered by the nutrition care teams if the time does not exceed two days.

Turnover is a hidden personnel cost. High levels of turnover can be indicative of problems. The cost related to turnover include orientation time, training, productivity (lack thereof when first hired), recruitment, and selection and retention of records. It is desirable to keep the yearly turnover rate under ten percent.

Direct cost of salaries should include the benefit package. For example if the monthly/yearly salary is $3,600/43,200, respectively, with a 25 percent benefit package, the monthly/yearly cost of that FTE is $4,500/54,000. If 7.5 FTEs make the same salary, the total personnel cost per month and year would be $33,750/405,000. This cost can be equated to the number of nutrition interventions and/or counseling per year.

Indirect Costs are resources that support the clinical nutrition care services, such as administrative overhead, space, or maintenance, depreciation/amortization, central supplies, data processing, and payroll. This cost can vary from 5 - 30 percent depending on how the facility manages overhead costs.

For example, a nutrition clinic within a hospital may not have overhead, space or maintenance allocated to its specific cost center but a freestanding clinic associated with the same facility may have an overhead cost. In this case, the unit recovery cost would vary greatly. If a 25 percent overhead cost is allocated to the clinic budget, the cost recovery per patient could vary as much as $30 to cover expenses. If all costs amounted to $200,000, then the average unit cost should be $100 per 2,000 patients. This represents an average one hour consultation; whereas, the average unit cost for the same number of patients would be less if an overhead charge did not exist. Revenue must cover expenses.

Building Operation and Maintenance:

Square feet of space used x cost per square foot x the percent time used by the clinic during the budget period equals the overhead cost.

Accounting is the third phase of the management control process. Financial services accumulates and records information on outputs and inputs. The information is provided along both program and responsibility lines. Responsibility cost information is used to determine the degree of compliance with budget projections. Program costs are used to assess the desirability of continuing a particular program at its present size and scope.

In the analysis and reporting phase, differences between actual costs and budgeted costs are reported. The method used in this step is referred to as variance analysis. By reporting the differences (actual versus budgeted), the probable cause of any deviations can be analyzed.

SALARY DETERMINATION

Salaries and wages are established in response to the basic organizational need to attract and retain competent employees. Two methods for determining salaries and wages are: fair market and internal equity and/or comparable worth.

Fair Market:

"Market pricing" as it is called is based on the going rate within the local labor market. The salary decision can be based on high wages or middle-of-the-road wages. Also, salaries can follow the law (economic principle) of supply and demand. Those in short supply and great demand benefit from fast-growing salary increases and status within the job market. An example is the nursing shortage phenomenon. The supply of nurses has been inadequate and accompanied by high turnover thus increasing the demand. Explanations for the nursing shortage include arrogant doctors, politics, red tape, fragmentation of patient care, bad hours, excessive bed making, low pay and lack of advancement opportunities. Nutrition professionals face some of the same frustrations so the question for the rest of the 90s and the next millennium is "will there be a shortage of nutrition professionals and will the salaries continue to lag behind?"

Short supply + Great demand = Higher salary

Fair market pricing is not without problems. The first is the difficulty determining the "going rate." Salary ranges vary greatly between geographic regions. Salaries can range from $18.00 per hour to $30.00 per hour.

This range does not give a complete representation of the market price. This presents the **second** problem; determining whether the salary range is the mean or median rate as well as considering other variables such as position longevity and comparable job title/responsibility. Nutrition professionals with longevity in the same institution can "top-out" their salary range. The **third** problem in this system is the difficulty comparing job titles and responsibilities. For example, a clinical dietitian, nutrition support dietitian and a clinical nutrition specialist might perform the same job functions in different facilities but receive different levels of pay. At the clinical management level, the difficulty comparing job worth may be greater. A clinical nutrition manager and a chief clinical dietitian may be benchmarked the same for salary. The chief clinical dietitian usually has direct patient care responsibilities, whereas the clinical nutrition manager may not perform any patient care.

The **fourth** problem is obtaining salary information in a timely fashion. Salary surveys frequently are obsolete by the time they are incorporated into the budget. Also, salary surveys may not indicate what encompasses the total salary package, such as health insurance, dental insurance, retirement, vacation, sick leave, education days, professional fees/registration payment, and subscriptions.

Internal Equity System:

The internal equity system attempts to measure the contribution of various employee groups to the organization. A systematic analysis of the duties and responsibilities of various positions is conducted. Salaries are determined according to the perceived or real contribution to the total organization. If a systematic analysis of duties and responsibilities of various positions is not utilized, the possibility of salary inequity may be a real problem. In healthcare this problem is sometimes related to gender segregation by position title. Most allied healthcare professionals are female, with possible exception of the pharmacist. In many facilities pharmacists (regardless of gender) receive a substantially higher salary than their female allied health counterparts.

Comparable worth is defined as "the provision of similar salaries for positions that require or impose similar responsibilities, judgment, knowledge and working conditions." Every job contains certain elements that can be defined, evaluated and compared for the purposes of establishing salaries.

A comparable worth advocacy movement developed with the purpose of overcoming discriminatory wage and salary practices and promoting equal pay or jobs of comparable worth. Pro-comparable worth actions have produced some significant court rulings, state laws and labor agreements.

Comparable worth studies indicate nutrition professionals are not receiving compensation equal to their responsibilities, judgment, knowledge and working conditions. Other considerations for salary increases should encompass the fact that nutrition intervention is cost effective and the salary increase would be less than the overall savings from nutrition intervention.

Ensuring salaries are commensurate with responsibilities, all nutrition professionals need to have a basic understanding of the salary negotiation process. Components of this process include:

A. Understanding the organizational policy and procedures by which the organization specifies salaries and wages.

B. Knowing how to write job descriptions, specifications and performance appraisal instruments. Learn to delineate job responsibilities accurately. The four factors to consider in writing a job description and job analysis are:

1. Knowledge and skill
   a. Job knowledge/comprehension/application
   b. Managerial skill
   c. Interpersonal/intrapersonal communications skills
   d. What must be accomplished to perform satisfactorily
   e. Education requirements

2. Mental demand
   a. Independent judgment
   b. Problem solving
   c. Perform mathematical calculations
   d. Analytical ability
3. Accountability
   a. Freedom to take action
   b. Size, nature and impact of the job
   c. Ability to organize and utilize time effectively
4. Working conditions
   a. Physical effort
   b. Hazards
   c. Discomfort
   4. Stress

The job description should include action verbs and action phrases:

Key Action Verbs

Maintain	Establish
Evaluate	Coordinate
Screen	Assess
Educate	Consult
Manage	Organize
Develop	Implement
Instruct	Supervise
Determine	Monitor

Without these key words assignment of the relative worth of the job might not reflect the scope of the position. The position requires a great deal of independent thinking and decision making with minimal or no supervision. It is necessary to maintain a high level of expertise in the field of nutrition and continuing education credits are mandatory to maintain professional registration and licensure.

Key Action Phrases

Practice independently

Bill through insurance

Responsible for supervision of

Exercise independent judgment

Responsible for

C. Conducting labor market surveys. Key jobs/benchmarks may be used to compare jobs or comparable positions in other facilities as a point of reference. If a key job in another profession is used, be sure the job has similar qualifications to prevent future inequities. (For example, do not use nurses because not all RNs have BS degrees nor internships. The pharmacist's education and training is similar to the dietitian.).

    D. Influence and negotiation skills are very important in assuring the job is priced to reflect skills, mental demands, accountability and working conditions necessary to the job.

Hardship of working conditions in a hospital should not be discounted. Clinical nutrition professionals are held accountable for the nutrition care and assessment of patients at nutritional risk, face stress with death and dying, may encounter confrontations with nurses, physicians and/or patients, and may be on their feet a lot.

Regionally, nutrition professionals need consensus on appropriate job descriptions, job titles and cleverly defined job responsibilities. Salary negotiation includes identifying levels of responsibility. Larger institutions may have several levels of nutrition professionals, such as an RD I, RD II, and RD III. RD I may be entry level with no experience; RD II may be two years experience and greater than fifty percent of time spent with high nutritional risk patients. RD III may be three to four years experience, especially in PN and TF, plus management skills and a Masters Degree. Criteria should be established for each level.

The following example can be used as a job description base for clinical dietitians in all patient areas:

Roles:

> Provide specialized medical nutrition therapy and education to patients identified at nutritional risk.

> Provide nutrition expertise and education to the interdisciplinary health care team.

Responsibilities:

> Perform initial nutrition assessment for all high nutritional risk patients.

> Develop quality medical nutrition therapy plans and goals; implement medical nutrition therapy and monitor status and effectiveness of the plan.

> Documentation of the outcome-based nutrition care plan in the medical records according to established clinical pathways.

> Provide effective nutrition education to patients and family member, physicians and other health care professionals.

> Actively participate in patient care conferences and medical rounds. Effectively communicate nutrition concerns and considerations to other health care team members.

> Provide nutrition expertise and serve as a resource person to other members of the health care team and the community.

> Maintain current knowledge in clinical practices of nutrition therapies and treatment protocols.

> Supervise dietetic technicians, students and support personnel.

REIMBURSEMENT/PAYMENT SYSTEMS

The negative effects of malnutrition, susceptibility to infections and other complications, recovery rate, functional status and general well being are well documented in the literature. Early nutrition intervention can make an indisputable contribution to cost-effective, quality care for patients by preventing or treating malnourished and disease specific patients. Appropriate documentation and billing can increase revenue from payers.

Reimbursement for nutrition services depends on documenting the outcome of nutrition intervention. Determine the cost effectiveness of services by evaluating these major areas:

- The effects of nutrition intervention on specific diseases: (e.g., decreased weight loss during chemotherapy or decreased muscle wasting post transplantation.)

- The effectiveness of nutrition education: (e.g., decreased drug use, control of blood pressure without medication, control of blood sugar without medication, lower cholesterol without medication, home tube feeding.)
- The impact of specific nutrition treatment regimens: (e.g., appropriate supplementation to meet nutritional goals, implementation of tube feeding instead of parenteral nutrition.)

Measurable and beneficial outcomes affecting both the patient and facility:

- Decreased length of stay.
- Increased community programs, outreach and ambulatory care.
- Increased reimbursement.
- Meeting accreditation standards.
- Decreased cost to both patient and facility by using enteral rather than parenteral nutrition.
- Improved nutritional status with a decrease rate of infection or other complications.

These outcomes are cost-efficient and outcome effective.

PAYMENT SYSTEMS

A hospital may have four or more different payment systems in effect at any given time. Each payment system has a different effect on the financial situation. The four major payment systems are historical cost reimbursement, specific services (charge payment), negotiated bids and DRGs.

A **Diagnostic Related Group** (DRG) is a grouping of services provided to patients based on diagnosis of patients illness. With approximately 492 DRG categories, every patient with an illness can be categorized into one of the DRGs.

Diagnostic related group (DRG) payment systems have influenced the hospitalized patient's length of stay. Health care professionals are asked to provide proof of cost-effective services. Comprehensive and timely nutrition intervention benefits the patient, lowers health costs and improves reimbursement under the DRG payment system. It is well known that lack of nutrition intervention in malnourished or nutritionally compromised patients can increase the possibility of serious complications, slow recovery, slow wound healing, increase the potential for infection, increase the costs and increase the length of stay while reducing the quality of life.

Under the DRG system, the facility receives a single payment for hospital services provided. The hospital receives the same payment for a patient who stays a short time and incurs few costs as it does for a patient with the same diagnosis who stays beyond the designated DRG days and requires more costly services. Payments are based on the average costs of caring for patients in each DRG. The factors that are considered are primary diagnosis, secondary diagnosis (complications or comorbid conditions), surgical procedure and patients age and sex. Exceptions are made for extraordinary cases (called outliers).

Secondary diagnosis are referred to as complications or comorbid conditions (CCs). Patients with CCs require longer hospitalization and therefore they consume more resources. The DRG systems include categories to cover groups that may include either uncomplicated or complicated cases. Also, many diagnoses are assumed to have complicating conditions, so CCs are not mentioned. Identification of an overlooked secondary diagnosis, malnutrition, can change a DRG category in some patients, thereby decreasing the payment to the hospital.

DRGs are assigned using the principal diagnosis, up to eight additional diagnoses, the principle procedure, plus up to five additional procedures codes, age, sex, and discharge status. One DRG is assigned to each inpatient stay. Factors suggesting nutritional risk include inadequate nutrient absorption; inadequate intake and susequent weight loss; decreased nutrient utilization (alcoholism); increased nutrient losses (abnormal metabolism, alcoholism, blood loss, diarrhea, draining abscesses, fistulas and wounds, dialysis, recurrent vomiting); and increased nutrient requirements (trauma, burns, infection, surgery).

A DRG study may be beneficial to identify patients who require nutrition intervention. Malnutrition can qualify as a comorbidity or complicating condition (CC). The CC could have existed at the time of admission (comorbidity) or developed during the hospitalization (complication) which could increase the length of stay. The DRGs are coded with a CC so the institution receives maximum payment. Previous studies have demonstrated the projected length of stay (LOS) for all DRGs managed by dietitians were 6.8 days; whereas the actual LOS for patients requiring nutrition intervention was 18 days and the patients managed by dietetic technicians average 12 days. Current studies indicate the LOS of stay is 6.1 days and the average length of stay for high nutrition risk patients is between 10 and 12 days.

A DRG study can be done by doing a prospective-retrospective chart study. The clinical nutrition staff can code the medical charts or keep detailed records of those patients receiving nutrition intervention. After discharge, medical records personnel can identify the patients and supply the following information: 1) DRGs receiving nutrition intervention, 2) the ten major DRGs receiving nutrition intervention, 3) percentage of patients who received nutrition intervention during that time period, 4) length of stay and projected length of stay for that DRG, 5) age, 6) sex, and 7) nursing unit. The number of patients assessed by each dietitian and dietetic technician can also be noted. Each would be assigned their own code number. An example of a DRG monitor is shown in Figure 12.

Figure 12: DRG Monitor

Admit Date	Patient Last and First Name	Med Record No	Disease State, Primary and Secondary	Feeding Modality	Dc Date

The DRG study allows the staff to quantify the extent of high risk patients, determine if selected variables can profile patients at nutritional risk and determine where high risk patients are concentrated, all have implications for staffing. Medical records can determine if these patients have CCs coded for them so the facility receives proper payment. According to Hospitals and Health Networks January 1997, the 20 most common DRGs are:

    5 - Extracranial vascular procedures
   14 - Specific cerebrovascular disorders except TIA
   79 - Respiratory infection & inflammations age > 17 with complications
   88 - Chronic obstructive pulmonary disease
   89 - Simple pneumonia and pleurisy age > 17 with complications
  106 - Coronary bypass with cardiac cath
  107 - Coronary bypass without cardiac cath
  112 - Percutaneous cardiovascular procedures
  116 - Other permanent cardiac pacemaker implant
  127 - Heart failure and shock
  148 - Major small and large bowel procedures with complications
  174 - GI hemorrhage with complications
  182 - Esophagitis, gastroenteritis and miscellaneous digestive disorders age > 17 with complications
  209 - Major joint and limb (lower) reattachment procedures

210 - Hip and femur procedures except major joint age > 17 with complications

296 - Nutritional and miscellaneous metabolic disorders age > 17 with complications

336 - Transurethral prostatectomy with complications

430 - Psychoses

462 - Rehabilitation

478 - Other vascular procedures with complications

Timely assessment, treatment and documentation of malnutrition is important for patients covered by the DRG systems. Thorough documentation of malnutrition in some patients can lead to increased hospital revenue as well as quality patient care.

HUMAN RESOURCES

Progressive management is the artful incorporation of people management skills. Cost-effectiveness and fiscal efficiency are top priorities. Health care is marked by ultracompetitiveness, alternative delivery systems, shrinking resources and increased public scrutiny. Nutrition professionals need to approach human resources with optimum efficiency and maximum effectiveness. Quality output is achieved through the intelligent use of human resources and sound human resource practices encourage maximum input and output from each health care employee. All personnel/staff need to provide premium productivity and high-level performance.

STAFFING

Clinical staffing requirements must be determined in order to provide daily nutrition coverage efficiently and cost-effectively. A productivity study and the identification of the population at risk helps determine the number and type of clinical staff needed to provide optimal nutrition care.

Clinical staffing should be based on the identified levels of care and must consider weekend staffing requirements. In determining professional staffing needs the following steps can be implemented:

Step 1 Develop the nutrition care matrix to determine the work hours for patient care.
- Determine levels of care and who provides care in each level.
- Determine number of patients in each level.
- Determine percent of time allocated to each level of care.
- Determine percent of time spent with each patient.
- Determine the acuity level.

Step 2 Determines work hours available.
- Estimate "non direct*" care.
- Estimate "non productive*" care.

Step One Plus Step Two Equals Total FTE Needed

*Terminology:

Direct Patient Care: Nutrition care process

Non-Direct Patient Care: Conferences (patient), meetings, medical rounds, students' education, administrative responsibilities, charging

Non-Productive Time: Coffee breaks, personal time, plus delays for records, patients, elevators

ACUITY LEVEL

A patient acuity measurement system can be a mechanism to categorize patients according to the amount of direct nutrition care required. Acuity should examine the care activities required, time required for each activity and the frequency with which the activities must occur to provide quality nutrition care. Acuity is not measured by the diagnosis nor the risk factors by themselves. Acuity measures the frequency of and time consumed by tasks/data collection.

Knowing the facility's patient population profile, an acuity level can be established. The benefits of such a system are twofold: the information derived from the system can be utilized to establish the nutrition personnel budget and to cost nutrition services accurately. By identifying the acuity of the patients, acuity-based staffing requirements can be used to support staffing decisions.

An acuity system is a mechanism to better utilize available staff and assign staff to appropriate nursing units. In current practice there could be a need to determine the time required to do a task and the expected frequency of the task. An analysis may be done to determine the acuity level of the patients assigned to each staff member. This is beyond the time management study. The results of this study may show whether the current job is matched to the knowledge, skills and abilities of the staff member. **Figure 13** is an acuity measurement for comprehensive/complex nutrition care. It measures time and frequency of tasks of performed and the documentation of the tasks. The acuity analysis is designed to follow the nutrition care process.

Figure 13: Acuity Measurement for Comprehensive Care

Patient _____ Diagnosis _____ Feeding Modality _____

Page ___ of ___	Day	Day	Day	Day	Day	Day	Total RVUs
RVUs/Frequency	R/F	R/F	R/F	R/F	R/F	R/F	Total R/F

Assessment/Evaluation of:
    Histories
    Drugs
    Functional status
    Clinical/physical
    Anthropometrics
    Labs/procedures							

Formulation of Plan							
Documentation							

Monitoring
    Hydration status
    Vital signs
    Diarrhea
    Residuals
    I & Os (TF/PN)
    Electrolytes
    Labs results
    ABGs
    Vent settings
    Drains, fistulas
    NIAs
    Weights
    Wound healing
    Skin grafts (burns)
    Swallowing							

Discharge Planning
    Implementation
    Referral							

Education
    Eval of readiness
    Eval of needs
    Instruction							

Total Daily RVUs							

With this system, the criteria or nutrition care process, associated with patient care are assigned RVUs or data points. The specific nutrition care criteria are identified and the sum of all the RVUs becomes the indicator of time required. The daily RVU frequency can change as the patient's medical condition changes.

KEY:			
RVU (data points)		**Frequency**	
1: 1 - 5 min	6: 26 - 30 min	1x	
2: 6 - 10 min	7: 31 - 35 min	2x	
3: 11 - 15 min	8: 36 - 40 min	3x	
4: 16 - 20 min	9: 41 - 45 min	4x	
5: 21 - 25 min	10: 46 - 50 min		

Directions:

1. Acuity records are to be completed for each high nutritional risk patient until discharge or nutrition status changes secondary to medical status change or a DNAR has been ordered. Records are to be completed daily and submitted at the end of admission or status change.

2. For each section of the acuity record, the nutrition professional determines which criteria accurately reflect the care given, the RVUs and frequency per day. The RVUs per patient would increase as the acuity level increases. The choice is indicated by inserting the letter/frequency by the process, for example under monitoring (ABGs) 2/2x would indicate the ABGs were evaluated twice and documented, which would represent approximately 12 to 20 minutes if this were the only part of the care process being addressed.

   The number of minutes to perform total activity can be converted to RVUs (data points). The higher the minutes the higher the RVUs, which results in a higher acuity level. The results can be analyzed daily or at the end of the study period. Staffing requirements and placement can be based on the acuity analysis.

Example:

• Minutes (RVUs) required to accomplish each activity.

• How many times (frequency) each activity will be performed during the length of stay.

• Multiply RVUs by frequency to estimate the total minutes per patient's length of stay.

• Total minutes for each activity to project the nutrition care minutes needed for each level of care.

Acuity level evaluation should be performed annually to determine staffing for the budget process. Nutrition care then can be further subdivided into four levels of care as shown in **Table 3**. The RD/patient ratio can be based on 80 percent of time in direct patient care. If other non-patient activities are assigned to the staff the patient/RD ratio should reflect this. For example, if 60 percent of the time is spent in patient care and 40 percent in operations, the ratio of RD/patient would be adjusted accordingly.

For Example: ICU patients can be on vents, have blood gases drawn several times a day, have medical status susceptible to change (organ dysfunction), multiple lines, drains, etc. The time spent assessing and implementing nutrition care is time/frequency intense. If the ICU patient consumes 0.6 RVUs for work-up, 0.3 every day of ICU care and stays in the ICU a week, the total time devoted to this patient should be .6 RVU + .3 x 4 = 1.8 RVUs (3 hours). Three hours per week per patient would allow time for approximately 10 to 15 patients, based on 80 percent time in direct patient care.

It is important to note, for simplicity sake, the estimation of time/frequency assumes the intensity is the same for each patient and each day of the week. In reality, the intensity could be greater on Tuesdays, Thursdays, Fridays and Saturdays. Schedules should be adjusted to accommodate the needs of the patients.

On the other hand, for general medical/surgical areas the time/frequency could be less. For the high nutritional risk patient, the total time devoted in a week could be .6 RVU (day one) + .3 x 2 (two follow-ups) = 1.2 RVUs (two hours). Two hours per week per patient would allow time for approximately 16 to 20 patients, based on 80 percent time in direct patient care.

Time calculated for a dietetic technician could be .3 RVU (day one) + .3 x 1 to 2 (follow-ups) = .6 (one hour). One hour per week per patient allows time for approximately 20 to 30 patients per week. Other job responsibilities (screening/supervision) would have to be analyzed prior to assigning 30 patients.

TABLE 3: Levels of Care

Level 4: Intensity	**Complex/In-depth**
RD/patient ratio care needs	1:10 - 15 daily or every other day
Level 3: Intensity	**Major/Advanced**
RD/patient ratio care needs	1:16 - 20 every 2 to 3 days
Level 2: Intensity	**Moderate/Intermediate**
RD/patient ratio care needs	1:20 - 25 every 4 to 5 days
Level 1: Intensity	**Basic**
RD/patient ratio care needs	1:50 every 6 to 7 days

Nutrition acuity levels can be a useful concept with practical application to the mission of the nutrition department. Acuity provides a means of documenting nutrition productivity and determining staffing needs based on the patient population.

Another approach to allocating workload is to assign 1.5 high nutritional risk patients per dietitian per hour. This would encompass new admits and established patients. For example, if productivity studies show that each staff member has one new high risk patient admitted each day, the time allocated would be .6 RVU (one hour) plus 32.4 RVUs (5.4 hours) left for follow-up care. That would allow for 12 patients daily or 24 patients with follow-up care every other day. The productivity study would also indicate the time, (according to the job analysis), devoted to patient care. This is based on a standard 80 percent time in patient care. If the standard time is not at 80 percent, the assignment of high nutritional risk patients has to be adjusted accordingly.

Existing systems used to determine the number and type of nutrition professionals may not be based on the number and types of tasks required for patients who are nutritionally compromised. Therefore, it may be imperative to evaluate the current staffing levels and requirements.

Staffing Model Example for the Dietitian:

Assumptions:		Policy is to screen in the first 24 hours.
		Reassessment with documentation every third day.

	RVU	screening	15 min
		assessment	60 min
		reassessment	30 min

Bed size:		**400**
% occupancy	80%	320
% at nutritional risk	50%	160
% at high risk	80%	128
% at moderate risk	20%	32

Number of admissions/day		**40**
% screened	95%	38
% at risk	50%/80%	15

Number of screens/assessments/follow-ups per day

% screened by RD	50%	4.75 hours
# of high risk assessments		19 per day/19 hours
# of follow-ups per day		36/18 hours
total hours needed		41.75
RDs need with 80% adjustment		6.5
RDs needed with 70% adjustment		7.5

The key approach/formula to determine staffing needs is **task x time x frequency**. This approach also can be applied to determine the number of dietetic technicians needed. Each medical service/nursing unit can be evaluated individually. ICUs/NICUs vary from general medical/surgical units in task/time/frequency.

PRODUCTIVITY

Declining patient days brings focus on doing the right things right. An evaluation of current practices is an integral part of the plan for an effective nutrition care program. Evaluations of current practices may indicate definite areas where role changes will improve the quality of nutrition care provided. The outcome may mean reassigning or eliminating some of the activities. Outcomes management is designed to continuously improve quality care delivered by providing complete data that enables the health care professional to develop the best practices. Outcomes management is doing things right and doing the right thing. Right things identify patient needs, convert needs into requirements (standards), then align processes to meet these requirements. Doing things right means executing processes to effectively meet the requirements.

Productivity can be qualitatively or quantitatively defined. A qualitative study documents services to accepted standards of care. A quantitative study requires selection of a method to accumulate data and is usually in the form of time studies. Time estimates can be obtained through time sampling procedures to define "normal" times for the performance of a specific task/nutrition care process. The studies have an identifiable beginning and end; characterize activities, not skills or knowledge; are performed by an individual staff member; differentiate between activities that involve different kinds of knowledge and skills; are neither too broad nor too specific; and are expressed in clear, unambiguous statements that means the same to all. The clinical productivity process is defined as the ratio of output divided by input.

$$\frac{\text{Nutrition Procedures}}{\text{Hours worked by the Clinical Staff}}$$

Productivity studies allow for intelligent, informed decisions regarding comprehensive nutritional care. Cost containment pressures make it imperative for clinical nutrition to document the demand for and impact of the procedures/services provided in terms of maximum efficiency for effectiveness. A time management study quickly documents the types of activities performed. The productivity study must be approached systematically, following eight steps.

Step 1. Staff Participation.

The staff must be involved in determining the codes, estimated time (Relative Value Unit, RVU) each task requires, the data, and any proposals for end results and/or actions.

RVUs can be used as a time measurement analysis for providing nutritional care. An RVU can have any relative value of time assigned (e.g., 0.1 RVU = 10 minutes), it is important that the value remains consistent.

Step 2. Preliminary Data Collection

Time estimates obtained through time sampling procedures can determine "normal" (or average) times per activity.

The RVU, in conjunction with uniform (standard) definitions, enables reporting qualification and output comparisons. RVUs can reflect the scope of care required in moderate and complex levels of nutrition care. The results provide information regarding the productivity of the entire clinical staff as well as each individual.

Figure 14 represents the RVUs for the initial nutrition assessment for high risk patients in an acute care facility. Follow-up care requires approximately .30 RVUs per high risk patient every one to two days. RVUs can be assigned to dietetic technicians for moderate nutritional risk patients.

Figure 14: RVUs for Initial Nutrition Assessment for High Risk Patients

Action	RVU's*
Screening	.10
Comprehensive Nutrition Assessment	.60 - .90
Education	.30 - .60
Total	1.0 - 1.5

*Relative Value Unit 0.1 RVU = 10 minutes

All tasks need to be sorted into activity types. **Figure 15** is an example of clinical productivity codes for the dietitian and technician. It is divided into direct and indirect patient care. The results usually demonstrate that of the total time spent in patient care, approximately ten percent is spent with the patient and the remainder of the time is spent in activities not conducted in the patient's presence. For example if 80 percent of the staff's time is spent in patient care, 10 percent would be in direct care and 70 percent in indirect care.

Figure 15: Clinical Productivity Codes

Code	Description
DPC	Procedures conducted in patient's presence: Patient interview Diet history Counseling Diet instruction

IPC	Procedures not conducted in patient's presence: Chart review/screening Formulating care plans Documentation Monitoring
SS	Support services: Medical rounds Patient care conferences Q.I. Literature review Menu changes/writing NX implementation Kardex/computer notes Billing Food service operations
SUPV	Supervision/Evaluations: Scheduling DTs, support personnel
TCH	Teaching - students (includes prep time)
CB	Coffee breaks
L	Lunch
ADM	Administrative: Sick leave Annual leave Educational conferences Professional activities

Another way to approach the productivity study can be done using the nutrition care process, utilizing the benchmarking units of service. Benchmarking should validate the productivity study and vise versa.

Comprehensive nutrition assessment: Screen, assess, implement, document	60 to 90 min
Reassessment: Monitor, change or adjust care plan document	30 min
Educate:	30 to 60 min

Step 3. Inservice Training

Each staff member must understand their code lists and how to complete their time logs. A trial period study should be conducted prior to the actual productivity study.

The time management log, **Figure 16**, tracks 15 minute increments (as the benchmarking units of service collection form). The time management log allocates space for ten hours. The activity codes are printed on the log to maintain uniformity. It also has a space for work not accomplished. The work not accomplished represents task/ activities not meeting the standards of care. The log needs to kept daily and the number of squares for each code recorded. This saves time when the analysis begins.

Figure 16: Time Management Form

NAME:_____ DATE:_____
POSITION: _____ DAY OF THE WEEK: _____

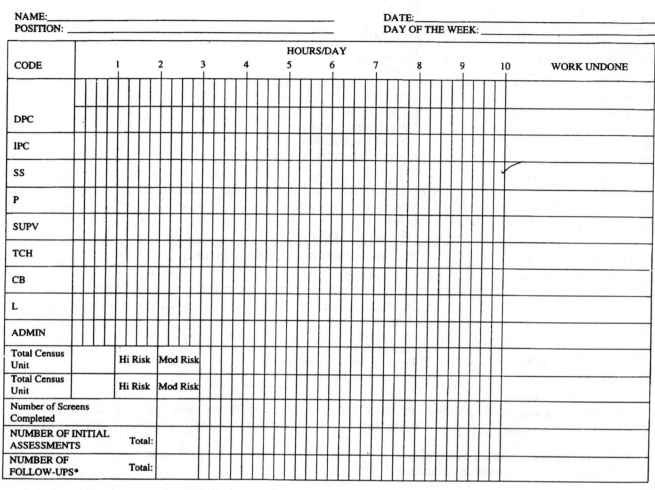

CODE	HOURS/DAY											WORK UNDONE
	1	2	3	4	5	6	7	8	9	10		
DPC												
IPC												
SS												
P												
SUPV												
TCH												
CB												
L												
ADMIN												
Total Census Unit		Hi Risk	Mod Risk									
Total Census Unit		Hi Risk	Mod Risk									
Number of Screens Completed												
NUMBER OF INITIAL ASSESSMENTS	Total:											
NUMBER OF FOLLOW-UPS*	Total:											

*Does not receive a chart entry (i.e., data collection, chart review, etc.).

Step 4. Collection Period

The timing of a productivity study is important. The activity needs to be planned around the time when the facility is in normal census/circumstances. The study should run at least three weeks if not four the first time. This enables a better calculation/evaluation of the number of times a task/activity is repeated. The collection also includes weekend activities. Then the study can be done quarterly for a period of one week. A similar productivity study can be done in the clinic area at the same time.

During the collection time, the daily census should be kept. An area for the number of initial assessments and follow-ups, census of the unit(s) covered, number of high/moderate patients and number of patients receiving nutrition care for that day is part of the daily record collection sheet.

Step 5. Evaluation of Data

The data for the entire evaluation period should be separated by position and by person. If a computer program is available, the data can be entered by each staff member and employee and designed to give percent time spent by each person and the total time spent by each position for the various activities. The program should be designed around the FTE's allocated. The analysis will show the individual's average FTE and the total plus can demonstrate what is actually needed by incorporating the work not accomplished, if applicable.

The week days should be separated from the weekend. When analyzing the weekend time, the level of care needs to be evaluated. If the activities are moderate or basic care, the staff assigned to the weekends should reflect that level of care. The time management form does not reflex designated time (i.e. 8:00 am) because of the flexibility of schedules.

   Evaluation of professional time includes:
   • The average amount of time for procedures conducted in the patient's presence
   • The average amount of time for procedures not conducted in the patient's presence
   • Determine the amount of time spent in support services
   • Evaluate all categories of time spent by each staff member, each job classification and as a total. Each staff position must be evaluated by job assignment(s) i.e., an ICU dietitian could spend more time assessing and managing less patients than a dietitian covering a normal medical/surgical unit
   • Cost of the services can be determined by the $\frac{\text{out-put}}{\text{in-put}}$ formula

The time spent in nutrition assessment can be compared to the RVUs assigned. This could validate the RVUs or suggest "short-cutting" is occurring due to lack of staff. When shortcutting occurs the quality of care must be evaluated. A performance evaluation can be used against the standard of care.

Step 6. Results/Outcomes

Results of the productivity study can help determine and identify specific tasks/activities needed to fulfill patient care responsibilities related to the established standards of care, mission statement and who the activity should be assigned to. Tasks/activities that require flexibility and judgment require greater knowledge and comprehension. Results may have the following outcomes:
   • Reduction and/or increase of FTE's
   • Better use of support personnel
   • Redesign of job descriptions
   • Reevaluate priorities in view of present staffing levels
   • Cost-control
   • Evaluation of peak days and staff accordingly

Results may reflect a need for flex scheduling, which puts the nutrition professional on the assigned work area at the most conducive time for patient care and interaction with other members of the health care team. Flex time can decrease overtime. If a staff members works over the hours assigned, the time needs to be flexed out within a given time period. The time should not be accumulated and flexed out by a whole day of work. Time not flexed out is lost.

If weekends and holidays are not worked by the clinical dietitian, there is a savings/reduction in FTEs. Relief FTE's may not be needed. One day of sick leave need not be covered. If the staff work in teams, the other dietitian(s) can respond to any "emergency."

An outcome productivity study can justify maintaining the current staffing level or justify more staffing to meet the mission statement of the department and facility and meet the standards of care. The end result also justify working within the allocated resources.

Goals of the study are to:
- Discover all tasks being performed
- Estimate and/or validate the time each task requires/takes
- Obtain objective data that permits/documents defensible staffing ratios

PERSONNEL SELECTION

Selection of essential staff is vital to achieving the goals and objectives of the mission statement. The person supervising, evaluating and hiring, along with the person orienting and training, should interview the candidate(s). Success is more likely with good planning.

Example: The manager of clinical nutrition and another clinical dietitian interview and hire the clinical dietitians. Clinical dietitians interview and hire the dietetic technicians and the dietetic technicians may interview and hire the dietary clerks and dietary aides.

This process has accountability and responsibility and it ensures candidate hired is compatible with their team members. Poor hiring processes can cost countless dollars in recruitment, training, benefits enrollment, and downtime. Turnover is also costly.

Interview: The interview provides an opportunity for the employer and applicant to assess whether the applicant's qualifications and skills with the department's goals and expectations are compatible.

In preparation for the interview the following needs to be addressed:

- Determine the questions will be asked each candidate. What you elicit from one, elicit from all. (**Figure 17** Example of Interview Questions). All questions should address work-related experience, training and skills. Each question should have "expected" answers that help rate each applicant appropriately.

- Review each application before the interview, marking any points needing clarification.

- Allow sufficient time for each interview. Interviews typically require one hour up to two hours, depending on the job, complexity of the work, amount of information required and interview styles.

- Develop valid criteria for evaluating the abilities and questions to elicit the necessary information. See (**Figure 18** Applicant Profile Evaluation Form).

Figure 17: Interview Questions

Applicant	Clinical Knowledge	Organizational Skills	Working Relationships	Analytical Skills
	1. How would you calculate fluid needs of a post op patient with multiple drain sites? Answer 2. What would your recommendations be for a patient who has a terminal illness and is not receiving nutrition support? Answer 3. An MD asks for help in formulating PN for an obese post op pt with a 25% wt loss (>30 BMI). Pt is septic and vent dependent. What information is needed, what would your recommendations be and how would you monitor the effectiveness of your care plan? Answer	1. How do you organize your day and set priorities? Answer 2. You have 2 hrs left in your Friday work day. You have 4 new (risk pts, 2 current pts being considered: for tube feeding and PN (the line is being placed on Sat). How will you organize the rest of your day and set priorities? Answer 3. You are in clinic for the day. You have two hours left. Situation: 2 return phone call to established pts; 2 return phone calls to MDs; charting and charging for 4 pts and a new client interview slated for an hour in the next 1/2 hr. How will you set your priorities? Answer	1. How would you make a negative situation positive? Answer 2. What kind of people irritate you and how do you respond to them? Answer 3. How do you manage stress? Answer 4. Under what style of supervision do you function most effectively? Answer 5. A nurse requests you see a pt. You walk into the room and the pt gets verbally abusive. How would you respond? Answer 6. How have you demonstrated flexibility and responsibility in your last/current job? Answer 7. What does success mean to you? Answer	1. An MD calls for information on placing an outpt on home tube feeding. What information do you need to gather? Answer 2. What impact does comp time and O/T have on FTEs and the overall department budget? Answer 3. What is the impact of health care reform on nutrition services? Answer 4. What can you do to demonstrate the cost effectiveness of nutrition intervention? Answer

Figure 18: Applicant Profile Evaluation Form

Name	Clinical Knowledge Gen Spec	Analytical Skills	Organizational Skills	Verbal/ Written Skills	Working Relationships	Confidence/ Response

Evaluate on a scale of 1 to 3; with 3 being the highest and 2 demonstrating basic knowledge

During the interview:

- Describe the job accurately and realistically.
- Share the job description and performance evaluation form.
- Show or describe the exact work setting.
- Be clear regarding quality of work expectations, performance evaluation, work schedules, benefits, vacation and sick leave and encourage the applicant to observe a clinical staff member in the work environment. Allow time for questions.

Outcome of the interview:

- Demonstrates good clinical knowledge/competency.
- Demonstrates effective communication skills (oral and written).
- Demonstrates analytical thinking.
- Demonstrates organizational skills.
- Demonstrates good working relationships (team player).
- Demonstrates being able to function independently while accountable to the mission of the facility/ department.
- Demonstrates enthusiasm.
- Demonstrates spontaneity.

Determine in advance what reference information is needed from employers.

- Be consistent in securing work-related, versus personality or personal habits, information on all candidates.
- Avoid inquiries that can be answered "yes" or "no" in favor of open-ended questions.
- Be wary of and pursue further general responses such as "left for personal reasons" or "would probably be more effective in another work setting than ours."
- Obtain telephone references whenever possible. Telephone inquiries are less time consuming and are more likely to generate valuable work performance information.
- Contact applicant's immediate supervisor, rather than the personnel office and record the person's name.
- Assure the former employer that answers to reference questions will be confidential and will not be shared with the applicant.
- Consider carefully the value of unsolicited letters of reference. They may conscientiously evade important work performance information.

A typical list of elements to cover in a reference check may be:

 Major responsibilities of the former position

 Quality of performance at the time of leaving

 Ability to work effectively with others (team player)

 Attendance

 Eligibility for rehire; if not, why ineligible for rehire.

After completing the interview and checking references, make the hiring decision and offer the job. After the job offer has been accepted, notify the other candidates that the job has been filled.

CRITERIA-BASED PERFORMANCE EVALUATIONS

A criteria-based performance evaluation is a systematic appraisal of an employee's performance based on measurable standards. Performance criteria describe expected performance related to various aspects of the job (fulfilling job requirements according to standards). A key element is the development of a criteria-based performance evaluation system by which an employee is made aware of expectations for successful job performance and observations of performance since last evaluation or in case of new employee at three and six month intervals. A well-designed system focuses on strengths and areas for improvement as they relate to job functions.

The performance evaluation entails factors from the job description (defines the parameters and expectations of the job), performance criteria (describes expected performance related to various parts of the job) and competency (measurable skills necessary to meet performance criteria, where an educational intervention would be used to alter/correct deficiencies).

Job performance evaluation usually are rated using the following criteria:

Quality of Work:
   • Demonstrates accurate, thorough outcome based nutrition care plans in a timely manner
   • Able to identify and analyze problems
   • Demonstrates and promotes high standards
   • Documentation is clear, concise, complete, and accurate

Quantity of Work:
   • Amount of work produced
   • Use of time
   • Volume
   • Productivity results
   • Able to effectively process multiple tasks simultaneously

Job Knowledge:
   • Demonstrates clinical knowledge and application of skills and abilities
   • Amount of supervision required/level of independent functioning

Working Relationships:
   • Cooperation
   • Teamwork; versatility
   • Able to work in a high-stress fast-paced work environment
   • Demonstrates effective oral communication skills
   • Demonstrates listening skills and responds in a positive, supportive manner
   • Develops clear, concise and complete written materials

Supervisory Skills:
- Selection
- Training
- Directing
- Evaluating personnel

Figure 19 is an example of an outcome based performance evaluation. A peer review, a self-evaluation and colleague (physician, nurse, social work or pharmacist) evaluation can be incorporated into the components of the final evaluation.

Figure 19: Performance Criteria (Clinical Dietitian)

Factors	Performance Expectations	Performance Measurements	Rating 1-3	Comment
Quality of work	• Effectively provide nutrition care/education	• The lack of variation	1 - 2 - 3	
		• Full compliance with standards	1 - 2 - 3	
	• Demonstrate the ability to comprehend interpret, and integrate medical condition vs nutrition needs	• Chart audit	1 - 2 - 3	
		• Peer review	1 - 2 - 3	
	• Demonstrate clinical knowledge/ skill and competency	• Colleague review	1 - 2 - 3	
		• Observation	1 - 2 - 3	
	• Written documentation is effective, appropriate and accurate			
	• All work is thorough and complete			
Quantity of work	• Effectively fulfills responsibilities of patient assignment	• Is accountable to assigned work-load	1 - 2 - 3	
	• Coordinates work to achieve maximum productivity and efficiency	• Adheres to established standards	1 - 2 - 3	
	• Manages time and prioritizes tasks effectively	• Completes projects on time	1 - 2 - 3	
		• Able to multitask	1 - 2 - 3	
	• Completes QI in a timely manner			
Job Knowledge	• Develops and implements sound nutrition care plans	• Completes outcome-based nutrition care plans efficiently and accurately	1 - 2 - 3	
	• Maintain current knowledge of and effectively applies current research while providing nutrition care	• Participates in journal club and inservices	1 - 2 - 3	
		• Attends and reports on educational conferences	1 - 2 - 3	
	• Maintain current knowledge of and adheres to departmental policies and procedures	• Follows established policies and procedures	1 - 2 - 3	

Factors	Performance Expectations	Performance Measurements	Rating 1-3	Comment
Working Relationships	• Create effective and positive relationships within the department and with other professionals • Positively promote and cooperate with facility and department plans, programs, and objectives • Exhibit the ability to adapt to different personalities and cultures; maintain calm, professional approach to pressure • Demonstrate effective verbal skills; express ideas freely and clearly • Practice good listening skills • Elicit input from others when presenting ideas and concepts • Is reliable and dependable; self-motivated and self-directive	• Demonstrates approachability to team members and others	1 - 2 - 3	
		• Interacts in a positive manner	1 - 2 - 3	
		• Practices good listening skills	1 - 2 - 3	
		• Actively contributes as a team member	1 - 2 - 3	
		• Remains calm and professional	1 - 2 - 3	
		• Adapts to change in a positive manner	1 - 2 - 3	
		• Serves as a resource person to team members	1 - 2 - 3	
		• Offers and receives feedback constructively	1 - 2 - 3	
		• Demonstrates respect of others' ideas and opinions	1 - 2 - 3	
		• Recognizes and performs activities not directly assigned	1 - 2 - 3	
Supervisory skills	• Demonstrate effective problem solving skills • Effectively delegate • Effectively provide direction and training to support personnel • Demonstrate decision making ability • Accept responsibility for decisions • Maintain confidentiality	• Provides assistance and support to others	1 - 2 - 3	
		• Recognizes problems, gathers facts and reaches sound decisions	1 - 2 - 3	
		• Accepts responsibility	1 - 2 - 3	
		• Follow-through is apparent	1 - 2 - 3	

Performance Rating Definitions

1. Performance does not consistently meet standards. Improvement is necessary.

2. Performance consistently meets standards.

3. Performance consistently meets standards and frequently exceeds performance expectations.

COMPETENCY

Competency is the demonstration of knowledge, interpersonal relationship skills, and critical thinking skills necessary to perform defined job functions. Competencies demonstrates the ability to:

- Define problems, collect data, establish facts, and draw valid conclusions. Ability to interpret an extensive variety of technical/medical treatments and deal with several variables.

- Work with mathematical concepts such as probability and statistical inference. Ability to apply concepts such as fractions, percentages, ratios, and proportions to practical situations.

- Demonstrates clinical knowledge and skills in specialty areas.

The nutrition professional is expected to demonstrate current nutrition information base for the following age groups: neonatal, pediatric, adolescent, adult and geriatric, given present skills, knowledge, abilities, training and education. These competencies should be part of the job description, interview process and performance evaluation.

Competency can be measured/evaluated during the interview process. The candidate must demonstrate the ability to integrate medical nutrition therapy into the planned medical therapy and goals of a specific patient population(s) or disease states. Continued measurement of competency can be reviewed through the performance evaluation process, which would include both peer and colleague evaluations. Competency also can be evaluated through inservices; journal club presentations; and reports from continuing education programs.

JCAHO STANDARDS

The Joint Commission on Accreditation for Hospitals (JCAHO) is a not-for-profit organization that sets standards and accredits hospitals and other health care organizations providing long-term, home, mental-health and ambulatory care. JCAHO accreditation standards have major impact on how health care organizations deliver care. JCAHO focus is on assessing an organizations overall performance and how well multidisciplinary patient care is being integrated. Decisions made by JCAHO affect nutrition in health care.

JCAHO re-focused accreditation from process and structure to patient-care outcomes and established means for monitoring key indicators. The indicators provide data about the relationship between performance and patient health outcomes. Clinical indicators are the tools used to monitor and evaluate the nutrition care of patients. The indicators focus on key functions, treatment processes and other high frequency, high risk and problem-prone aspects of care. They describe events, complications, or outcomes.

Clinical indicators are not meant to be used as direct measurements of quality. Indicators are simple flags that signal potential problems that warrant further review. Indicators include items such as identification of patients who require nutrition intervention, timeliness of nutrition intervention, appropriateness of diet order versus diagnosis, appropriateness of enteral/parenteral nutrition and accurate implementation of the diet order, plus more.

ASSESSMENT AND CARE OF PATIENTS

Assessment and Care of Patients describes everything that must be considered in patient assessment (i.e., physical, psychological and social needs; assessment of nutritional risk; and the assessment of functional status). The goal

---

of patient assessment is to determine what kind of care is required to meet patients' initial needs as well as their needs as they change in response to care; in other words, to provide the right care at the time it is needed.

Nutrition status is assessed when warranted by patients' needs or condition. Nutrition screening/assessment should occur within 24 hours of admission if the patients nutritional status warrants it.

Intent: In the initial assessment, patients who are at nutritional risk are identified according to the criteria developed by the Food and Nutrition Department. A multidisciplinary patient assessment form would be beneficial. If a standardized clinical/critical pathway is used, all staff involved work from the same form, thus eliminating duplication of information. The facility should define assessment activities in policies and procedures or protocols. Assessment polices and procedures define the data gathered to assess patient needs; the scope of assessment by each discipline; the processes used to analyze these data to determine the approach to the care needed; and the framework for making decision on the analysis of information. The plan also identifies measurable goals and actions to achieve them.

Reassessment: Standards state a patient must be reassessed per the established care plan in response to treatment or when there is a significant change in the patient's medical condition.

Intent: Patients are reassessed throughout the care process according to established policies and procedures and/or the clinical pathway. Nutrition care monitoring is a collaborative process involving integration of care with the health care team.

JCAHO standard states that nutrition care practices are standardized throughout the organization.

Intent: The medical staff, nutrition department, and other disciplines collaborate in developing and maintaining standard approaches to nutrition care. A Nutrition Advisory/Care Committee can help develop and/or approve the nutrition care and education processes. This committee also approves the Nutrition Care Manual. The manual is reviewed and revised at least every three years to reflect advances in nutrition knowledge. The manual should be a complete and representative selection of diets and serve as a basis for all diet orders and nutrition products including enteral and parenteral nutrition.

Evidence of Performance: Includes policies and procedures addressing nutrition screening and assessment including criteria for identifying patients at nutritional risk, interviews with clinical staff during JCAHO inspections, and documentation in the medical records.

EDUCATION

The Joint Commission education recommendations state:

- Patient and/or significant other is provided with appropriate education and training to increase knowledge of the patient's illness and treatment needs and learn skills and behaviors that promote recovery and improve function.

Intent: Educating the patient is integral to providing patient care. A positive outcome of a patient's care is often dependent on the instructions given to the patient before care or treatment, the patient's activities subsequent to the patient's discharge from the health care organization, and information given about the patient's health maintenance.

- Patient and/or significant other receive education specific to the patient's assessed needs, abilities, and readiness, as appropriate to the patient's length of stay.

Intent: The organization identifies the responsibilities of patients and their families and educates them accordingly. Patient responsibilities may include but need not be limited to provision of information, compliance with instruction and refusal of treatment.

- Any discharge instructions given to the patient/family are provided to the organization or individual responsible for the patient's continuing care.

Intent: The discharge instructions are communicated to anyone responsible for the patient's health care needs; that is a copy of the discharge summary and instructions are forwarded to the patient's primary care provider.

JCAHO requires a defined assessment process that is current and comprehensive. In a subacute area screening and assessment completed within 48 hours of admission and reviewed every two weeks for the first quarter. In home care the process is developed by the home care providers. The screening requirements for all patients admitted for home care should be completed during the admitting process. The screening includes nutrition-related problems, open wounds, medically prescribed diets, and the elderly who live alone without family support. Reassessment at designated intervals throughout the care according to the patient is specific nutrition care plan. Patients not compromised, a simple nutrition screen every 60 days is required to detect any changes in nutrition status.

Some of the key questions that may be asked on a JCAHO site visit may include:

- How are each patient's learning needs assessed?
- How is a teaching plan prepared specific to the knowledge and skills needed for each patient and family?
- How are patients and families ensured proper education on desired topics?
- What resources are used to review the content and appropriateness of the education material used?
- What resources and references are used to guide education plans?
- Who participates in planning and development of education?
- What ensures patients understand what is taught?
- Where is patient/family teaching documented?
- What is emphasized when documenting patient and family education?
- How is outcome learning documented?
- What information is included in providing follow-up instructions?
- How are follow-up instructions communicated to the patient and family and to the health care provider(s) responsible for continuing care?
- How do you measure, assess, and improve patient education?

QUALITY IMPROVEMENT

Quality Improvement (QI) is a planned systematic process designed to evaluate patient care, identify, analyze and correct any deficiencies and improve the patient care process. Mission, vision, values, and strategic goals form the frame-work of a QI program.

The Joint Commission on Accreditation for Hospitals Organizations (JCAHO) has a QI standard statement, which reads: "There shall be evidence of a well defined, organized program to enhance patient care through the ongoing objective assessment of important aspects of patient care and the correction of identified problems." This requires an ongoing comprehensive quality assurance and quality improvement program to regularly assess all aspects of patient care and implement recommendations to provide more efficient and optimal care.

Quality improvement can also be a way to monitor nutrition assessment and care. The QI process utilizes medical records to evaluate and improve in delivery of nutritional care based on predetermined criteria.

Quality patient care is demonstrated mainly by the clinical competence of practitioners and their performance. Acceptable quality is the specific desired level of achievement or goal against which actual practice can be measured.

Monitors also may be initiated to:

- Compare quality, cost and efficiency of different therapy modalities (e.g., TF versus PN; type of TF versus cost versus outcomes; cost in hours, dollars and resources to operate at this level).

- Collect baseline of performance.

- Determine if a service or an element of care is important. (Determine the outcome each way and then whether to do or not to do it).

Data on the above items may be collected once or infrequently whereas other performance levels (department or staff specific) may be so critical as to warrant regular data collection whether problems are detected or not.

Enough data should be collected so the department manager feels confident making estimates and drawing conclusions from summary reports. The amount of data should not exceed what can be collected and analyzed efficiently within the context of the staff's usual activities. The appropriateness is demonstrated by answering yes to the following questions.

- Is it needed?
- Is it the right timing?
- Is it the right level of care?
- Is it delivered with consideration for alternate types of service?

The aspects or elements of patient care should reflect the overall care/services provided by clinical nutrition. High Priority Clinical indicators should be selected. They will generate the information the institution and department most urgently need to determine quality as well as efficiency and cost. A quality indicator is a measurable variable that can be used as a guide to monitor and evaluate the quality of important patient care. A clinical indicator measures what happens to the patient after something is done to the patient.

The basics for developing clinical indicators are:

- A clinical indicator must be valid (measure what it intends to measure)
- It must be meaningful (detects cases in which actual quality of care problems exist)
- It is designed to examine what that problem is a symptom of
- It collects data elements not just data points
- Analysis of data must be incorporated into the care process

Figure 20 A clinical indicator reflecting a direct relationship to the key function/aspect of care provided by nutrition professionals.

Figure 20: Nutrition Intervention for High Risk Patients

A patient's nutritional status is maintained and/or improved as indicated by the following preselected measurable outcomes(s):

1. Weight maintained and/or dry weight gain and/or weight loss minimized.

2. Appropriate/adequate intake of nutrients (includes tube feeding and parenteral nutrition) according to the clinical nutrition pathways/care plans.

3. Improved hydration and electrolyte status.

4. Protein repletion and/or minimizing protein depletion as designated by improvement and/or maintenance in lab values (accounts for wound healing and decreased infection).

5. Appropriate education provided with learning outcomes.

Instruction for data collection:

1. Record all *new* high nutritional risk patients for two weeks. Do not include the current patient population.

2. Select top measurable outcome(s)/goals for each patient and list them by number.

3. At the time of discharge, score the outcomes as I = maintained/improved; Ø = decreased/compromised.

4. Monitoring of the selected patients occurs for two weeks past the cut off date.

If the patient transfers during the study, treat the patient as though they have been discharged.

Figure 21 offers a Nutrition Intervention Data Collection Form that can be used to collect the data.

Figure 21: Nutrition Intervention Data Collection Form

Patient Name	Admit Date	Diagnosis	Diet	Scrn Date	Ass. Date	Measureable Outcome Selected	Goal I M	Outcome At Dc I Ø N/A	Dc Date	Cause/ Reason For Ø Score

I = Improve   M = Maintain   Ø = Decreased/compromised   N/A = Data not available

The collected data need to be summarized using narrative form, graphs, tables or diagrams. The primary focus in evaluating data is to determine if the desired outcome/established standards are met. Resolution of the identified problem(s) can be addressed in a cause and effect diagram. This type of reporting can be addressed in storybook form:

Objective Statement: To increase the percent of at high nutritional risk patients with improved outcomes following nutrition intervention.

A patient's nutritional status is maintained and/or improved as indicated by the following preselected measurable outcomes(s):

Initial Process: When screening criteria identify a patient at nutritional risk, the patient will have a documented outcome-based nutrition care plan.

Quality Performance Measures: measures to monitor process behaviors and increase the percent of measurable outcomes.

The following is a graphical display of cause and effect. Causes must be identified. The effect is patients at high nutritional risk are not consistently meeting their desired outcome-based nutritional care plan at discharge and/or transfer.

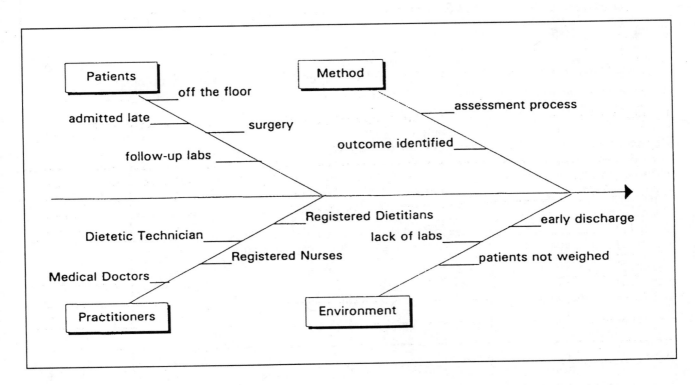

The outcomes are analyzed and solutions are implemented to improve process performance. Variances can be reported using the following criteria: severity of illness, change in the medical condition, patient/family decision, non-compliance, and/or availability of treatment in a timely fashion. The results can be reported on a trend chart as shown below.

Process Indicator: measures important steps in the patient care process; the best process indicators focus on processes of care that are closely linked to patient outcomes. More examples of process indicators are discussed in the benchmarking section of this chapter.

JCAHO expects QI to be meaningful and have a demonstrable impact on patient care over a period of time. Preparation and organization are of key importance during a JCAHO survey. Surveyors will evaluate the capability to assure the quality and appropriateness of nutrition services as it relates to patient care. Surveyors will ask the department to show them what is being done about quality improvement. They will want to see quality related monitors that access direct patient care issues, not simply management related monitors.

The goal of QI should be directly related to the department mission statement. For example, the mission statement of the Food and Nutrition department may be to provide optimal nutrition care and quality food service. Therefore, the QI monitor/survey should reflect that statement. If the results show variances, these must be acted upon. Variances may be an opportunity to improve the patient care process. It is important and necessary to do "things" better today and constantly be on the lookout for ways to correct problems, prevent problems and make improvements.

BENCHMARKING

According to the Webster's dictionary benchmarking is something that serves as a standard by which others may be measured. In industry/healthcare benchmarking is the search for the best practices that will lead to exceptional performance through their implementation of the best practices. In comparing data with like facilities, similar data collection techniques and methods of analysis need to be used. Benchmarking is a process of identifying and learning from the best practices. There are two types of benchmarking: comparative and process.

COMPARATIVE

Comparative benchmarking measures organizational performance against that of competing organizations by focusing on key measures and indicators. The purpose is a self assessment and to identify the best performers. The uses of comparative benchmarking are for cost containment initiatives, annual budgeting, comparison against peers, and productivity monitoring and improvement.

Comparative benchmarking can be accomplished across the country for comparative analysis of like institutions. Common problems with comparative benchmarking of the Food and Nutrition department are how meals are counted, patient acuity, definition of consults, outpatient services/outreach services and how meal trays are passed out and picked up.

A unit of service study can be done quarterly and/or daily to define how many nutrition consults are done by the Food and Nutrition department per year. The first step is to define a consult in terms of its components and time. A consult is a professional service performed by dietitians and dietetic technicians and the unit of time for the consult is 30 minutes. This type of benchmarking does not measure quality.

Figure 22 represents a quarterly unit of service study based on the nutrition care process for high and moderate nutritional risk patients. It is important to be cognizant of the time required for the care process and the definition of each term. This study should validate the nutrition care process.

Figure 22: Unit of Service Study for High Nutritional Risk Patients

Date	Units Billed	Units Non-billed*	Total Units*	Hours Worked	% time in Patient Care	Number of High Risk Patients

If the units are performed daily, the following form can be used to collect information. The staff can record daily units of service monthly, weekly, or daily by email. A computer data analysis program can't determine total units of service, percent time in patient care and the number of high nutrition risk patients. This information then can be analyzed for reasonable, equitable work loads.

*Units of service are measured in 15 minutes

PROCESS

Process benchmarking measures discrete process performance and functionality against organizations that lead in those processes. It seeks best practices for conducting a particular operational or clinical process and the purpose is to analyze processes and identify the best/better performers. First, the process has to be validated as the best.

The steps in process benchmarking are 1) planning, 2) analysis, 3) discovery, 4) implementation, and 5) change.

Planning:

The process and methodology needs to be defined. Who will participate in the study?

Analysis:

What is the current process and how does it work? How will it be measured? How well is it performing? What is the process's performance goals? What data needs to be collected for comparisons? What criteria should be used to identify benchmarks?

Discovery:

Which organization(s) performs this process better? Which organization is performing this process best? What can be learned from this organization? How well does their process perform over time? What is the basis for comparing processes from one facility to another? What is the magnitude of the performance gap? What is the nature of the performance gap? What characteristics distinguish the other process as superior? What activities in the current process can be improved?

Implementation:

How does knowledge of their process help improve ours? Where should the future effectiveness of their process performance be projected? Should our process be redesigned or should performance goals be reset based on their benchmark? What goals need to be set for process improvement and how to implement the changes in the current process.

Monitoring:

How will future performance of the process be monitored? What mechanism will be used? How will we report this information and to whom? With whom will we continue to compare with our organization?

The screening and assessment process should be considered for this type of benchmarking (**Figure 23**).

Figure 23: Clinical Nutrition Intervention QI

Patient	Med No	Admit Date	Scrn Date	Risk Status No Mod	Risk Date	Assess Date	F/U Date	2nd F/U Date	3rd F/U Date

Directions:
1. Record all assigned patients.
2. Assign appropriate level of care.
3. List admit date.
4. List screen date, if different from initial assessment date.
5. List assessment date.
6. List follow-up (F/U) dates.

The results of this process indicator indicate the percent of patients identified at nutritional risk within the first 24 hours of admission; the percent of patients identified at nutritional risk who are documented according to the standards; and the percent of patients documented who meet the standards of charting.

Another process indicator is the evaluation of high nutritional risk patients who are NPO or on clear liquids diets. Do they remain NPO and on clear liquids longer than three days? (See **Figure 24**).

Figure 24: Patients NPO or on Unsupplemented Clear Liquids Longer than 3 Days

Date _____ Unit _____ Census _____ Auditor _____

Patient	MD	Risk	CI Date	NPO Date	Diet 3 Days	Variance M S Pro	Action	Comment

Directions:

1. Review for NPOs and clear liquids.
2. List all patients NPO and/ or clear liquid.
3. List total unit census.
4. Identify MD service.
5. Identify risk category.
6. Record diet order 72 hours later.
7. If patient's diet has not changed, identify the variance as procedural, medical or surgical and the plans/ actions.
8. List actions taken.
9. Comment on reasons for the variances.

Exceptions: DNAR, TF, PN

(Note: NPO to clear liquid needs a follow-up)

The results of this process indicator will indicate the percent of patients who are NPO and/or on clear liquids, their service/diagnosis, the length of time without nutrition support, their primary nutritional risk category, the outcome(s) if any, and documented nutrition intervention and/or appropriate diet advancement.

Another process indicator is the patient needing drug-nutrient interaction counseling prior to discharge. Counseling should be given to those patients receiving drugs with a high risk for drug-nutrient/food interactions, patients with chronic diseases receiving long-term drug treatment, and patients receiving high-dosage regimens, such as chemotherapy. The following QI improvement form (**Figure 25**) demonstrates the type of drug administered, the type of counseling given/needed, patient comprehension, and the action taken if the patient cannot comprehend and or adhere to the instruction.

Figure 25: Clinical Quality Improvement

Drug/Nutrient Interactions

Patient Name	Diagnosis	Drug(s)	Counseling Given	Comprehension	Action/ Comments

The results demonstrates the patient/care-giver can describe appropriate food choices and/or feeding regimens consistent with the counseling received.

Benchmarking helps to create a healthy discomfort with the current state of excellence, determine what to change/not to change, define the desired results after the change and accelerate innovation. Benchmarking helps reengineering decisions. Issues to address are:

- Does the function need to be done?
- Is there a duplication of effort?
- Is it performed by the appropriate level of care?
- Is it done at the most effective time?
- Is there a more efficient, cost-effective way to do it?

Benchmarking can be used in the budget process. It can be used to project units of service (UOS) for both inpatient and outpatient consults with the FTEs needed for that level of care. It can demonstrate the labor dollar, time utilized and revenue for each UOS. The future budgets then can be benchmarked against that data. Some questions that will need answer in this type of process are: What process improvements are being made? What changes are being made? What is being done today to be successful in operating future budgets? How will changes be sustained?

Benchmarking is a never-ending journey – not a destination.

AMBULATORY CARE MANAGEMENT

The need for nutrition education and consultation, brought about by shortened length of stay; increased incidence of chronic disease in an aging population and increased public interest in nutrition, are contributing factors to expanding ambulatory nutrition services. The nutrition education process consists of screening, assessment, implementation and/or education, documentation and communication, and reassessment/monitoring.

NUTRITION EDUCATION PROCESS

Screening

Screening should occur in the ambulatory/clinic settings. Policies for screening vary amongst settings. A facilities' policy may indicate that screening could be a referral from a physician, nurse, social worker, pharmacist, lab technician, acute care dietitian, any other member of the health care team or the patient.

Screening in ambulatory care consists of the following:

- Physical and medical history
- Diagnosis/disease state that are known to have adverse effects on nutritional status
- Weight – 5 percent loss in one month, 10 percent loss in six months, or a BMI greater than 30
- Labs – albumin of 3.0 gm/dL or less and a prealbumin of 10 mg/dL or less
- Age greater than 70 years or less than 16 years
- Feeding modality (tube feeding and parenteral nutrition)
- Chewing and swallowing problems
- Drug/nutrient interaction – chronic drug use by the elderly and known drugs identified as impacting nutritional status and/or having drug/nutrient implications
- Diet history indicating limited food choices and/or limited access to adequate nutrition

Figure 26 can be used as a screening tool. **Figure 27** can be used as a screen for education purposes.

Figure 26: Nutrition Screening in Ambulatory Care

1. Age: **Assign Point Score as Follows:**

50 - 60 years	0
60 - 70 years	1
70 - 80 years	2
80+ years	3

2. Weight History:

Current Weight _____   % Usual Weight _____   3 mo.   6 mo.   1 yr.

Usual Weight _____   % Wt loss/gain _____   3 mo.   6 mo.   1 yr.

Ideal Body Weight _____   % Ideal Body Weight _____

During the past two weeks: wt ↑   wt ↓   no change

% weight loss (3 mo)	Points
0 - 10 %	1
10 - 20 %	2
< 20 %*	3

3. Diet History

Food frequency, 3 to 7 day food record or a 24 hour recall.

Food intake over past one to two months:

☐ Unchanged   ☐ > Usual

☐ Changed   ☐ < Usual

Assign Point Score:	Points
100% RDA	1
75 - 100% RDA	2
50 - 75% RDA	3

4. Lab Data

Assign Point Score:		Points
Albumin:	3.5 or >	1
	3.5 - 3.0	2
	<3.0	3

5. Nutritional Status:

Points	Nutritional Status
3 - 4	not compromised
5 - 7	moderately compromised
8 -12	compromised

* if labs are not available, recalibrate form accordingly

Functional Status: past one to two months activity

☐ Normal with no limitations

☐ Not normal; able to be up with some limitations

☐ In a chair or bed half the day

☐ In a chair or bed most of the day

☐ Rarely out of bed

Figure 27: Nutrition Screen for Education

Name _____ Date _____

Age _____ Height _____ Weight _____ Desired Weight _____

Please answer the following questions:

1. How would you describe your eating habits? ☐ Good ☐ Fair ☐ Poor

2. Please check any of the following you have:

   ☐ Nausea ☐ Diarrhea ☐ Swallowing Problems

   ☐ Vomiting ☐ Constipation ☐ Chewing Problems

3. Please check the following meals you eat:

   ☐ Breakfast ☐ Lunch ☐ Dinner

4. Do you have any food allergies or intolerances? Please list: _____

   _____

5. How often do you eat out? _____ times per week

   Which meals? _____

   What type of restaurants? _____

6. How many caffeinated beverages do you drink daily?

   _____ Cups of coffee (regular)

   _____ Colas (cans)

   _____ Cups of tea (regular)

7. Do you take any vitamin/mineral supplements? Please list: _____

   _____

8. Do you routinely exercise? Please describe: _____

9. Are you now following or have you ever followed a special diet? What type? _____

   Who did you receive the instruction from? _____

   Were you able to implement the suggested changes into your daily food habits? _____

10. Do you think you need more information to incorporate a healthy diet into your lifestyle? _____

Assessment

Chart Review

1. Histories: medical and social

2. Physical exam

3. Anthropometrics: documented height and weight

4. Laboratory evaluation of:
   a. Hematological data
   b. Fluid and electrolyte balance
   c. Transport protein levels
   d. Lipid profile
   e. Others as appropriate

5. Clinical Assessment
   a. Assess nutritional status
   b. Evaluate degree of malnutrition
   c. Evaluate patient's functional status
   d. Determine potential drug/nutrient interactions
   e. Evaluate factors that may affect intake
   f. Assess for evidence of maldigestion and/or malabsorption

Patient Interview

1. Weight patterns

2. Perceived appetite change

3. Chewing and swallowing problems

4. Chronic medication use; including over-the-counter drugs

5. Diet
   a. Determine patient's diet/nutrition history
   b. Identify/diagnosis deficits/imbalances
   c. Evaluate intake and output: fluids and solids
   d. Calculate nutrient requirements
   e. Determine diet/nutrition plan needed

Implementation/Education

1. Formulate the care plan
   a. Specify goal of therapy and desired outcome(s)
   b. Determine/recommend modality of feeding
   c. Determine/recommend vitamin/mineral supplements
   d. Specify macro/micro nutrients
   e. Recommend electrolytes as appropriate

2. Counsel patient and/or significant other

3. Provide for continuity of care

Documentation/Communication

1. Document the care plan in the medical record; include statement on instruction given, who was instructed (if not the patient), comprehension, expected adherence, goals and outcomes expected.

2. Communicate the care plan to other health care professionals.

3. The SOAPE style can be implemented. (Refer to education for components to include in the documentation).

Reassessment/Monitoring

1. Monitor the effectiveness of the nutrition plan
2. Monitor changes in medical status
3. Monitor for complications of feeding modalities
4. Revise the plan if condition/need of the patient changes
5. Reeducate the patient and significant other
6. Document follow-ups
7. Communicate follow-ups

JCAHO IN AMBULATORY CARE

Joint Commission on Accreditation for Hospitals Organization in the ambulatory area states the following for nutrition care:

Assessment of Patients

- Nutritional status is assessed when warranted by the patient's need or condition.
- The facility has defined patient assessment activities in writing.
- The facility defines the scope of assessment performed by each discipline.

Nutrition - Care of Patients

- Care is planned to meet all identified needs and is documented in the medical records.
- Patient's progress is evaluated periodically against care goals and the plan or goals are revised as necessary.
- Each patient's nutrition care is planned.
- Interdisciplinary nutrition therapy plan is developed and periodically updated for patients at nutritional risk.
- Each patient's response to nutrition care is monitored.
- Nutrition care practices are standardized throughout the organization.

Education

- The patient's learning needs, abilities, preferences, and readiness to learn are assessed.
- The assessment considers cultural and religious practices, emotional barriers, desire and motivation to learn, physical and cognitive limitations, language barriers, and the financial implications of care choices.
- Patients are educated about potential drug-food interactions, and are provided counseling on nutrition and modified diets.
- Patients are informed about access to additional resources.
- The patient and family educational process is collaborative and interdisciplinary, as appropriate to the plan of care.

DISEASE STATE MANAGEMENT/PROTOCOLS OF CARE

Disease state management (or protocols of care) is an approach that contributes to cost control and quality care. Outcomes are evaluated by continuous quality improvement measures such as decreased blood sugars, decreased cholesterol, weight management/control, decreased medication use and decreased hospitalization.

Protocols provide for equitable quality care for the various disease/diagnosis states encountered in practice. Protocols define medical nutrition therapy in concrete terms, increase effectiveness of care by promoting consistency, are easier to measure for quality and effectiveness of care and are compatible with current trends in health-care financing. Protocol development can help provide cost-effective nutrition care. They should be flexible working models and should provide guidelines to ensure patients receive quality nutrition counseling and education. The following is an example protocol for weight management.

Protocol of Care for Weight Management:

I. Counseling Session/length: #1/60 minutes

  Assessment:

  A. Chart Review/clinical data
  1. History: medical, social and drug
  2. Physicians goals and patient goals
  3. Pertinent lab data
  4. Weight/BMI

  B. Patient Interview
  1. Weight/weight patterns history
  2. Nutrition history, including meals away from home
  3. Patient goals/expected outcomes
  4. Psychosocial and economic issues
  5. Exercise/activity pattern – type, frequency, duration
  6. Knowledge/readiness to learn

  C. Intervention
  1. Diet prescription
  2. Meal planning/food record/food pyramid
  3. Label reading
  4. Dining out
  5. Exercise program

  D. Documentation and Communication
  1. Place nutrition progress note in the medical record
  2. Send copy of nutrition assessment to referring MD
  3. Instruct patient to call with questions

  E. Follow-up:
  1. Schedule next counseling session in two to three weeks
  2. Call and/or send postcard prior to next appointment

  F. Expected Outcomes:
  1. Meet desired goals
  2. Lose one pound per week
  3. Complete food records
  4. Increase exercise

II. Counseling Session/length: #2/30 minutes

  A. Assessment:
  1. Clinical Data
    Current weight
    Current exercise regimen
    Food records

  B. Outcomes: change in patient
  1. Change in weight
  2. Change in eating habits
  3. Exercise program

REIMBURSEMENT/CHARGING

Coding practices for nutrition services vary across the United States and from insurer to insurer. Nutrition professionals can use the diagnosis or diagnosis code that has been designated by the physician. When a health care provider submits a claim for nutrition services to an insurance company, the provider completes an insurance claim form describing the patient's condition, services rendered, and charges for these services.

To receive payment for professional services rendered, a billing system has to be implemented. The Physicians' Current Procedural Terminology (CPT) is a coding system that can be important for the nutrition services provided in the outpatient environment. Also, The International Classification of Diseases, Clinical Modification (ICD-9-CM) clearly describes particular procedures for the patient.

ICD-9-CM system lists diseases, diagnosis codes and inpatient procedures codes. Diagnoses and procedures as designated by ICD-9-CM codes can be used to distinguish the type of malnutrition.

Using proper codes for nutrition services facilitates efficient claims processing. The following are Nutrition-Related ICD-9-CM Codes that can be used in the billing process.

Codes qualifying as a substantial comorbidity or complication

260	Kwashiorkor: nutritional edema with dyspigmentation of skin and hair
261	Nutritional marasmus: nutritional atrophy, severe calorie deficiency, severe malnutrition NOS*
262	Other severe protein-calorie malnutrition: malnutrition of third degree (weight for age <60% of standard), nutritional edema without mention of dyspigmentation of skin and hair
263.0	Malnutrition of moderate degree: malnutrition of second degree (weight for age 75% to <90% of standard)
263.2	Arrested development following protein-calorie malnutrition: nutritional dwarfism, physical retardation due to malnutrition
263.8	Other protein-calorie malnutrition
263.9	Unspecified protein-calorie malnutrition: dystrophy due to malnutrition, malnutrition (calorie) NOS. Excludes nutritional deficiency NOS (269.9)
269.0	Deficiency of vitamin K. Excludes deficiency of coagulation factor due to vitamin K deficiency and vitamin K deficiency in newborns
276.0	Hyperosmolality and/or hypernatremia: sodium excess, sodium overload
276.1	Hypo-osmolality and/or hyponatremia: sodium deficiency
276.2	Acidosis: acidosis NOS, lactic, metabolic, respiratory. Excludes diabetic acidosis
276.3	Alkalosis: alkalosis NOS, metabolic respiratory
276.4	Mixed acid-base balance disorder: hypercapnia with mixed acid-base disorder
276.5	Volume depletion: dehydration, depletion of volume of plasma or extracellular fluid, hypovolemia
276.6	Fluid overload: fluid retention. Excludes ascites, localized edema
276.7	Hyperpotassemia: hyperkalemia, potassium excess, intoxication or overload
276.8	Hypopotassemia: hypokalemia, potassium deficiency
276.9	Electrolyte and fluid disorder not elsewhere classified: electrolyte imbalance, hypo- or hyperchloremia
277.00	Cystic Fibrosis: fibrocystic disease of pancreas, mucoviscidosis, without mention of meconium ileus
277.01	Cystic Fibrosis: with meconium ileus

279.10   Deficiency of cell-mediated immunity with predominant T cell defect unspecified

279.3   Unspecified immunity defect

279.9   Unspecified disorder of immune mechanism

280.0   Iron-deficiency anemia secondary to blood loss (chronic). Excludes acute posthemmorrhagic anemia

281.4   Protein-deficiency anemia: amino-acid deficiency anemia

281.8   Anemia associated with other specified nutritional deficiency: scorbutic anemia

285.1   Acute posthemorrhagic anemia: anemia due to acute blood loss

286.7   Other and unspecified coagulation defects

305.00   Alcohol abuse, unspecified

305.01   Alcohol abuse, continuous

305.02   Alcohol abuse, episodic

307.1   Anorexia nervosa

425.7   Nutritional and metabolic cardiomyopathy

536.0   Achlorhydria

536.1   Acute dilation of stomach: acute distention of stomach

564.3   Vomiting following gastrointestinal surgery: vomiting (bilious) following gastrointestinal surgery

579.3   Other and nonspecified postsurgical nonabsorption: hypoglycemia or malnutrition following GI surgery

Codes Not Qualifying as a Substantial Comorbidity or Complication

536.2   Persistent vomiting: habit vomiting, uncontrollable vomiting

783.0   Anorexia

783.1   Obesity

783.2   Abnormal weight loss

783.3   Feeding difficulties or mismanagement: elderly or infant

783.4   Lack of expected normal physiological development. Failure to gain weight, failure to thrive, lack of growth, physical retardation, short stature

783.5   Polydipsia

783.9   Other symptoms concerning nutrition, metabolism, and development

988   Toxic effects of noxious substance eaten as food

990   Effects of radiation, unspecified: complication of radiation therapy

994.2   Effects of hunger: deprivation of food, starvation

994.3   Effects of thirst: deprivation of water

*NOS = not otherwise specified.

The most significant problems associated with coding for nutrition services are 1) no CPT codes that uniquely describe nutrition services; 2) absence of nutrition code may contribute to nonpayment by insurers; 3) general codes used do not specifically describe nutrition services and 4) lack of uniformity in coding practices for nutrition services.

Figure 28 is an example of a charge form used in an outpatient nutrition department.

Figure 28: Ambulatory Care Charge Form

X	CHRG CODE	MIN	VISITS DESCRIPTION
			NEW PATIENTS
	200	15	Brief Service
	210	30	Limited Service
	215	45	Intermediate Service
	220	60	Comprehensive Service
	217	75	Initial Extended
	225	90	Extended Comprehensive
			ESTABLISHED PATIENTS
	240	15	Brief Service
	250	30	Limited Service
	260	45	Intermediate Service
	270	60	Extended Service
	280	75	Comprehensive Service
	285	90	Extended Comprehensive

CHARGE CODE DESCRIPTION

X	CHRG CODE	CPT CODE	MISC. CHRG. DESCRIPT - WRITE CLEARLY	CHRG AMOUNT
	299			$.
				$.
				$.
				$.

#	ICD9 CODE	DIAGNOSIS - INDICATE PRIORITY: 1- PRIMARY 2- SECONDARY
	042.9	AIDS
	693.1	Allergy - Food
	335.2	ALS
	280.9	Anemia - Iron Deficiency
	307.1	Anorexia Nervosa
	414.0	Arteriosclerotic Heart Disease
	174.0	Breast Cancer
		Cancer - Malignant Neoplasm (Site)
	425.4	Cardiomyopathy
	496	Chronic Obstructive Pulm. Dis.
	571.9	Cirrhosis
	428.0	Congestive Heart Failure
	555.9	Crohn's Disease
	277.0	Cystic Fibrosis
	250.00	Diabetes Mellitus
	558.9	Diarrhea
	562.10	Diverticulosis
	977.9	Drug Interaction, GI
	564.2	Dumping Syndrome
	787.2	Dysphagia
	783.3	Feeding Problem
	564.9	Functional Bowel
	575.9	Gallbladder Disease
	648.8	Gestational Diabetes
	044.9	HIV
	573.3	Hepatitis
	272.0	Hypercholesterolemia
	401.1	Hypertension
	251.2	Hypoglycemia
	244.9	Hypothyroidism
	564.1	Irritable Bowel
	176.9	Kaposi's Sarcoma
	573.9	Liver Disease
	710.0	Lupus
	579.9	Malabsorption
	263.9	Malnutrition
	648.9	Malnutrition Complicating Pregnancy
	386.00	Meniere's Disease
	270.1	PKU
	410.9	Myocardial Infarction
	278.0	Obesity
	733.0	Osteoporosis
	269.9	Other Nutritional Deficiency
	V22.1	Prenatal Care
	593.9	Renal Disease
	579.2	Short Bowel
	V42.1	Transplant - Heart
	V42.0	Transplant - Kidney
	V42.7	Transplant - Liver
	V42.6	Transplant - Lung
	V42.8	Transplant - Pancreas
	531.90	Ulcer - Gastric

#	MISC. DIAGNOSIS - WRITE CLEARLY & INDICATE ICD9 CODE IF AVAILABLE	
	ICD9 CODE	DESCRIPTION
	ICD9 CODE	DESCRIPTION

NUTRITIONIST

NUTRITIONIST

_____ PATIENT REFERRAL SOURCE _____ _____ PATIENT DISPOSITION

ORDERING / REFERRING PHYSICIAN — PHYSICIAN NO.

PERFORMING PHYSICIAN — PHYSICIAN NO.

ATTENDING PHYSICIAN NAME & SIGNATURE (M.D.) — PHYSICIAN NO. — ☐ NOT PRESENT

DATE

ORD.STA.NO.

PT.NO.

NAME

HUMAN RESOURCES

The size of the staff depends on the number of enrollees, clients and/or members (covered lives) and the type of facility. For instance, specialty clinics (cystic fibrosis, organ transplants, radiation oncology, high-risk pregnancy, virology, and others) may need more staffing than a family medicine clinic secondary to patient disease state complexity and health care team meetings.

In free-standing clinics the nutrition professional to enrollee/member ratio is one full-time equivalent to approximately 20,000 to 25,000 enrollees. A ratio of new versus established clientele will impact on the hours available for nutrition counseling.

Staffing needs are determined by the following key elements:

- Percent time in direct patient contact.
- Percent time allotted for initial and follow-up sessions.
- Percent time allotted for documentation/dictation, chart reviews.
- Percent time in program planning and development, meetings, patient care conferences, education days, vacation and sick leave.
- Number (percent) of no shows and cancellations.
- Scheduling and calling prior to appointments and follow-up calls.
- Number of scheduled classes and time allocated for preparation.

If 60 percent of time is allocated for direct patient contact and follow-up, the following could apply for one FTE/day.

60% x 8 hrs	=	4.8 hours
2 new consults per day	=	2.0 hours
6 follow-ups per day	=	3.0 hours

260 days/year with adjustments for cancellations/no shows, vacation, sick days and holidays = ~1200 - 1500 billable patients per FTE. These numbers do not represent services provided without charging.

Performance Evaluation

The same type of performance evaluation can be used in the clinic setting with an adaptation of outpatient personnel. **Table 4** can be used for chart review.

Table 4: Clinic Evaluation - Medical Record Review

Dietitian _____ Patient _____ Instruction Given _____

Date _____ Diagnosis _____

Initial Documentation	Yes	No	Comments
Statement of who has been instructed			
Statement of type of instruction			
Evaluation of nutritional status			
(wts, labs, intakes drugs)			
Evaluation of nutritional needs			
Statement on evidence of learning			
Statement of expected goals/outcomes			
Statement on adherence/compliance			
Statement of drug/nutrient interaction, if appropriate			
Statement on acknowledgment of culture, lifestyle, if appropriate			
Statement on continuum of care			
Follow-up care address:			
Review of compliance			
Review of comprehension, if necessary			
Review of labs, wt, intake as appropriate			
Statement on progress/goals			

Productivity

The same type of productivity study can be done in the clinic setting with an adaptation to outpatient.

BENCHMARKING

A unit of service/consult study based on the nutrition education process for clinic/ambulatory patients is similar to the benchmarking for inpatient services. It is important to be cognizant of the time required for the education process and the definition of each term. (See previous education process terminology.) This study should validate the nutrition education process. **Figure 29** is a unit of service study based on the nutrition education process for clinic/ambulatory service patients.

Benchmarking also can be used as a productivity study in the clinics and can be used in the budget process to maintain/increase current staffing. It helps verify productivity data; shows charging may not demonstrate services provided, and documents the need for standardized units of service.

Figure 29: Units of Service - Ambulatory Care

NUTRITION CLINIC

UNITS OF SERVICE

Patient Name	Diagnosis	Medical Service	New	Return	Assess	Educate	Document

*each small square represents 15 minute intervals

QUALITY IMPROVEMENT

Quality Improvement (QI) monitoring must be done in the ambulatory service area. QI can be accomplished through a patient questionnaire, diet instruction indicator, or by an appropriateness of diet orders for condition/diagnosis and/or consult requested by the physician. QI can also indicate whether nutrition goals have been met.

QI patient satisfaction survey can be accomplished through a Quality Improvement Questionnaire (**Figure 30**).

Figure 30: Quality Improvement Questionnaire

1. Were you given enough information to make the recommended changes?

   Comments:

2. What results do you want from changing your usual eating habits?

   Comments:

3. List the changes you have made.

4. Do you have difficulty following the recommendations?

   If Yes, check the following:

   _____ Unable to find the suggested food items.

   _____ Too many other conflicts or stresses at this time.

   _____ Do not understand the benefit of the diet.

   _____ More difficult to make changes than I thought it would be.

   _____ Made some changes but need to make more.

   _____ Other _____

Results Outcome:

The goal is to educate and counsel the patient. Patient or care-givers demonstrate/describe appropriate food choices and/or feeding regimens consistent with the diet counseling.

The outcomes are patient comprehension of the main instruction principle, identify food choices, plan a day's menu that is appropriate for the counseling given and indicate how their present food habits can be altered to the recommendations presented.

QI for monitoring follow-up is demonstrated by **Figure 31**.

Figure 31: Nutrition Goals on Reassessment

Patient Name	Diagnosis	Nutrition Goals Met Yes No	Action Plans	Comments

Results Outcome

The intent is to evaluate whether the patient was able to meet the established goals determined at the time of instruction.

The outcome may mean reeducation of the patient or establishing more realistic goals.

Appropriateness of diet orders and/or consult requested by the ambulatory care physician can be done by using **Figure 32**.

Figure 32: Appropriateness of Diet Order/Consult

Patient Name	Diagnosis/ Condition	Diet Order	Appropriate Yes No	Action Plans	Comments

Results Outcome:

The goal is an appropriate diet order for the patient's disease state.

The outcome results in the education of the physician in writing appropriate diet orders for disease states.

Quality management in the ambulatory care can be accomplished through the PCDA cycle:

Plan: The mission statement and goals expected to be achieved through quality performance.

Do: Implement a cost-effective, outcome-based education process.

Check: The outcomes through quality improvement measures.

Act: Implement changes/programs as needed.

Ambulatory services is a growing area in the health care arena. Nutrition plays a pivotal role in maintaining health. Good nutritional status may prevent or delay a catastrophic event or help speed the recovery process. Optimal nutritional status is critical for good health at any age.

TERMINOLOGY

Accreditation	Formal process by which an agency or organization evaluates an institution as meeting certain predetermined criteria or standards.
Acute	Care rendered for an illness, injury, or condition marked by a sudden onset or abrupt change of health status and requiring prompt attention, which is of limited duration (30 days or less).
Adjusted Case Mix	A unit of measurement that takes into account Value Unit (ACMVU) inpatient and outpatient volumes plus the DRG case mix index; ACMUV = (total patient revenue/inpatient revenue) x admissions x case mix index.
Ambulatory Care	Health services rendered to persons who are not confined overnight in a health care institution (also referred to as outpatient services).
Allowable Cost	Cost incurred by the provider in the course of providing service that is recognized as payable by a third party.
Available Beds	Health facility beds that are maintained and staffed for the provision of care.
Average Daily Census	Average number of inpatients (based on the daily census) present each day for a given period of time.
Average Length of Stay	The average number of days of service rendered to each inpatient discharged during a given period.
Bed Turnover Rate	The number of times a health facility bed, on the average, changes occupants during a given period of time.
Benefits	Healthcare services covered by a particular healthcare plan; benefits may vary significantly from contract to contract within a plan.
Budget	A financial plan serving as an estimate of and providing control over future operations or a work program which involves unit of service, revenue and expense, cash flow and capital expenditures; a budget year is a fiscal period, usually 12 months, for anticipated expenses and revenues.
Capital Allowance	The portion of the institution's total approved new capital requirements for construction, equipment and approved capital increases.
Capital Budget	A plan for major capital expenditures for new equipment or facilities, along with sources of funding for the expenditures.
Capital Reserves	Current assets to support the maintenance and purchase of equipment and fixtures.
Capitation	Method of payment for health services in which individual or institutional provider is paid a fixed, per capita per month amount for each person served without regard to the actual number or nature of services provided.

Case Mix	Categories of patients, classified by disease, procedure, method of payment or other characteristics, in an institution at a given time, usually measured by counting or aggregating groups of patients sharing one or more characteristics.
Charges	Fees billed for services rendered, including cost percent markup.
Clinical Indicator	An instrument used to assess a measurable aspect of patient care by assessing performance of the health care organization or individual practitioner; serves as a means for measuring what is done.
Costs	Expenses incurred: direct - labor, supplies, materials, benefits.
Cost Center	An organizational division, department, or unit performing functional activities within a facility; for each center, cost accountability is maintained for revenue produced and for controllable expenses incurred
Daily Census	The number of inpatients present at the daily census-taking time each day (usually census is taken at midnight).
Depreciation	The allocation of a capital asset's cost over its beneficial useful life.
Direct Cost	The cost of any good or service that contributes to and is readily ascribable to product or service output.
Expense	Expired cost: any item cost of (or loss from) performing an activity; a present or past experience defraying a present operating cost or representing an irrecoverable cost or loss.
Fee for Service	A method of reimbursing providers on the basis of a charge (fee) for each service rendered.
Fixed Cost (or Expense)	An operating expense that does not vary with the business volume.
Flexible Budgeting	A method that provides a means of adjusting estimates on the basis of changes in activity levels and costs; tailors a budget after the fact.
FTE	Full-time equivalent employee. An objective measurement of the personnel in term of full-time labor capability.
Indirect Cost	A functional cost not attributed to the production of a specific good or service but to an activity associated with production.
Medicaid	Federally-aided, state operated and administered program which provides medical benefits for certain indigent persons in need of health and medical care; covers persons who are eligible for welfare cash payment programs – the aged, the blind, the disabled and members of families with dependent children where one parent is absent, incapacitated or unemployed; states control the benefits.
Medicare	A third-party reimbursement program administered by the social security administration that underwrites the medical costs of person 65 and over and some qualified persons under 65; part A covers hospital services and Part B covers physicians services.

Non-Revenue Producing These are overhead units such as nutrition and plant operations and maintenance, that provide necessary service.

Occupancy Rate Used to compare actual inpatient utilization to the maximum possible utilization if every bed was full every day; can be calculated on licensed or on available set-up beds.

Outcome (of care) Complications, adverse events, short-term results of specific procedures and treatment, and long-term status of patient's health and functioning.

Outcome Indicator Measures what happens (or does not happen) to a patient after something is done (not done).

Process (of care) Functions by practitioners, including assessment, treatment planning, technical aspects of performing treatment, management of complications, as well as the indications for treatments and procedures.

Productive Hours The number of hours dedicated to the activity of a department.

Revenue Center An account for accumulating revenue consistent with the functional definition of the matching cost center.

Semi-Fixed Expense An operating expense(s)or operating expenses such as an FTE that change with the volume but not in direct proportion.

Semi-Variable Expense An operating expense(s) or operating expenses such as an FTE that vary in direct relation to the volume after a minimum level of activity has been reached.

Staffed Beds The daily average complement of beds fully staffed during the reporting period; staffed beds are set up, staffed, equipped, and in all respects ready to use.

Standards Standardized process of developing criteria for care incorporating the best scientific evidence of effectiveness.

Revenue Monies received for services given; gross revenue ÷ total revenue received = net revenue ÷ gross revenue - direct and indirect costs.

Revenue To Cost Ratio Gross revenue divided by total cost.

Units of Service A unit of measure commonly accepted for determining average cost, time or efficiency.

Variable Expense Operating expense(s) or operating expenses such as a FTE that vary in direct relation with the business volume.

References

• DeHoog, SJ: The Assessment of Nutritional Status. In: Krauss, M, Mahan K, eds. Food, Nutrition and Diet Therapy. Philadelphia: W.B. Saunders, 1996.

• Krauss, M and Mahan, K: The Nutritional Care Process. Food, Nutrition and Diet Therapy. Philadelphia: W.B. Saunders, 1996.

• Ford, DA and Fairchild, MM: Managing inpatient clinical nutrition services: a comprehensive program sssures accountability and success. J Am Diet Assoc 1993; 90:695.

• Applegren, KN and Dean, RE: Enteral Feeding in Long Term Care. Chicago: Precept Press, 1990.

• Nutrition Screening Initiative. AAFP, ADA, National Council on Aging. Washington, DC: 1992.

• Breslow, RA and Bergstrom N: Nutritional prediction of pressure ulcers. J Am Diet Assoc. 1994; 94: 1301.

• Walker, A and Hendricks, K: Manual of Pediatric Nutrition. Phildelphia: W.B. Saunders, 1985.

• Wade, R: Risk Management: Hospital Professional Liability Primer. Columbus: Hospital Insurance Publications, 1983.

• Reilly, J et al: Economic impact of malnutrition: a model system for hospitalized patients. JPEN 1988; 12:371.

• Cost-Benefits of Nutrition Service. A Literature Review. J Am Diet Assoc 1989 (suppl); April.

• Clinical Nutrition Management Dietetic Practice Group. Study in progress.Chicago: American Dietetic Association, 1996.

• Nagel, MR. Nutrition screening: identifying patients at risk for malnutrition. Nutr in Clin Prac 1993; 8:171.

• Farfaglia, PG, and Rosow, P: Automating clinical dietetics documentation. J Am Diet Assoc. 1995; 95:687.

• Charney, P: Nutrition assessment in the 1990's: where are we now? Nutr in Clin Prac 1995; 10:131.

• Dwyer, JT and Coleman, KA: Errors in dietary data. Am J Clin Nut 1997; 65 (suppl): 1132S.

• Howat, PM et al: Validity and reliability of reported dietary intake data. J Am Diet Assoc 1994; 94:2.

• Potosky, AL, Block, G and Hartman, A: The apparent validity of diet questionnaires is influenced by number of diet-record days used for comparison. J Am Diet Assoc 1990; No 6.

• Bergman, EA, Boyungs, JC and Erickson, ML: Comparison of a food frequency questionnaire and a 3-day diet record. J Am Diet Assoc 1990; No 10.

• Zulkfli, SN and Yu, SM: The food frequency method for dietary assessement. J Am Diet Assoc 1992; No 6.

• Feskanich, D et al: Reproducibility and validity of food intake measurements from a semiquantitative food frequency questionnaire. J Am Diet Assoc 1993; No 7.

• Cleverley, WO: Essentials of Health Care Finance. Silver Spring: ASPEN, 1992.

• Ellwood, PM: Outcomes management: a technology of patient experience. N. Eng J Med 1988; 318:1549-56.

• St. Anthony's DRG Guidebook. Reston: St. Anthony's Publishing,1997.

• DeHoog, SJ: Benchmarking clinical nutrition services. Future Dimen in Clin Man 1996; Vol 15, No 1.

• Health Care Benchmarks: Amer Health Consult 1996; No 11.

• MECON Benchmark Reporting., San Ramon: MECON Associates, 1992.

• Auton, G: Managing for competitiveness: benchmarking nutrition services. Clinical Nutrition Management meeting (presentation). Atlanta GA, 1996.

- Shetselaar, LG: Nutrition Counseling Skills: Assessment, Treatment and Evaluation. Silver Spring: ASPEN, 1989.

- DeHoog, S: Determining high nutritional risk patients and clinical productivity. J Am Diet Assoc 1985; No 12.

- Ford, DA, and Fairchild MM: Applied nutrition practice guidelines for patient screening and interventions in hospitals. Dietetic Currents 1993; No 4.

- Nelson, J: The impact of health care reform on nutrition support- the practitioner's perspective. Health Care in Transit 1995; Vol. 10, No 2, ASPEN, 1995.

- Spencer, RA: In defense of dietetics. CNM 1987; No 8.

- Position of the American Dietetic Association: issues in feeding the terminally ill adult. J Am Diet Assoc 1992; No 8.

- Position of the American Dietetic Association: Nutrition services in health maintenance organizations and other forms of managed care. J Am Diet Assoc 1993; No 10.

- Laramee, SH: Case Management: An overview. CNM 1995, No 4.

- Michaels, FG: Effective use of nutrition services in a managed care environment – the food service perspective. Nutr and the MD 1996; No 4.

- Fischbach, FT: Documenting Care: Communication, the Nursing Process and Documentations Standards. Philadelphia: F.A. Davis, 1991.

- Maxey, C et al: Approaches to wage and salary determination: J Am Diet Assoc 1979; No 3.

- Financial Managment. Hospital Nutrition and Food Service. Silver Spring: ASPEN, 1993.

- Schatz, GB: Coding for nutrition services: challenges, opportunities, and guidelines. J Am Diet Assoc 1993; No 4.

- Price, J and Schofield, M: Criteria based performance appraisals. CNM 1989, No 2.

- Alford, M: Using productivity data in evaluating dietitian peformance. CNM 1994, No 4.

- 1997 Accreditation Manual for Hospitals. Oakbrook Terrace: The Joint Commission on Accreditation for Healthcare Organizations, 1997.

- Westbrook, NH: Applying the 1995 JCAHO standards for clinical practice in home Care. J Am Diet Assoc 1996; No 4.

- Robinson, GE: Applying the 1996 JCAHO nutrition standards in long term care setting. J Am Diet Assoc 1996; No 4.

- Medical Nutrition Therapy Across the Continuum of Care. Chicago: American Diet Association, 1996.

- Bartlett, BJ: Nutrition and aging: quality of life in the later years. Columbus: Ross Products Division, 1996.

- The Omnibus Budget Reconciliation Act. Oct. 1990.

- Business success in dietetics: generating revenue and cost savings. The Ross Development Series, 1990.

Tables and Figures

ANTHROPOMETRIC ASSESSMENT

Anthropometry provides a fast, inexpensive method of evaluating body composition. It is commonly used in one of three ways. First, to compare a subject's protein and energy content to that of an appropriate, healthy reference population. Second, anthropometric measures repeated over time allow documentation of changes in body composition, perhaps in response to disease or a program of therapy. Thirdly, they can indicate if a patient is at risk of having or developing certain complications. For example, undernutrition is associated with infection, sepsis, wound breakdown, and cardiac arrhythmias. Overnutrition is associated with hypertension, coronary artery disease, gallstones, hypoxia, pulmonary hypertension, congestive heart failure, and some cancers.

Sources of error in anthropometric measures can be several. Variability in measurements made by different measurers can be reduced by using the same measurer each time for a specific subject. Variability in measurements repeated over time by the same measurer can be reduced by marking the site with indelible ink. More measurement variability occurs with inaccurate equipment. Whenever possible, good quality equipment should be used and calibrated periodically. Inaccurate measurements can also result from changes in hydration. This is most likely in subjects with heart or liver failure, or who are receiving high sodium intravenous fluids. For most reliable results, anthropometric measures should probably be omitted in these subjects. Total body water also increases with semi-starvation and hydration varies with the menstrual cycle.

Multiple skinfold measurements are more reliable than a single measure because of differences in fat distribution. Equations which allow estimation of total body fat are most valid when used in the same type of population from which the equations were derived, usually lean, healthy subjects. Techniques and reference standards for a number of anthropometric indices, both measured and calculated, are presented in this chapter.

STATURE

Stature is a major component of body size and important in evaluating growth and body weight. Heights are frequently not available in the medical records of hospitalized patients. When they are, it's often unclear whether they are reported or measured. And if asked, patients often don't remember. Persons tend to overstate their height an average 1.5 cm. Men overreport their height more than women. The extent of overreporting increases with age. When used to calculate body surface area and basal energy expenditure, however, differences between reported and measured heights are not clinically important.

Measurement of Stature

Accurate measurement requires a "stadiometer" – a nonstretch tape or measuring stick attached to a vertical board with a moveable horizontal headboard. Alternately, anthropometers can be used to measure stature. They consist of a vertical graduated rod with a moveable horizontal rod. They can be freestanding or attached to a wall. The freestanding ones tend to yield lower measurements. If stature must be measured against a wall, there should be no baseboard and the floor should not be carpeted. The measuring rods on platform scales are not recommended as many of them are inaccurate. Subjects should be barefoot or in thin socks and wearing minimal clothing so that body alignment can be seen.

1. Have subject stand erect with weight equally distributed on both feet and the heels together and touching the vertical board. If the legs are of unequal length, boards should be placed under the short limb to make the pelvis level. Where possible the head, shoulder blades, buttocks and heels should all touch the vertical board. Arms should hang free at the sides with palms facing the thighs.

2. Have subject "look straight ahead" (so that the line of vision is perpendicular to the body), take a deep breath, and hold that position while the horizontal headboard is brought down firmly on top of the head. Measurer's eyes should be level with the headboard. Record the measurement to the nearest 0.1 cm.

Recumbent Length

Recumbent length is measured on infants, children less than 2 to 3 years and others unable to stand without assistance. A recumbent length table has a fixed headboard, a moveable footboard, and a measuring tape along the side. Shoulders and legs should be flat against the tabletop with the arms at the sides. The head firmly touches the headboard while the line of vision is perpendicular to the table. The soles of the feet are vertical and the footboard should exert enough pressure to compress the soft tissues. Length is recorded to the nearest 0.1 cm.

Recumbent Bed Height

For institutionalized patients who are comatose, critically ill or unable to be moved, a recumbent bed height may be possible.

1. Remove the pillows and make the bed level.
2. Straighten the patient out in bed but with the feet flexed.
3. With a clipboard or ruler, extend perpendicular lines from the top of the head and the bottom of the feet out to the side of the bed.
4. Mark the two positions on the sheet and measure the distance between them to the nearest 0.5 centimeter.

When compared to standing height, bed height is significantly greater by 3.68 cm (a 2% difference). Results are not altered by lying on an eggcrate mattress. The authors believe there is a true difference in length in the supine versus standing position since others have shown similar results.

Stature from Arm Span

Arm span is the distance between the tips of the middle fingers (excluding fingernails) when both arms are extended maximally to the side at shoulder level. It is highly correlated with stature and may be used to estimate height when stature or recumbent length cannot be measured. Arm span must be done supine between birth and two to three years of age.

The subject is positioned with the feet together and the back against a flat surface, usually a wall. The arms are extended maximally at shoulder level, with the palms facing forward. A tape two meters (6.5 feet) or longer is placed along the wall at shoulder level between the tips of the middle fingers. This usually requires two operators. For ease of measuring subjects of different heights, one end can be attached to a vertical sliding board which is then attached to the wall. The measurement is recorded to the nearest 0.1 cm.

Anthropometers have also been used for supine measurements of arm span. The fixed end is placed at the tip of one middle finger and the moveable end at the other with the rods passing over the clavicles. If deformity or contracture is present, arm span can be estimated by measuring the distance from the "notch" at the top of the sternum to the fingertips of the normal arm and the value doubled.

In early adulthood arm span and stature are nearly equal and arm span does not change significantly with age. Arm span can be used in the elderly to estimate maximum stature at maturity before age related bone loss occurred. Arm span can be difficult to measure in elderly subjects as they may be unable to stretch out their arms adequately, and chest measurements can be altered by lung disease, kyphosis, and osteoporosis.

Total Arm Length

Mitchell and Lipschitz report a highly significant correlation between total arm length and height in both the young and the elderly. Total arm length is the distance between the acromial (the highest point on the acromial process) and the dactylion (the most distal point on the middle finger). It is measured with the subject in the standard erect position. It does not decrease significantly with age and is easy to measure in both elderly and bedridden subjects. At this time there are no formulas or nomograms allowing derivation of height from total arm length. This method also needs further testing in a larger population sample to determine its reliability.

Stature from Knee Height

Knee height provides a method of assessing stature for those with spinal deformities or who cannot stand to be measured. It correlates better with stature than total arm length or other limb measurements and decreases little with age. Knee height is more accurate when taken in a recumbent rather than sitting position. Sliding calipers can be obtained from:

Medical Express, 5150 West Griffith Drive, Beaverton, OR 97005

or

Ross Laboratories, Columbus, OH 43216

Chumlea has derived age, gender, and race-specific equations to estimate stature from recumbent knee height.

TABLE 1: Estimation of Stature from Knee Height

White Male		Factor
6-18 years	(2.22) (knee height) + 40.54	± 8.42 cm*
18-60 years	(1.88) (knee height) + 71.85	± 7.94 cm*
60-80 years	(2.08) (knee height) + 59.01	± 15.68 cm*
Black Male		
6-18 years	(2.18) (knee height) + 39.60	± 9.16 cm*
18-60 years	(1.79) (knee height) + 73.42	± 7.2 cm*
60-80 years	(1.37) (knee height) + 95.79	± 16.8 cm*
White Female		
6-18 years	(2.15) (knee height) + 43.21	± 7.8 cm*
18-60 years	(1.87) (knee height) + 70.25 - .06 age)	± 7.2 cm*
60-80 years	(1.91) (knee height) + 75 - (0.17 age)	± 17.64 cm*
Black Female		
6-18 years	(2.02) (knee height) + 46.59	± 8.78 cm*
18-60 years	(1.86) (knee height) + 68.10 - (.06 age)	± 7.6 cm*
60-80 years	(1.96) (knee height) + 58.72	± 16.5 cm*

The stature of an individual will have a 95% chance of falling within the boundaries represented by the formula with the appropriate correction factor.

Adapted from: Chumlea, W. et al: Prediction of stature from knee height for black and white adults and children with application to mobility-impaired or handicapped persons. J. Am. Diet. Assn. 94:1385, 1994.

FRAME SIZE

Weight varies with age, stature, body width, bone thickness, muscularity, and length of trunk relative to height. It is appropriate to obtain some estimate of body size that reflects these factors to aid in the evaluation of weight. Frame size may also help distinguish between those who have a large fat-free mass and those who are overweight because of excess fat. Methods of estimating frame size from wrist circumference and elbow breadth have been proposed.

Frame Size from Wrist Circumference

Grant measured height and wrist circumference on 100 men and 100 women at Duke University Medical Center and related these two measurements to determine an "r" value for estimating frame size.

Measurement of Wrist Circumference

1. Have subject face measurer with the right arm flexed at the elbow and the palm up.
2. Place a narrow (0.7 cm or less) measuring tape around the smallest part of wrist distal (towards the fingers) to the styloid process of radius and ulna ("wristbone"). The tape should fit into the depression just in front of the wristbone and touch the skin all around but not compress the soft tissue. Record to the nearest 0.1 cm.

FIGURE 1: Measurement of Wrist Circumference

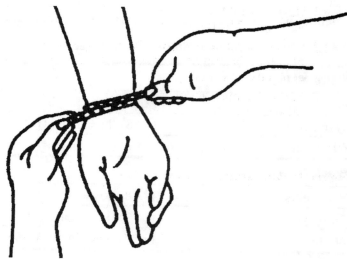

Frame Size from "r" Value

The 25% with the smallest "r" values were classified as large-framed, the middle 50% as medium-framed and those with the 25% largest "r" values as small-framed.

Calculation of "r" value is as follows:

$$\text{"r"} = \text{height (cm)} \div \text{wrist circumference (cm)}$$

TABLE 2: Body Frame Size from "r" Value

Men		Women	
"r" Value	Frame Size	"r" Value	Frame Size
> 10.4	Small	> 11.0	Small
9.6- 10.4	Medium	10.1 - 11.0	Medium
< 9.6	Large	< 10.1	Large

Frame Size from Elbow Breadth

Frisancho notes that frame size based on wrist circumference is influenced to some extent by soft tissue and fatness but elbow breadth is a good index of skeletal or frame size and is less affected by fatness than wrist circumference. It is also closely associated with lean body mass as well. Elbow breadth is the distance between the epicondyles of the humerus and can be measured with either sliding or spreading calipers. The former are recommended because they are less likely to slide off the epicondyles.

Sliding calipers can be obtained from:

Laffayette Instrument
P.O. Box 5729
3700 Sagamore Parkway North
Lafayette, IN 47903
(800) 428-7545
(765) 423-4111 (fax)
rehab@licmef.com (e-mail)

Measurement Of Elbow Breadth

1. Have subject face measurer with the right arm extended and the forearm bent upwards at a 90° angle. The fingers should be straight and the inside of the wrist turned towards the body.
2. Locate the epicondyles of the humerus, the 2 prominent bones on either side of the elbow. Place the blades of the sliding caliper (blades pointing up) or the tips of the spreading caliper on the epicondyles. (Figure 2)
3. Exert firm pressure to compress the soft tissues and record the measurement to the nearest 0.1 cm.

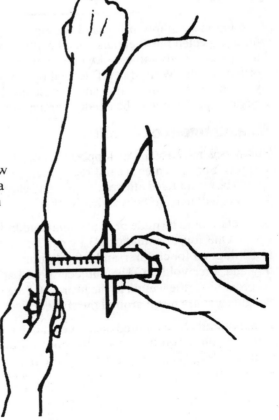

Figure 2: Measurement of Elbow Breadth

Frisancho has developed an index of frame size based on elbow breadth, height, and age. "Frame Index 2" was derived using data from NHANES data. and accounts for age related changes in weight and height. He emphasizes that elbow breadth is best done with calipers.

Frame index 2 = elbow breadth (mm) ÷ height (cm) x 100

Values below the 25th percentile are designated small, values from the 25th to 75th percentile are medium frame, and values greater than 75th percentile are large frame.

TABLE 3: Frame Size Based on Stature and Age

Age	Small	Male Medium	Large	Small	Female Medium	Large
18-25	< 38.4	38.4-41.6	> 41.6	< 35.2	35.2-38.6	> 38.6
25-30	< 38.6	38.6-41.8	> 41.8	< 35.7	35.7-38.7	> 38.7
30-35	< 38.6	38.6-42.1	> 42.1	< 35.7	35.7-39.0	> 39.0
35-40	< 39.1	39.1-42.4	> 42.4	< 36.2	36.2-39.8	> 39.8
40-45	< 39.3	39.3-42.5	> 42.5	< 36.7	36.7-40.2	> 40.2
45-50	< 39.6	39.6-43.0	> 43.0	< 36.7	37.2-40.7	> 40.7
50-55	< 39.9	39.9-43.3	> 43.3	< 37.2	37.2-41.6	> 41.6
55-60	< 40.2	40.2-43.8	> 43.8	< 37.8	37.8-41.9	> 41.9
60-65	< 40.2	40.2-43.6	> 43.6	< 38.2	38.2-41.8	> 41.8
65-70	< 40.2	40.2-43.6	> 43.6	< 38.2	38.2-41.8	> 41.8
70-75	< 40.2	40.2-43.6	> 43.6	< 38.2	38.2-41.8	> 41.8

Adapted from: Frisancho, AR: Anthropometric Standards for the Assessment of Growth and Nutritional Status. University of Michigan Press: Ann Arbor, MI, 1990.

WEIGHT

A common assumption is that a weight above a standard or desirable weight equals obesity, or that a weight within expected limits equals good health is misleading. A muscular individual may be above a weight standard but have low body fatness. An undernourished person with low muscle mass may have edema and still have a normal weight. Weight is influenced by a number of factors including the presence of edema, ascites, altered hydration, tumor, and frame size. These need to be kept in mind when evaluating weight. Other paramteres of body composition may be needed for a more reliable assessment of body weight.

Measurement of Weight

Subjects who can stand unsupported should be weighed on a leveled platform scale with a beam and moveable weights. Spring scales are not recommended but accurate electronic scales are acceptable. Scales with wheels should be recalibrated after each move and checked with standard weights two to three times a year. Nonambulatory subjects will need to be weighed with a wheelchair balance beam scale or a bed scale.

Subjects should be nude or in minimal underclothing or wear standardized lightweight clothing such as a paper gown. One-fourth pound or 0.1 kg can be subtracted for undergarments. Because of diurnal weight variations (1.0 kilogram for children and 2.0 kilograms for adults), subjects should ideally be weighed at the same time of day and after voiding. The subject should stand still with weight evenly distributed on both feet while the recorder notes the weight to the nearest 0.1 kg or 1/4 lb. The recorder should stand behind the beam to adjust the weights and not reach around the subject.

Infants should be weighted on a leveled pan scale with a beam and moveable weights. It should be calibrated to zero with only a quilt on it and the quilt should remain on it for all weights. Weight should be measured to the nearest 0.1 kg. Three repeated measurements should be averaged. The weight of a diaper (if worn) should be subtracted.

Adjustment for Amputation

When there is loss of body parts, estimation of desired body weight becomes more difficult. Osterkamp has reviewed available data on relative proportion of body weight contributed by individual body parts. She notes that most recent data show evolutionary changes from the earliest data. She also reports that studies of living subjects show that males and females are similar in the percent of total weight contributed by individual parts. As children grow to adults body proportions change in relation to their percent of body weight. Head mass decreases as a proportion of total weight as extremity weight increases. There appear to be further changes that occur with aging. There are also reported ethnic differences in body proportions. After pooling the most recent data she suggests the following percentages be used for adjusting body weight and estimating nutrient requirements in amputees.

TABLE 4: Percent Total Body Weight by Individual Body Parts

Body Part	Percent
Head	8.0
Trunk	50
Upper Arm	2.7
Forearm	1.6
Hand	0.7
Entire Arm	5
Thigh	10.1
Calf	4.4
Foot	1.5
Entire Leg	16

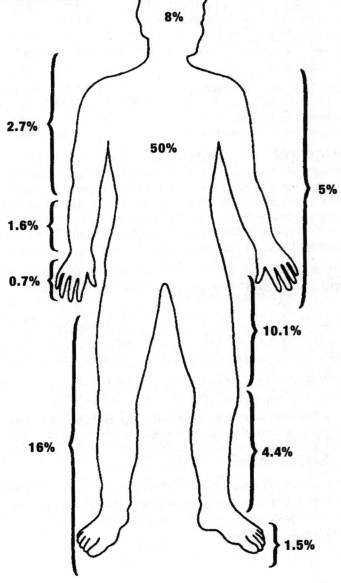

Figure 3: Percent Total Body Weight Contributed by Individual Body Part

WEIGHT STANDARDS

Weight Standards for Children

The National Center for Health Statistics growth curves for children are included with the pediatric chapters. Comparison of a child's head circumference, stature, and weight to the growth curves allows determination of whether growth is appropriate for age. The growth curves, however, do not account for the contribution of parental height to the child's stature. If, for example, a child is near the 5th or 95th percentile this could be due to genetic, environmental or pathological causes. Himes et al have developed adjustment factors which allow adjustment for parental stature. If, after adjustment, a child is still at the extremes of growth, further invesigation is needed to determine the reason.

Metropolitan Height and Weight Tables

The Metropolitan Life Insurance Company Height-Weight Tables are frequently used as a source of ideal or desirable weights upon which to base goals of nutritional therapy. The 1959 tables are based on the 1959 Build Study which included approximately five million insurance policy holders of 26 companies between 1935 and 1953. Subjects were followed for periods of one to 20 years. Those with heart disease, cancer or diabetes were excluded to determine the effects of weight alone on mortality.

The weight ranges for each height are those associated with the lowest mortality and are statistically divided according to frame size to allow for variation in body build. Frame size was based on self-appraisal. Eighty percent of the subjects were actually weighed and measured. Heights and weights for the remaining twenty percent are self-reported. Clothing weight was assumed to be four pounds for women and seven for men. Shoe heights were assumed to be two inches for women and one for men.

The 1983 tables are based on data from the 1979 Build Study which included approximately four million policy holders of 25 companies between 1950 and 1971. As with the 1959 study those with significant disease were screened out. Weight ranges were determined for each frame size but frame size was not actually measured on individual subjects. Instead, the elbow breadths of the subjects in NHANES 1 were statistically divided into three groups with the middle fifty percent of the population designated medium frame while the remaining 50% were divided equally between large and small frame. These frame sizes were then superimposed upon the Metropolitan data resulting in the weight ranges as shown in the 1983 tables.

Approximately 90 percent of the subjects were actually weighed and measured. The remaining 10 percent of heights and weights were self-reported. Weight of clothing was assumed to be three pounds for women and and five pounds for men. Shoe heights were assumed to be one inch for both sexes.

In the 20 years between the 1959 and 1979 studies the weights associated with the lowest mortality increased. The increases were greatest among short men and woman and least among the tall. Although desirable weights increased they still remained below average weights.

Both the 1959 and 1983 tables have been criticized as a source of "ideal" or "desirable" weights. In fact those labels are deleted from the 1983 tables. Criticism of these tables includes the following:

- Subjects were measured and weighed in shoes and clothes. Clothing weights and shoe heights were assumed and not standardized.

- Ten to twenty percent of the data is self-reported and subject to under or overstatement.

- Only ages 25 to 59 are included. The elderly are excluded.

- The data does not represent the population as a whole and is weighted towards Caucasians and the upper income levels.

- Some subjects are represented more than once as multiple policy holders. Smokers are included.

Irregardless of which tables are used, the weights presented are associated only with the lowest mortality. They are not necessarily weights at which people look their best, perform their best, or are healthiest. The original intent of the tables was to provide actuarial information to insurance underwriters. They should be used cautiously and in conjunction with other parameters by health care professionals in setting nutritional goals.

TABLE 5: 1959 Metropolitan Desirable Weight Tables for Men

Height			Frame Size Small		Medium		Large	
in	cm	sq m	lb	kg	lb	kg	lb	kg
61	155	2.40	105-113	47.7-51.4	111-122	50.4-55.5	119-134	54.1-60.9
62	157	2.48	108-116	49.1-52.7	114-126	51.8-57.3	122-137	55.4-62.3
63	160	2.56	111-119	50.5-54.1	117-129	53.2-58.6	125-141	56.8-64.1
64	163	2.64	114-122	51.8-55.4	120-132	54.6-60.0	128-145	58.2-65.9
65	165	2.73	117-126	53.3-57.3	123-136	55.9-61.8	131-149	60.0-67.7
66	168	2.81	121-130	55.0-59.1	127-140	57.7-63.6	135-154	61.4-70.0
67	170	2.90	125-134	56.8-60.9	131-145	59.6-65.9	140-159	63.6-72.3
68	173	2.98	129-138	58.6-62.7	135-149	61.4-67.7	144-163	65.4-74.1
69	175	3.07	133-143	60.5-65.0	139-153	63.2-69.5	148-167	67.3-75.9
70	178	3.16	137-147	62.3-66.8	143-158	65.0-71.8	152-172	69.1-78.2
71	180	3.25	141-151	64.1-68.6	147-163	66.8-74.1	157-177	71.4-80.4
72	183	3.34	145-155	65.9-70.4	151-168	68.8-76.4	161-182	73.2-82.7
73	185	3.44	149-160	67.7-72.7	155-173	70.5-78.6	166-187	75.4-85.0
74	188	3.53	153-164	69.5-74.6	160-178	72.7-80.9	171-192	77.7-87.3
75	190	3.63	157-168	71.4-76.4	165-183	75.0-83.2	175-197	79.6-89.6

These tables correct the 1959 Metropolitan tables to nude weight and height without shoe heels

TABLE 6: 1959 Metropolitan Desirable Weight Tables for Women

Height			Frame Size Small		Medium		Large	
in	cm	sq m	lb	kg	lb	kg	lb	kg
56	142	2.02	88-94	40.0-42.7	92-103	41.8-46.8	100-115	45.5-52.3
57	145	2.10	90-97	40.9-44.1	94-106	42.7-48.2	102-118	46.4-53.6
58	147	2.17	92-100	41.8-45.5	97-109	44.1-49.6	105-121	47.7-55.0
59	150	2.25	95-103	43.2-46.8	100-112	45.5-50.9	108-124	49.1-56.4
60	152	2.32	98-106	44.5-48.2	103-115	46.8-52.3	111-127	50.5-57.7
61	155	2.40	101-109	45.9-49.5	106-118	48.2-53.6	114-130	51.8-59.1
62	157	2.48	104-112	47.2-50.9	109-122	49.5-55.5	117-134	53.2-60.9
63	160	2.56	107-115	48.6-52.3	112-126	50.9-57.3	121-138	55.0-62.7
64	163	2.64	110-119	50.0-54.1	116-131	52.7-59.6	125-142	56.8-64.5
65	165	2.73	114-123	51.8-55.9	120-135	54.6-61.4	129-146	58.6-66.4
66	168	2.81	118-127	53.6-57.7	124-139	56.4-63.2	133-150	60.4-68.2
67	170	2.90	122-131	55.4-59.6	128-143	58.2-65.0	137-154	62.3-70.0
68	173	2.98	126-136	57.3-61.8	132-147	60.0-66.8	141-159	64.1-72.7
69	175	3.07	130-140	59.1-63.6	136-151	61.8-68.6	145-164	65.9-74.5
70	178	3.16	134-144	60.0-65.4	140-155	63.6-70.9	149-169	67.7-76.8

These tables correct the 1959 Metropolitan tables to nude weight and height without shoe heels

TABLE 7: 1983 Metropolitan Height and Weight Tables for Men

| | | | Frame Size | | | | | |
| | Height | | Small | | Medium | | Large | |
in	cm	sq m	lb	kg	lb	kg	lb	kg
61	155	2.40	123-129	55.9-58.6	126-136	57.3-61.8	133-145	60.5-65.9
62	157	2.48	125-131	56.3-59.5	128-138	58.2-62.7	135-148	61.4-67.3
63	160	2.56	127-133	57.7-60.5	130-140	59.1-63.6	137-151	62.3-68.6
64	163	2.64	129-135	58.9-61.4	132-143	60.0-65.0	139-155	63.2-70.4
65	165	2.73	131-137	59.5-62.3	134-146	60.9-66.4	141-159	64.1-72.3
66	168	2.81	133-140	60.4-63.6	137-149	62.3-67.7	144-163	65.5-74.1
67	170	1.90	135-143	61.4-65.0	140-152	63.6-69.1	147-167	66.8-75.9
68	173	2.98	137-146	62.2-66.4	143-155	65.0-70.5	150-171	68.2-77.7
69	175	3.07	139-149	63.2-67.7	146-158	66.4-71.8	153-175	69.6-79.6
70	178	3.16	141-152	64.1-69.1	149-161	67.7-73.2	156-179	70.9-81.4
71	180	3.25	144-155	65.4-70.5	152-165	69.1-75.0	159-183	72.3-83.2
72	183	3.34	147-159	66.8-72.3	155-169	70.4-76.8	163-187	74.1-85.0
73	185	3.44	150-163	68.2-74.1	159-173	72.3-78.6	167-192	75.9-87.3
74	188	3.53	153-167	69.5-75.9	162-177	73.6-80.5	171-197	77.7-89.5
75	190	3.63	157-171	71.4-77.7	166-182	75.4-82.7	176-202	80.0-91.8

These tables correct the 1959 Metropolitan tables to nude weight and height without shoe heels

TABLE 8: 1983 Metropolitan Height and Weight Tables for Women

| Height | | | Frame Size | | | | | |
| | | | Small | | Medium | | Large | |
in	cm	sq m	lb	kg	lb	kg	lb	kg
57	145	2.10	99-108	45.0-49.1	106-118	48.2-53.6	115-128	52.3-58.2
58	147	2.17	100-110	45.5-50.0	108-120	49.1-54.5	117-131	53.2-59.5
59	150	2.25	101-112	45.9-50.9	110-123	50.0-55.9	119-134	54.1-60.9
60	152	2.32	103-115	46.8-52.3	112-126	50.9-57.3	122-137	55.5-62.3
61	155	2.40	105-118	47.7-53.6	115-129	52.3-58.6	125-140	56.8-63.6
62	157	2.48	108-121	49.1-55.0	118-132	53.6-60.0	128-144	58.1-65.5
63	160	2.56	111-124	50.5-56.4	121-135	55.0-61.4	131-148	59.5-67.3
64	163	2.64	114-127	51.8-57.7	124-138	56.4-62.7	134-152	60.9-69.1
65	165	2.72	117-130	53.2-59.1	127-141	57.7-64.1	137-156	62.2-70.9
66	168	2.81	120-133	54.5-60.5	130-144	59.1-65.5	140-160	63.6-72.7
67	170	2.90	123-136	55.9-61.8	133-147	60.5-66.8	143-164	66.4-75.9
68	173	2.98	126-139	57.3-63.2	136-150	61.8-68.2	146-167	65.0-74.6
69	175	3.07	129-142	58.6-64.6	139-153	63.2-69.5	149-170	67.7-77.3
70	178	3.16	132-145	60.0-65.9	142-156	64.5-70.9	152-173	60.1-78.6
71	180	3.24	135-148	61.4-67.3	145-159	65.9-72.3	155-176	70.5-80.0

These tables correct the 1959 Metropolitan tables to nude weight and height without shoe heels

NHANES weight percentiles. Frisancho has published weight tables based on measurements from a cross-sectional multiracial sample of 4340 subjects aged 18 to 24 and 21,752 subjects aged 25 to 74 from NHANES-1 and NHANES-11. Subjects and are representative of the noninstitutionalized U.S. population. Weight and elbow breadth were measured on all subjects according to standard procedures. Clothing weight ranged from 0.2 to 0.6 pounds (0.1 to 0.3 kg) and is included in the weights. Heights were measured in rubber slippers.

Weight percentiles are established according to age, sex, height and frame size. Values are omitted where the number of subjects of a specific height, age, sex and frame size are too small to give reliable values. While there are significant differences between black and white populations when only age and height are considered, differences were minor when comparisons included frame size as well. For this reason data from all races was combined.

Subjects with weights in the highest and lowest percentiles can be further evaluated by determining skinfold thickness and arm muscle area. An obese person would be expected to have excess fat tissue along with excess body weight. A muscular person would not. A subject with low body weight secondary to undernutrition would be expected to have a low level of lean and fat tissue as well.

TABLE 9: Weight Percentiles for US Men Aged 18 to 25

Frame	\multicolumn{9}{c}{Percentiles}
	5	10	15	25	50	75	85	90	95
Small	54.5	57.4	59.0	62.3	68.3	76.1	80.5	83.8	89.8
Medium	57.5	60.6	62.3	65.3	71.5	80.3	86.0	91.6	99.6
Large	58.2	61.3	62.6	67.4	74.7	85.0	91.2	95.0	104.9

Adapted from: Frisancho, R.: Anthropometric Standards for the Assessment of Growth and Nutritional Status. University of Michigan Press, 1990

TABLE 10: Weight Percentiles for US Women Aged 18 to 25

Frame	Percentiles								
	5	10	15	25	50	75	85	90	95
Small	44.0	46.1	48.0	50.3	55.1	60.9	64.4	66.9	71.5
Medium	46.0	48.4	50.0	52.5	58.1	64.4	69.5	72.8	78.4
Large	48.9	51.3	53.1	56.3	62.9	76.2	83.8	89.0	102.7

Adapted from: Frisancho, R.: Anthropometric Standards for the Assessment of Growth and Nutritional Status. University of Michigan Press, 1990

TABLE 11: Height Percentiles for US Men and Women Aged 18 to 25

	Percentiles								
	5	10	15	25	50	75	85	90	95
Men	165.4	167.8	169.5	171.9	176.6	181.2	183.7	185.5	188.6
Women	152.3	154.8	156.4	158.8	163.1	167.1	169.6	171.0	173.6

Adapted from: Frisancho, R.: Anthropometric Standards for the Assessment Growthand Nutritional Status. U. Michigan Press, 1990

TABLE 12: Weight Percentiles for US Men Aged 25 to 54 with Small Frames

Height		Percentiles						
in	cm	5	10	15	50	85	90	95
62	157	46	50	52	64	71	74	77
63	160	48	51	53	61	70	75	79
64	163	49	53	55	66	76	76	80
65	165	52	53	58	66	77	81	84
66	168	56	57	59	67	78	83	84
67	170	56	60	62	71	82	83	88
68	173	56	59	62	71	79	82	85
69	175	57	62	65	74	84	87	88
70	178	59	62	67	75	87	86	90
71	180	60	64	70	76	79	88	91
72	183	62	65	67	74	87	89	93
73	185	63	67	69	79	89	91	94
74	188	65	68	71	80	90	92	99

Heights are without shoe heels. Allow 0.1 to 0.3 kg for clothing. Adapted from: Frisancho, R. AJCN 40:808, 1984.

TABLE 13: Weight Percentiles for US Women Aged 25 to 54 with Small Frames

Height		Percentiles						
in	cm	5	10	15	50	85	90	95
58	147	37	43	43	52	58	62	66
59	150	42	43	44	53	63	69	72
60	152	42	44	45	53	63	65	70
61	155	44	46	47	54	64	66	72
62	157	44	47	48	55	63	64	70
63	160	46	48	49	55	65	68	79
64	163	49	50	51	57	67	68	74
65	165	50	52	53	60	70	72	80
66	168	46	49	54	58	65	71	74
67	170	47	50	52	59	70	72	76
68	173	48	51	53	62	71	73	77
69	175	49	52	54	63	72	74	78
70	178	50	53	55	64	73	75	79

Heights are without shoe heels. Allow 0.1 to 0.3 kg for clothing. Adapted from: Frisancho, R. AJCN 40:808, 1984.

TABLE 14: Weight Percentiles for US Men Aged 25 to 54 with Medium Frames

Height		Percentiles						
in	cm	5	10	15	50	85	90	95
62	157	51	55	58	68	81	83	87
63	160	52	56	59	71	82	85	89
64	163	54	60	61	71	83	84	90
65	165	59	62	65	74	87	90	94
66	168	58	61	65	75	85	87	93
67	170	62	66	68	77	89	93	100
68	173	60	64	66	78	89	92	97
69	175	63	66	68	78	90	93	97
70	178	64	66	70	81	90	93	97
71	180	62	68	70	81	92	96	100
72	183	68	71	74	84	97	100	104
73	185	70	72	75	85	100	101	104
74	188	68	76	77	88	100	100	104

Heights are without shoe heels. Allow 0.1 to 0.3 kg for clothing. Adapted from: Frisancho, R. AJCN 40:808, 1984

TABLE 15: Weight Percentiles for US Women Aged 25 to 54 with Medium Frames

Height		Percentiles						
in	cm	5	10	15	50	85	90	95
58	147	41	46	50	63	77	75	79
59	150	47	50	52	66	76	79	85
60	152	47	50	52	60	77	79	85
61	155	47	49	51	61	73	78	86
62	157	49	50	52	61	73	77	83
63	160	49	51	53	62	77	80	88
64	163	50	52	54	62	76	82	87
65	165	52	54	55	63	75	80	89
66	168	52	54	55	63	75	78	83
67	170	54	56	57	65	79	82	88
68	173	58	59	60	67	77	85	87
69	175	49	58	60	68	79	82	87
70	178	50	54	57	70	80	83	87

Heights are without shoe heels. Allow 0.1 to 0.3 kg for clothing. Adapted from: Frisancho, R. AJCN 40:808, 1984

TABLE 16: Weight Percentiles for US Men Aged 25 to 54 with Large Frame

Height		Percentiles						
in	cm	5	10	15	50	85	90	95
62	157	57	62	66	82	99	103	108
63	160	58	63	67	83	100	104	109
64	163	59	64	68	84	101	105	110
65	165	60	65	69	79	102	106	111
66	168	60	65	75	84	103	106	112
67	170	62	70	71	84	102	111	113
68	173	63	74	76	86	101	104	114
69	175	68	71	74	89	103	105	114
70	178	68	72	74	87	106	112	114
71	180	73	78	82	91	113	116	123
72	183	73	76	78	91	109	112	121
73	185	72	77	79	93	106	107	116
74	188	69	74	82	92	105	115	120

Heights are without shoe heels. Allow 0.1 to 0.3 kg for clothing. Adapted from: Frisancho, R. AJCN 40:808, 1984

TABLE 17: Weight Percentiles for US Women Aged 25 to 54 with Large Frame

Height		Percentiles						
in	cm	5	10	15	50	85	90	95
58	147	56	63	67	86	105	110	117
59	150	56	62	67	78	105	109	116
60	152	55	62	66	87	104	109	116
61	155	54	64	66	81	105	117	115
62	157	59	61	65	81	103	107	113
63	160	58	63	67	83	105	109	119
64	163	59	62	63	79	102	104	112
65	165	59	61	63	81	103	109	114
66	168	55	58	62	75	95	100	107
67	170	58	60	65	80	100	108	114
68	173	51	66	66	76	104	105	111
69	175	50	57	68	79	105	104	111
70	178	50	56	61	76	99	104	110

Heights are without shoe heels. Allow 0.1 to 0.3 kg for clothing. Adapted from: Frisancho, R. AJCN 40:808, 1984

TABLE 18: Weight Percentiles for US Men Aged 55 to 74 with Small Frames

Height		Percentiles						
in	cm	5	10	15	50	85	90	95
62	157	45	49	56	61	68	73	77
63	160	47	49	51	62	71	71	79
64	163	47	50	54	63	72	74	80
65	165	48	54	59	70	80	90	90
66	168	51	55	59	68	77	80	84
67	170	55	60	61	69	79	81	88
68	173	54	54	58	70	79	81	86
69	175	56	59	63	75	81	84	88
70	178	57	61	63	76	83	86	89
71	180	59	62	65	69	85	87	91
72	183	60	64	66	76	86	89	92
73	185	62	65	68	78	88	90	94
74	188	63	67	69	77	89	92	95

Heights are without shoe heels. Allow 0.1 to 0.3 kg for clothing. Adapted from: Frisancho, R. AJCN 40:808, 1984.

TABLE 19: Weight Percentiles for US Women Aged 55 to 74 with Small Frames

Height		Percentiles						
in	cm	5	10	15	50	85	90	95
58	147	39	46	48	54	63	65	71
59	150	41	45	48	55	66	68	74
60	152	43	45	47	54	67	70	73
61	155	43	43	45	56	65	70	71
62	157	47	49	52	58	67	69	73
63	160	42	45	49	58	67	68	74
64	163	43	47	49	60	68	70	75
65	165	43	47	49	60	69	72	75
66	168	44	48	50	68	70	72	76
67	170	45	48	51	61	71	73	77
68	173	45	49	51	61	71	74	77
69	175	46	49	52	62	72	74	78
70	178	47	50	52	63	73	75	79

Heights are without shoe heels. Allow 0.1 to 0.3 kg for clothing. Adapted from: Frisancho, R. AJCN 40:808, 1984.

TABLE 20: Weight Percentiles for US Men Aged 55 to 74 with Medium Frames

Height		Percentiles						
in	cm	5	10	15	50	85	90	95
62	157	50	54	59	68	77	81	85
63	160	51	57	60	70	80	82	87
64	163	55	59	62	71	82	83	91
65	165	56	60	64	72	83	86	89
66	168	57	62	66	74	83	84	89
67	170	59	64	66	78	87	89	94
68	173	62	66	68	78	89	95	101
69	175	62	66	68	77	90	93	99
70	178	62	68	71	80	90	95	101
71	180	68	70	72	84	94	97	101
72	183	66	65	69	81	96	97	101
73	185	68	72	79	88	93	99	103
74	188	69	73	76	95	98	101	104

Heights are without shoe heels. Allow 0.1 to 0.3 kg for clothing. Adapted from: Frisancho, R. AJCN 40:808, 1984.

TABLE 21: Weight Percentiles for US Women Aged 55 to 74 with Medium Frames

Height		Percentiles						
in	cm	5	10	15	50	85	90	95
58	147	40	44	49	57	72	82	85
59	150	47	49	52	62	74	78	86
60	152	47	50	52	65	76	79	86
61	155	49	51	54	64	78	81	86
62	157	49	53	54	64	78	82	88
63	160	52	54	55	65	79	83	89
64	163	51	54	57	66	78	81	87
65	165	54	56	59	67	78	84	88
66	168	54	57	57	66	79	85	88
67	170	51	59	61	72	82	85	89
68	173	52	56	59	70	83	86	90
69	175	53	57	60	72	84	87	91
70	178	54	58	61	73	85	88	92

Heights are without shoe heels. Allow 0.1 to 0.3 kg for clothing. Adapted from: Frisancho, R. AJCN 40:808, 1984

TABLE 22: Weight Percentiles for US Men Aged 55 to 74 with Large Frame

Height		Percentiles						
in	cm	5	10	15	50	85	90	95
62	157	54	59	63	77	91	95	100
63	160	55	60	64	80	92	96	101
64	163	57	62	65	77	94	97	102
65	165	58	63	73	79	89	98	103
66	168	59	67	73	80	101	102	105
67	170	65	71	73	85	103	108	112
68	173	67	71	73	83	95	98	111
69	175	65	70	74	84	96	98	105
70	178	68	73	77	87	102	104	117
71	180	65	70	70	84	102	109	111
72	183	67	76	81	90	108	112	112
73	185	68	73	76	88	105	108	113
74	188	69	74	78	89	106	109	114

Heights are without shoe heels. Allow 0.1 to 0.3 kg for clothing. Adapted from: Frisancho, R. AJCN 40:808, 1984

TABLE 23: Weight Percentiles for US Women Aged 55 to 74 with Large Frame

Height		Percentiles						
in	cm	5	10	15	50	85	90	95
58	147	53	59	63	92	95	99	104
59	150	54	59	63	78	95	99	105
60	152	54	65	69	78	87	88	105
61	155	64	68	69	79	94	95	106
62	157	59	61	63	82	93	101	111
63	160	61	65	67	80	100	102	118
64	163	60	65	67	77	97	102	119
65	165	60	66	69	80	98	102	111
66	168	57	60	63	82	98	105	109
67	170	58	64	68	80	105	104	109
68	173	58	64	68	79	100	104	110
69	175	59	65	69	85	101	105	110
70	178	60	65	69	85	101	105	111

Heights are without shoe heels. Allow 0.1 to 0.3 kg for clothing. Adapted from: Frisancho, R. AJCN 40:808, 1984

Desirable Weights for the Elderly

Masters et al have published provisional weight standards for those aged 65 to 94 years of age. These tables are based on a survey of 5619 ambulatory, apparently healthy elderly Caucasion males and females representing all social, economic and geographical areas of the US. Subjects were weighed and measured in underclothes and without shoes.

Average weights were calculated for each 5 year age range according to height and sex. The authors further calculated a weight range based on the average weight ± 10%. and ± 20%. The authors believe that ± 10% limits are more desirable for this age group than the ± 20% limits generally accepted for younger populations. Only the average weights ± 10% are presented here.

After 84 years the tallest and shortest categories were omitted due to small sample size. The tables show a 15 to 20 pound decrease in average weight in those past age 65 in both sexes and at all heights. The authors suggest this is a result of changing body composition (loss of protein, water , calcium and fat) and a decrease in the proportion of overweight subjects due to increased mortality. They believe this suggests a more favorable survival rate for thinner persons.

TABLE 24: Average Weights (± 10%) of Men Aged 65 to 94

Height		Age					
in	cm	65-69	70-74	75-79	80-84	85-89	90-94
61	155	128-156	125-153	123-151			
62	157	130-158	127-155	125-153	122-148		
63	160	131-161	129-157	127-155	122-150	120-146	
64	163	134-164	131-161	129-157	124-152	122-148	
65	165	136-166	134-164	130-160	127-155	125-153	117-143
66	168	139-169	137-167	133-163	130-158	128-156	120-146
67	170	140-172	140-170	136-166	132-162	130-160	122-150
68	173	143-175	142-174	139-169	135-165	133-163	126-154
69	175	147-179	146-178	142-174	139-169	137-167	130-158
70	178	150-184	148-182	146-178	143-175	140-172	134-164
71	180	155-189	152-186	149-183	148-180	144-176	139-169
72	183	159-195	156-190	154-188	153-187	148-182	
73	185	164-200	160-196	158-192			

Heights are without shoe heels. Weights include light underwear.
Adapted from: Master and Lasser. J.A.M.A. 172:658, 1960

TABLE 25: Average Weights (± 10%) of Women Aged 65 to 94

Height		Age					
in	cm	65-69	70-74	75-79	80-84	85-89	90-94
58	147	120-146	112-138	111-135			
59	150	121-147	114140	112-136	100-122	99-121	
60	152	122-148	116-142	113-139	106-130	102-124	
61	155	123-151	118-144	102-141	109-133	104-128	
62	157	125-153	121-147	118-144	112-136	108-132	107-131
63	160	127-155	123-151	121-147	115-141	112-136	107-131
64	163	130-158	126-154	123-151	119-145	115-141	108-132
65	165	132-162	130-158	126-154	122-150	120-146	112-136
66	168	136-166	132-162	128-157	126-154	124-145	116-142
67	170	140-170	136-166	131-161	130-158	128-156	
68	173	143-175	140-170				
69	175	148-180	144-176				

Heights are without shoe heels. Weights include light underwear.
Adapted from: Master and Lasser. J.A.M.A. 172:658, 1960

Weight for Stature in the Elderly

Extremes of leanness and fatness are important health problems in the elderly and can aid in predicting survival on admit to the hospital. Chumlea et al developed percentile values for weight divided by stature squared as an index of obesity and leanness (Body Mass Index).

$$W/S^2 = \text{weight (kg)} \div \text{stature (sq m)}$$

Example:

Weight = 65 kg
Height = 150 cms or 1.5 m
$$W/S^2 = 65 \div (1.5)^2 = 65 \div 2.25 = 28.8$$

The tables are based on data from 269 ambulatory, free-living Caucasion men and women, 62 to 104 years of age living in Southwest, Ohio. No health questionaires or physical exams were done. The authors state that, while the sample size is limited, stature and weights do not differ significantly from available data from other studies of the same age group. Because of racial differences these reference values should be used with caution in non-Caucasion populations.

TABLE 26: Percentiles for W/S² in Men and Women Aged 65 to 90

Age	Men			Women		
	5	50	95	5	50	95
65	21.9	27.6	34.5	33.5	44.5	66.4
70	21.0	26.6	33.6	33.0	44.1	65.9
75	20.1	25.7	32.6	32.6	43.6	65.5
80	19.1	24.8	31.7	32.2	43.2	65.1
85	18.2	23.9	30.8	31.8	42.8	64.7
90	17.3	22.9	29.8	31.3	42.4	64.2

Adapted from: Chumlea et al: Some anthropometric indices of body composition for elderly adults. J. Geront. 41:36, 1986.

Weight Goals in Health

In February of 1985 the National Institute of Health sponsored a consensus development conference on the health implications of obesity. The panel evaluated the data on the health implications of increased body weight. Data from NHANES 1 (1971-1974) and NHANES 2 (1976-1980) showed a strong association between weight equal to or greater than the 85th percentile and hypertension, diabetes, and hypercholesterolemia, especially in those aged 20 to 44. The Framingham heart study found increased risk of coronary artery disease with obesity, independent of other risk factors. An American Cancer Society study of over 3/4 million subjects found higher rates of certain cancers in the obese, regardless of smoking habits. Obese men had greater mortality from colon, rectal, and prostate cancers. Obese women had higher mortality from cancers of the gall bladder, biliary passages, breast, uterus, endometrium, cervix, and ovaries. Minimun mortality was found in subjects whose weights were 75 to 105 percent of average.

Bray plotted Body Mass Index (BMI) versus mortality for subjects in the American Cancer Society study and found the minimum mortality at a BMI of 22 to 25. Manson et al, after reviewing all major studies on the association between weight and longevity, conclude that the evidence shows minimum mortality when weight is at least 10% below the US average.

For adults 20 plus years of age, the panel recommended two indices of body composition, relative weight (RW) and body mass index (BMI), for use in clinical practice and public health studies.

RW = actual weight ÷ midpoint for medium frame (1959 or 1983 tables)

BMI = weight in kg ÷ height (sq. m.)

While health risks increase continually with increasing relative weight, the panel agreed that a relative weight of 120% or more is associated with a health risk significant enough to justify intervention and weight reduction. Increases in mortality rates with increasing duration of obesity are greater for those less than age 50. Although the panel did not specify which Metropolitan tables to use, it advised using the 1959 tables for lower weight goals when any of the following complications are present:

- Noninsulin dependent diabetes (NIDDM) or a family history of NIDDM or gestational diabetes.

- Hypertension, hypertriglyceridemia, hypercholesterolemia, or coronary heart disease.

- Gout, chronic obstructive pulmonary disease, or osteoarthritis of the hip, spine or knees.

Body Mass Indexes corresponding to a Relative Weight of 120 or the 85th percentile are shown below.

	Men	**Women**
NHANES 1 and 11	27.8	27.3
1959 Metropolitan Tables	26.4	25.8
1983 Metropolitan Tables	27.2	26.9

More recent studies have focused on the pattern of fat distribution (i.e., ratio of waist to hip circumference (WHR) and its relation to health risk. A higher WHR is associated with stroke, insulin resistance, diabetes mellitus, hypertension, gall bladder disease, and menstrual abnormalities. In men a greater risk of stroke and ischemic heart disease occurs at a WHR of 0.9 or greater. The risk increases sharply after 1.0. In women, increasing insulin resistance is associated with a WHR of 0.85. Risk of ischemia heart disease and stroke increase sharply after 0.8. Waist circumference should be taken at the natural waistline or where the circumference is smallest. Hip circumference should be taken at the maximum circumference of the buttocks.

Weight Goals in Illness

Height and weight tables best serve as goals for either weight loss or weight maintenance for healthy persons. When setting weight goals for nutritional repletion of the malnourished or seriously ill, compare a patient's usual or premorbid weight with his or her current weight to determine percent of weight loss. Where possible, the duration of the weight loss should also be noted. Sudden weight loss is mainly loss of body fluid. Chronic weight loss includes fluid loss as well as loss of fat and protein. Rapid weight loss, especially, is associated with protein catabolism. Loss of more than 5% of usual body weight the previous month or more than 10% loss the previous 6 months indicates protein malnutrition and a need to check other parameters.

Percent weight loss = (usual weight - current weight) ÷ usual weight x 100

Percent usual weight = current weight ÷ usual weight x 100

Weight gain is often a symbol of the reversal of the disease process, or else a desired goal of nutritional support. Restoration of premorbid or usual weight is a reasonable goal in most patients with malnutrition secondary to illness, except those at the extremes of population standards. When asked, many patients are able to state a weight or weight range at which they feel their best. For those who cannot give reliable information, height and weight tables provide a guide for setting goals of nutritional therapy.

Weight increase can be slow despite optimum nutritional support. More than 2 to 3 pounds per week (0.9 to 1.4 kilograms) should not be expected from successful nutritional support. Weight stabilization alone may be adequate along with correction of nutrient deficiencies, and may reduce the risk of overfeeding. In the obese, the goal is repletion of protein loss without weight gain.

BODY CIRCUMFERENCES

Body circumferences, alone or in combination with other anthropometric measures, can be an index of growth or nutrition status. When combined with skinfold thickness at the same site, cross-sectional arm fat area or muscle area can be derived. These measures can be monitered for changes during physical or nutritional therapy.

Measurement tapes should be nonstretch and less than 0.7 cm or 1/4" wide. The tape should be held snugly around the body part but should not indent the skin. The zero end of the tape is held in the left hand above the rest of the tape which is held in the right hand. Any gaps between the skin and the tape can be ignored as tightening the tape is not recommended. The length of the tape should be held parallel to the floor. Measurement errors are mainly due to the position and tension of the tape.

Measurement of Head Circumference

Measurement of head circumference is an important measure of growth in infancy and early childhood. When head circumference is abnormal, parental head circumference should also be measured. Reference values for children are found in the NCHS Growth curves at the end of the Pediatrics chapter. Reference values for adults are found in the references by Churchill and Churchill and White.

1. Subjects less than 36 months will need to be measured supine or seated in the lap. Remove any objects from the hair first.

2. While facing the left side of the head, place a nonstretch tape about 0.7 cm (1/4 in wide) around the head. In the front, the tape should rest just above the eyebrows. In the back, the tape should be placed so that the maximum circumference is measured. The tape should be at the same level on both sides of the head. Hold the tape so that the zero end is below the measure to be recorded.

3. Pull tape tight to compress the hair. Avoid large clumps of hair (e.g., braids). Record to the nearest 0.1 cm or mm.

Figure 4: Measurement of Head Circumference

Measurement of Arm Circumference

Arm circumference is an index of fat stores and muscle mass. Generally it is combined with triceps skinfold to estimate arm muscle circumference, arm muscle area, and arm fat area.

1. Have subject stand with the right arm bent at a 90° angle and the palm up. Clothing should be without sleeves so that the entire arm is exposed.

2. Place the end of a nonstretch tape on the lateral tip of the acromial process and extend it along the side of the upperm arm below the elbow to the olecranon process. Mark the midpoint on the side of the arm.

3. Next have subject release the arm to hang loosely at the side of the body with the palm forward.

4. Place the tape around the arm at the marked midpoint, parallel to the floor. The tape should touch the skin but not compress the soft tissue. Record to the nearest 0.1 cm or mm or mm.

Figure 5: Measurement of Arm Circumference

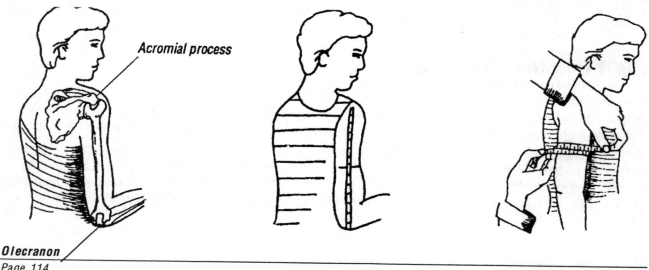

Acromial process

Olecranon

SKINFOLD THICKNESS

Measurement of skinfold thickness or "fatfold" is a frequent component of nutrition surveys. It involves measuring a double fold of skin and fat tissue at a specific body site. Skinfold thicknesses provide an index of body fatness although the degree of correlation with total body fat will vary with age, body site, the individual and the population group. The sum of several skinfolds can be used to estimate percent of body weight that is fat. Skinfolds can also be an indication of the pattern of fat distribution. Increased concentrations in certain areas are associated with increased health risk.

Compressibility of fat folds varies with hydration, age, size, and the individual. It is greater in the young because of greater hydration. Thicker skinfolds in the obese reduce reproducibility. In subjects who have lost a lot of weight, repeated skinfold values become increasingly lower.

Reliable Skinfold calipers should exert a constant pressure of ten grams/mm², provide a range of at least 2 to 40 mm, a contact surface of 20 to 40 mm and be accurate to 0.1mm. Calipers meeting these requirements are:

Lange Skinfold Calipers. Cambridge Scientific Industries, Inc. 101 Virginia Avenue, Cambridge, MD 21613.

Harpenden Skinfold Calipers. British Indicators, Ltd. St. Albans Hertfordshire, England.

Triceps skinfold is measured most often because of easy accessability in both men and women. It correlates closely with total body fat. The site is midline on the back of the arm over the triceps muscle midway between the acromial process of the scapula and the olecranon process of the ulna. Except for infants and the nonambulatory, subjects should be standing. Infants can be measured while held in the lap. Obese and muscular subjects are more difficult to measure because of the difficulty in picking up the fatfold. Increasing age and degree of fatness increase measurement error.

Measurement of Triceps Skinfold

1. Have subject stand with the right arm bent at a 90° angle and the palm up. Clothing should be without sleeves so that the entire arm is exposed. Place the end of a nonstretch tape on the lateral tip of the acromial process and extend it along the side of the upper arm below the elbow to the olecranon process. Mark the midpoint on the side of the arm. Now mark the site on the midline of the back of the arm over the triceps at the same level.

2. Have subject release the arm to hang loosely at the side with the palm forward. Stand behind subject and pick up the skinfold firmly between the thumb and index finger of the left hand (assumes the measurer is right handed) one centimeter above the marked level.

3. Place the calipers over the fatfold at the marked level at a point where the sides of the skinfold are approximately parallel, (at about one-half the depth of the skinfold). The jaws of the calipers should be parallel to the floor. Release the calipers gently. Do not release the pinch. Wait three to four seconds, and take the reading to the nearest 0.1 cm or mm. Repeat twice and average the values.

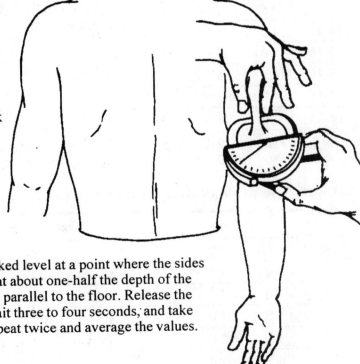

Figure 6: Measurement of Triceps Skinfold

Reference Values for Triceps Skinfold

Reference values in Tables 27 and 28 for triceps skinfolds were derived from measurements of 18,878 subjects in NHANES I and II aged 1 to 25 years. Reference values in Tables 29 through 40 were derived from measurments of 21,752 subjects in NHANES I and II aged 25 to 74 years.

TABLE 27: Triceps Skinfolds (mm) for US Males Aged 1 to 25

	Percentiles								
age	5	10	15	25	50	75	85	90	95
1-2	6.5	7.0	7.5	8.0	10.0	12.0	13.0	14.0	15.5
2-3	6.0	6.5	7.0	8.0	10.0	12.0	13.0	14.0	15.0
3-4	6.0	7.0	7.0	8.0	9.5	11.5	12.5	13.5	15.0
4-5	5.5	6.5	7.0	7.5	9.0	11.0	12.0	12.5	14.0
5-6	5.0	6.0	6.0	7.0	8.0	10.0	11.5	13.0	14.5
6-7	5.0	5.5	6.0	6.5	8.0	10.0	12.0	13.0	16.0
7-8	4.5	5.0	6.0	6.0	8.0	10.5	12.5	14.0	16.0
8-9	5.0	5.5	6.0	7.0	8.5	11.0	13.0	16.0	19.0
9-10	5.0	5.5	6.0	6.5	9.0	12.5	15.5	17.0	20.0
10-11	5.0	6.0	6.0	7.5	10.0	14.0	17.0	20.0	24.0
11-12	5.0	6.0	6.5	7.5	10.0	16.0	19.5	23.0	27.0
12-13	4.5	6.0	6.0	7.5	10.5	14.5	18.0	22.5	27.5
13-14	4.5	5.0	5.5	7.0	9.0	13.0	17.0	20.5	25.0
14-15	4.0	5.0	5.0	6.0	8.5	12.5	15.0	18.0	23.5
15-16	5.0	5.0	5.0	6.0	7.5	11.0	15.0	18.0	23.5
16-17	4.0	5.0	5.1	6.0	8.0	12.0	14.0	17.0	23.0
17-18	4.0	5.0	5.0	6.0	7.0	11.0	13.5	16.0	19.5
18-25	4.0	5.0	5.5	6.5	10.0	14.5	17.5	20.0	23.5

Adapted from: Frisancho, A.:Anthropometric Standards for the Assessmentof Growth and Nutritional Status. University of Michigan Press, 1990

TABLE 28: Triceps Skinfolds (mm) of US Females Aged 1 to 25

	Percentiles								
age	5	10	15	25	50	75	85	90	95
1-2	6.0	7.0	7.0	8.0	10.0	12.0	13.0	14.0	16.0
2-3	6.0	7.0	7.5	8.5	10.0	12.0	13.5	14.5	16.0
3-4	6.0	7.0	7.5	8.5	10.0	12.0	13.0	14.0	16.0
4-5	6.0	7.0	7.5	8.0	10.0	12.0	13.0	14.0	15.5
5-6	5.5	7.0	7.0	8.0	10.0	12.0	13.5	15.0	17.0

6-7	6.0	6.5	7.0	8.0	10.0	12.0	13.0	15.0	17.0
7-8	6.0	7.0	7.0	8.0	10.5	12.5	15.0	16.0	19.0
8-9	6.0	7.0	7.5	8.5	11.0	14.5	17.0	18.0	22.5
9-10	6.5	7.0	8.0	9.0	12.0	16.0	19.0	21.0	25.0
10-11	7.0	8.0	8.0	9.0	12.5	17.5	20.0	22.5	27.0
11-12	7.0	8.0	8.5	10.0	13.0	18.0	21.5	24.0	29.0
12-13	7.0	8.0	9.0	11.0	14.0	18.5	21.5	24.0	27.5
13-14	7.0	8.0	9.0	11.0	15.0	20.0	24.0	25.0	30.0
14-15	8.0	9.0	10.0	11.5	16.0	21.0	23.5	26.5	32.0
15-16	8.0	9.5	10.5	12.0	16.5	20.5	23.0	26.0	32.5
16-17	10.5	11.5	12.0	14.0	18.0	23.0	26.0	29.0	32.5
17-18	9.0	10.0	12.0	13.0	18.0	24.0	26.5	29.0	34.5
18-25	9.0	11.0	12.0	14.0	18.5	24.5	28.5	31.0	36.0

Adapted from: Frisancho, A.:Anthropometric Standards for the Assessment of Growth and Nutritional Status. University of Michigan Press, 1990

TABLE 29: Triceps Skinfolds (mm) for US Men Aged 25 to 54 with Small Frame

Height					Percentile			
in	cm	5	10	15	50	85	90	95
62	157				11			
63	160			6	10	17		
64	163		5	5	10	16	18	
65	165	4	5	6	11	17	19	21
66	168	5	6	6	11	18	18	20
67	170	5	6	6	11	18	20	22
68	173	5	6	6	10	15	16	20
69	175		6	6	11	17	20	
70	178			7	10	17		
71	180			7	10	16		
72	183				10			
73	185							
74	188							

Adapted from: Frisancho R.: AJCN 40:808, 1984

Table 30: Triceps Skinfolds (mm) for US Women Aged 25 to 54 with Small Frames

Height		Percentile						
in	cm	5	10	15	50	85	90	95
58	147		12	13	24	30	33	
59	150	8	11	14	21	29	36	37
60	152	8	11	12	21	28	29	33
61	155	11	12	14	21	28	31	34
62	157	10	12	14	20	28	31	34
63	160	10	11	13	20	27	30	36
64	163	10	13	13	20	28	30	34
65	165	12	13	14	22	29	31	34
66	168			12	19	30		
67	170				18			
68	173				20			
69	175							
70	178							

Adapted from: Frisancho R.: AJCN 40:808, 1984

TABLE 31: Triceps Skinfolds (mm) of US Men Aged 25 to 54 with Medium Frames

Height		Percentile						
in	cm	5	10	15	50	85	90	95
62	157				15			
63	160				11			
64	163		6	6	12	18	20	
65	165	5	7	8	12	20	22	25
66	168	5	6	7	11	16	18	22
67	170	5	7	7	13	21	23	28
68	173	4	5	7	11	18	20	24
69	175	5	6	7	12	18	20	24
70	178	5	6	7	12	18	20	23
71	180	4	5	7	12	19	21	25
72	183	5	7	7	12	20	22	26
73	185	6	7	8	12	20	24	27
74	188		6	9	13	21	23	

Adapted from: Frisancho R.: AJCN 40:808, 1984

TABLE 32: Triceps Skinfolds (mm) of US Women Aged 25 to 54 with Medium Frames

Height		Percentile						
in	cm	5	10	15	50	85	90	95
58	147			20	25	40		
59	150	15	19	21	30	37	40	40
60	152	14	15	17	26	35	37	41
61	155	11	14	15	25	34	36	42
62	157	12	14	16	24	34	36	40
63	160	12	13	15	24	33	35	38
64	163	11	14	15	23	33	36	40
65	165	12	14	15	22	31	34	38
66	168	11	13	14	22	31	33	37
67	170	12	13	15	21	29	30	35
68	173	10	14	15	22	31	32	36
69	175		11	12	19	29	31	
70	178				19			

Adapted from: Frisancho R.: AJCN 40:808, 1984

TABLE 33: Triceps Skinfolds (mm) of US Men Aged 25 to 54 with Large Frames

Height		Percentile						
in	cm	5	10	15	50	85	90	95
62	157							
63	160							
64	163							
65	165				14			
66	168			9	14	30		
67	170		7	7	11	23	27	
68	173		9	10	14	22	23	
69	175	6	7	8	15	25	29	31
70	178	7	7	7	14	23	25	30
71	180	6	8	10	15	25	27	31
72	183	5	6	7	12	20	22	25
73	185	5	6	7	13	19	22	31
74	188			8	12	19		

Adapted from: Frisancho R.: AJCN 40:808, 1984

TABLE 34: Triceps Skinfolds (mm) of US Women Aged 25 to 54 with Large Frames

Height		Percentile						
in	cm	5	10	15	50	85	90	95
58	147							
59	150				36			
60	152				38			
61	155		25	26	36	48	50	
62	157	16	19	22	34	48	48	50
63	160	18	20	22	34	46	48	51
64	163	16	20	21	32	43	45	49
65	165	17	20	21	31	43	46	48
66	168	13	17	18	27	40	43	45
67	170	13	16	17	30	41	43	49
68	173		16	20	29	37	40	
69	175			21	30	42		
70	178				20			

Adapted from: Frisancho R.: AJCN 40:808, 1984

TABLE 35: Triceps Skinfolds (mm) of US Men Aged 55 to 74 with Small Frames

Height		Percentile						
in	cm	5	10	15	50	85	90	95
62	157			6	9	12		
63	160		5	5	10	16	17	
64	163	4	4	4	9	20	21	22
65	165	5	6	7	11	18	19	24
66	168	5	6	7	11	16	20	20
67	170	5	6	6	10	15	17	25
68	173		5	5	10	15	17	
69	175			8	10	15		
70	178				11			
71	180				9			
72	183							
73	185							
74	188							

Adapted from: Frisancho R.: AJCN 40:808, 1984

TABLE 36: Triceps Skinfolds (mm) of US Women Aged 55 to 74 with Small Frames

Height		Percentile						
in	cm	5	10	15	50	85	90	95
58	147		14	16	21	31	34	
59	150	11	13	15	21	30	31	33
60	152	10	11	13	20	29	31	35
61	155	10	12	14	22	29	29	32
62	157	1	11	12	21	29	30	32
63	160		12	13	20	29	30	
64	163		12	13	21	27	29	
65	165				18			
66	168				23			
67	170							
68	173							
69	175							
70	178							

Adapted from: Frisancho R.: AJCN 40:808, 1984

TABLE 37: Triceps Skinfolds (mm) of US Men Aged 55 to 74 with Medium Frames

Height		Percentile						
in	cm	5	10	15	50	85	90	95
62	157			5	12	25		
63	160		7	7	11	20	23	
64	163	5	6	6	10	17	20	26
65	165	5	6	7	11	17	19	24
66	168	6	6	7	12	18	19	22
67	170	5	6	7	12	18	20	23
68	173	6	7	8	12	18	21	23
69	175	5	6	7	12	19	22	25
70	178	6	7	7	11	18	19	21
71	180	5	6	6	11	16	17	20
72	183		6	8	11	19	20	
73	185			8	13	16		
74	188				11			

Adapted from: Frisancho R.: AJCN 40:808, 1984

TABLE 38: Triceps Skinfolds (mm) of US Women Aged 55 to 74 with Medium Frames

Height					Percentile			
in	cm	5	10	15	50	85	90	95
58	147	5	13	17	28	40	40	41
59	150	12	15	18	26	34	38	41
60	152	13	15	18	25	33	34	38
61	155	13	16	18	25	35	37	42
62	157	13	15	17	24	33	36	39
63	160	12	14	16	24	32	35	38
64	163	12	14	16	25	33	34	37
65	165	14	16	17	24	33	35	39
66	168	12	13	16	24	33	33	36
67	170		17	17	27	35	35	
68	173				25			
69	175							
70	178							

Adapted from: Frisancho, R.: AJCN 40:808, 1984.

TABLE 39: Triceps Skinfolds (mm) of US Men Aged 55 to 74 with Large Frames

Height					Percentile			
in	cm	5	10	15	50	85	90	95
62	157							
63	160				15			
64	163				21			
65	165			11	14	22		
66	168		7	8	13	21	25	
67	170	6	8	9	16	21	25	27
68	173	6	7	8	13	20	21	23
69	175	6	7	8	12	18	20	23
70	178	5	6	8	14	22	25	31
71	180		6	6	13	18	22	
72	183		8	8	13	23	26	
73	185				11			
74	188				12			

Adapted from: Frisancho R.: AJCN 40:1984.

TABLE 40: Triceps Skinfolds (mm) of US Women Aged 55 to 74 with Large Frames

Height		Percentile						
in	cm	5	10	15	50	85	90	95
58	147				45			
59	150				36			
60	152		25	26	35	44	45	
61	155	18	22	24	33	40	44	46
62	157	19	24	24	32	40	43	50
63	160	20	24	25	33	41	43	45
64	163	18	22	23	29	42	46	50
65	165	15	17	20	30	43	44	46
66	168		18	18	27	35	40	
67	170			22	32	44		
68	173				26			
69	175							
70	178							

Adapted from: Frisancho R.: AJCN 40:808, 1984

RECUMBENT ANTHROPOMETRIC MEASURES

Handicapped or incompetent subjects, and those confined to bed or wheelchair, are best measured recumbent. Measurements taken on subjects in wheelchairs are prone to error. Techniques for recumbent measurement of arm circumference and triceps skinfold are described below.

Measurement of Recumbent Arm Circumference

1. Have subject lie on the back with the elbow bent at a 90° angle across the middle of the body, palm down. Place the end of a nonstretch tape on the lateral tip of the acromial process and extend it along the side of the upper arm below the elbow to the olecranon process. Mark the midpoint on the side of the arm.
2. Extend the arm along the trunk with the palm up. Raise the arm slightly with a sandbag under the elbow. Place the tape around the arm at the marked midpoint with the tape perpendicular to the length of the arm. The tape should touch the skin but not compress the soft tissue. Record to the nearest 0.1 cm or mm.

Measurement of Recumbent Triceps Skinfold

1. Have subject lie on the side with the trunk straight and the knees bent up slightly. The bottom arm is extended out at a 45° angle and the upper arm lies along the trunk with the forearm bent at a 90° angle across the middle of the body.
2. Place the end of a nonstretch tape on the lateral tip of the acromial process and extend it along the side of the upper arm below the elbow to the olecranon process. Mark the midpoint on the side of the arm. Now mark the site on the midline of the back of the upper arm over the triceps at the same level.

3. Extend the arm along the trunk with the palm down. Grasp a skinfold firmly between the thumb and index finger of the left hand one centimeter above the marked level. Place the calipers over the fatfold at the marked level at a point where the sides of the skinfold are approximately parallel, about one-half the depth of the skinfold. Bend down to take the reading. Release the calipers gently. Wait three to four seconds, and take the reading to the nearest 0.1 cm or mm. Repeat twice and average the values.

Figure 7: Position for Recumbent Triceps Skinfold

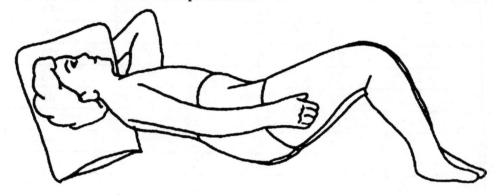

Figure 8: Measurement of Recumbent Triceps Skinfold

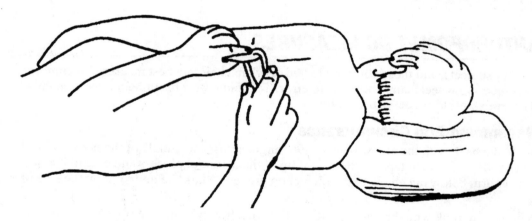

Refererence Values for Recumbent Measurements

Reference data for recumbent anthropometric measurements is limited. Chumlea et al have published percentile values for recumbent triceps skinfolds and arm muscle circumference in a group of 65 to 90 year olds. The values were derived from a sample of 269 ambulatory Caucasian men and women living in southwest Ohio. While they are not necessarily representative of the US population they do not differ significantly from values published by the National Center for Health Statistics for this age group. Values greater than the 95th percentile or less than the 5th percentile or else rapid changes in percentiles are of concern and suggest a need for further testing.

These measures were taken from a Caucasion population and cannot necessarily be used for other races. Still, repeated measures on an individual can be used to monitor changes over time or else response to nutritional intervention regardless of race.

TABLE 41: Recumbent Triceps Skinfold in Men and Women Aged 65 to 90

	Percentiles					
Age	Men			Women		
	5	50	95	5	50	95
65	8.6	13.8	27.0	13.5	21.6	33.0
70	7.7	12.9	26.1	12.5	20.6	32.0
75	6.8	12.0	25.2	11.5	19.6	31.0
80	6.0	11.2	24.3	10.5	18.6	30.0
85	5.1	10.3	23.4	9.5	17.6	29.0
90	4.2	9.4	22.6	8.5	16.6	28.0

Adapted from: Chumlea et al: J. Nutr. for the Elderly 4:39, 1985.

ARM MUSCLE AREA

Depletion of muscle mass is an important indicator of protein-calorie malnutrition. Estimation of arm muscle area is an inexpensive, practical method of assessing the degree of depletion. Repeated measurements over time can be used to monitor response to nutritional intervention.

Determination of Arm Muscle Area

Calculation of Arm Muscle Area (AMA) is based on the assumption that the mid upper arm and mid upper arm muscle are circular, that the triceps skinfold is two times the average diameter of the fat layer, and that bone atrophies in proportion to muscle in malnutrition. Computerized tomography has shown that these assumptions lead to a 20 to 25% overestimation of AMA, thus underestimating the degree of muscle atrophy.

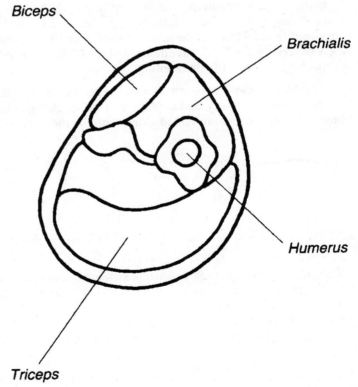

**Figure 9: Cross-Sectional View
            of Mid Upper Arm**

Heymsfield et al (28) has developed revised equations to correct for the bone area, the neurovascular bundle, and the noncircular shape of muscle. These equations were derived from a study of 26 individuals aged 20 to 70 years and within 90 to 115% of their ideal body weight according to the Metropolitan height-weight tables. Previous studies showed that anthropometric measurement of muscle mass is very inaccurate when ideal body weight is greater than 125% and obese subjects should probably be excluded. These revised equations are shown below:

$$\text{AMA (male)} = [\text{AC (cm)} - (\pi \times \text{TSF (cm)})]^2 \div 4\pi - 10$$
$$\text{AMA (female)} = [\text{AC (cm)} - (\pi \times \text{TSF (cm)})]^2 \div 4\pi - 6.5$$

Example:

arm circumference (AC) = 25 cm (male)
triceps skinfold = 6 mm or 0.6 cm
$\pi = 3.14$

$$
\begin{aligned}
\text{AMA (cm}^2) \quad &= [25 - (3.14 \times 0.6)]^2 \div 4\pi - 10 \\
&= [25 - 1.88]^2 \div 12.56 - 10 \\
&= [23.12]^2 \div 12.56 - 10 \\
&= 534 \div 12.56 - 10 \\
&= 42.5 - 10 \\
&= 32.5
\end{aligned}
$$

When the corrected equations were tested on another group of 33 subjects for accuracy, resulting AMA values were an average 7.7% greater than values determined by computerized tomography.

Minimal Arm Muscle Area

Heymsfield has also determined the "minimal AMA" that is compatible with survival. This is the amount of muscle tissue that remains at death from protein-calorie malnutrition, and which is metabolically unavailable. It is between 9 and 11 cm². This allows calculation of "available AMA" which is total AMA less that mimimum AMA described above. An available AMA of 0 to 5 cm² indicates severe protein calorie malnutrition. Values approaching zero are life threatening.

Since AMA is derived from arm circumference and triceps skinfold, accurate measurement of these is important. For increased sensitivity and detection of small changes in AMA, frequently repeated measurements by the same observer are recommended along with the the exclusion of obese subjects.

Reference Values for Arm Muscle Area

The Arm Muscle Area reference tables which follow do not include adjustments for bone area for those less than 18 years of age.

TABLE 42: Arm Muscle Area (cm²) in US Males Aged 2 to 11

Height	Percentile								
cm	5	10	15	25	50	75	85	90	95
87-92	9.3	10.4	10.6	11.2	12.9	14.2	15.0	15.8	16.5
93-98	10.2	10.9	11.2	12.1	13.5	15.3	15.9	16.5	17.0
99-104	10.9	11.7	12.2	13.0	14.5	15.9	16.5	17.1	18.4
105-110	12.0	12.8	13.3	14.1	15.4	17.0	17.8	18.6	19.8
111-116	12.6	13.6	14.3	15.0	16.6	18.1	18.9	19.6	20.7
117-122	14.1	14.5	15.0	16.1	17.7	19.7	20.7	21.6	23.4
123-128	15.0	15.9	16.3	17.4	19.2	21.2	22.3	23.2	24.2
129-134	16.1	17.3	18.4	19.3	21.1	23.2	24.7	25.3	27.9
135-140	17.2	18.12	18.9	20.4	22.6	24.9	26.1	27.2	30.2
141-146	19.3	20.1	20.8	21.9	24.0	27.2	29.0	30.5	34.0
147-152	21.2	22.4	23.3	24.8	27.0	29.8	31.8	32.9	34.4
153-158	22.3	23.2	24.3	25.4	28.4	32.2	34.8	36.9	40.1
159-164	23.7	24.5	25.3	27.5	31.9	35.6	39.7	41.4	44.5

Heights are without shoe heels. Values were not adjusted for bone area using the revised equations as they have not been tested on children. Adapted from: Frisancho, A.: Anthropometric Standards for the Assessment of Growth and Nutritional Status. University of Michigan Press, 1990.

TABLE 43: Arm Muscle Area (cm²) in US Males Aged 11 to 17

Height	Percentile								
cm	5	10	15	25	50	75	85	90	95
141-146	20.7	21.4	22.7	24.1	25.6	30.3	32.8	33.9	36.3
147-152	22.4	23.4	24.1	25.6	27.5	30.2	33.1	34.2	36.1
153-158	22.7	24.9	26.1	27.5	30.4	34.1	36.4	39.1	41.5
159-164	23.7	26.7	27.8	30.2	34.1	38.6	41.5	44.3	48.4
165-170	28.1	29.7	31.5	34.2	40.0	45.6	49.0	52.9	58.9
171-176	32.8	35.2	36.6	39.5	45.8	52.6	56.0	59.1	66.0
177-182	36.1	38.7	40.8	43.4	49.5	56.4	59.4	62.6	65.9
183-188	38.3	41.3	42.8	46.1	52.6	57.8	63.0	67.5	74.3
189-194	41.4	44.2	45.7	48.9	53.9	60.3	65.0	68.5	74.0

Heights are without shoe heels. Values were not adjusted for bone area using the revised equations as they have not been tested on children. Adapted from: Frisancho, A.: Anthropometric Standards for the Assessment of Growth and Nutritional Status. University of Michigan Press, 1990.

TABLE 44: Arm Muscle Area (cm²) in US Females Aged 2 to 11

Height	Percentile								
cm	5	10	15	25	50	75	85	90	95
87-92	9.5	10.1	10.5	11.0	12.6	14.2	14.8	15.5	16.2
93-98	10.1	10.7	11.0	11.8	13.2	14.4	15.3	15.8	16.9
99-104	10.6	11.2	11.7	12.5	14.0	15.5	16.4	16.9	18.0
105-110	11.3	11.9	12.4	13.2	14.6	16.3	17.3	17.9	18.9
111-116	12.3	13.0	13.5	14.2	15.7	17.4	18.4	19.1	20.3
117-122	13.0	13.9	14.4	15.2	16.7	18.5	19.6	20.3	21.4
123-128	14.2	15.0	15.5	16.2	17.9	19.6	20.8	21.6	22.9
129-134	15.3	16.1	16.8	17.6	19.7	21.7	22.9	23.8	25.4
135-140	16.1	17.4	18.1	19.2	21.1	23.8	24.8	26.3	27.9
141-146	17.6	18.5	19.5	20.5	23.0	25.8	27.9	28.8	30.6
147-152	18.5	20.0	20.7	21.7	24.4	27.8	30.0	31.2	32.9
153-158	19.4	20.1	22.4	23.0	25.4	29.2	31.8	34.0	38.2

Heights are without shoe heels. Values were not adjusted for bone area using the revised equations as they have not been tested on children. Adapted from: Frisancho, A.: Anthropometric Standards for the Assessment of Growth and Nutritional Status. University of Michigan Press, 1990.

TABLE 45: Arm Muscle Area (cm²) in US Females Aged 11 to 17

Height	Percentile								
cm	5	10	15	25	50	75	85	90	95
141-146	17.1	19.3	19.5	21.0	23.4	25.5	27.9	28.6	33.4
147-152	18.5	19.7	20.9	22.0	24.3	28.0	29.8	30.3	34.4
153-158	20.8	22.0	23.0	24.7	28.3	32.9	35.0	37.5	39.2
159-164	23.3	24.8	26.0	27.7	31.2	35.7	38.0	40.1	43.5
165-170	25.0	26.6	27.8	29.5	33.2	37.6	40.2	42.8	46.9
171-176	25.9	27.1	28.0	29.9	33.7	38.0	41.2	43.5	47.6
177-182	28.6	29.5	30.5	31.7	35.9	41.1	45.9	47.8	58.2

Heights are without shoe heels. Values were not adjusted for bone area using the revised equations as they have not been tested on children. Adapted from: Frisancho, A.: Anthropometric Standards for the Assessment of Growth and Nutritional Status. University of Michigan Press, 1990.

Table 46: Bone-Free Arm Muscle Area (cm²) of US Men Aged 18 to 25

	Percentile								
Frame	5	10	15	25	50	75	85	90	95
Small	30.8	33.8	35.8	38.7	44.6	51.3	55.2	58.1	63.2
Medium	35.5	38.2	40.8	43.6	49.5	56.5	60.8	63.2	69.3
Large	37.6	40.8	43.0	47.3	54.6	63.5	67.0	71.6	76.7

Heights are without shoe heels. Values werederived from the revised AMA equations. Adapted from: Frisancho, A.: Anthropometric Standards for the Assessment of Growth and Nutritional Status. University of Michigan Press, 1990.

TABLE 47: Bone-Free Arm Muscle Area (cm²) of US and Women Aged 18 to 25

	Percentile								
Frame	5	10	15	25	50	75	85	90	95
Small	18.2	19.6	20.7	22.5	25.5	29.2	31.2	32.8	36.2
Medium	19.8	21.9	23.2	24.9	28.4	32.8	35.2	37.2	40.7
Large	21.9	23.8	25.3	27.3	31.9	38.7	43.9	47.5	55.8

Heights are without shoe heels. Values were derived from the revised AMA equations. Adapted from: Frisancho, A.: Anthropometric Standards for the Assessment of Growth and Nutritional Status. University of Michigan Press, 1990.

Table 48: Bone-Free Arm Muscle Area (cm²) in US Men Aged 25 to 54 with Small Frames

Height		Percentile						
in	cm	5	10	15	50	85	90	95
62	157				52			
63	160			32	148	54		
64	163		37	38	49	58	63	
65	165	31	35	37	47	60	63	71
66	168	31	36	38	49	60	62	71
67	170	35	39	41	49	58	60	62
68	173	33	37	40	49	59	62	69
69	175		36	40	58	61	63	
70	178			35	48	57		
71	180			39	47	52		
72	183				45			
73	185							
74	188							

Heights are without shoe heels. Values were derived from the revised AMA equations.
Adapted from: AJCN 40:808 1984

TABLE 49: Bone-Free Arm Muscle Area (cm²) in US Women Aged 25 to 54 with Small Frames

Height					Percentile			
in	cm	5	10	15	50	85	90	95
58	147		22	24	29	36	44	
59	150	17	20	22	28	38	39	43
60	152	19	21	22	28	36	40	44
61	155	20	21	23	28	38	39	42
62	157	20	21	21	27	33	35	37
63	160	20	21	22	27	33	35	38
64	163	22	23	23	28	34	38	42
65	165	21	22	23	28	37	39	47
66	168			23	27	35		
67	170				26			
68	173				25			
69	175							
70	178							

Heights are without shoe heels. Values derived from the revised AMA equations. Adapted from: AJCN 40:808 1984:

TABLE 50: Percentiles for Bone-Free Arm Muscle Area (cm²) in US Men Aged 25 to 54 with Medium Frames

Height					Percentile			
in	cm	5	10	15	50	85	90	95
62	157				58			
63	160				55			
64	163		43	47	56	67	71	
65	165	40	43	45	56	67	69	70
66	168	38	42	44	55	69	72	78
67	170	39	42	44	53	66	69	73
68	173	41	44	45	55	67	71	76
69	175	38	41	44	54	66	69	73
70	178	39	42	43	55	65	68	72
71	180	37	41	44	54	67	68	73
72	183	40	42	44	56	65	67	74
73	185	39	42	43	55	67	69	73
74	188		43	43	55	62	63	

Heights are without shoe heels. Values are derived from the revised AMA equations.
Adapted from: Am. J. Clin. Nutr. 40:808 1984

TABLE 51: Bone-Free Arm Muscle Area (cm²) in US Women Aged 25 to 54 with Medium Frames

Height		Percentile						
in	cm	5	10	15	50	85	90	95
58	147			24	35	42		
59	150	23	24	26	33	43	45	49
60	152	22	25	25	32	42	45	49
61	155	21	24	25	31	42	45	51
62	157	21	23	25	31	40	43	48
63	160	22	23	25	32	41	43	50
64	163	21	23	24	31	40	43	48
65	165	21	23	24	31	40	43	49
66	168	21	23	24	30	39	41	44
67	170	22	24	25	30	40	43	48
68	173	22	24	25	30	37	38	39
69	175		23	24	30	36	39	
70	178				32			

Heights are without shoe heels. Values were derived from the revised AMA equations
Adapted from: Am. J. Clin. Nutr. 40:808 1984

TABLE 52: Bone-Free Arm Muscle Area (cm²) in US Men Aged 25 to 54 with Large Frames

Height		Percentile						
in	cm	5	10	15	50	85	90	95
62	157							
63	160							
64	163							
65	165				62			
66	168			48	58	76		
67	170		50	52	61	73	78	
68	173		51	53	65	78	86	
69	175	46	48	49	61	73	78	83
70	178	43	47	50	61	75	77	86
71	180	47	48	50	62	75	81	83
72	183	45	48	50	61	77	80	86
73	185	47	49	51	66	79	83	
74	188			53	66	78		

Heights are without shoe heels. Values were derived from the revised AMA equations. Adapted from: Am. J. Clin. Nutr. 40:808 1984

TABLE 53: Bone-Free Arm Muscle Area (cm²) in US Women Aged 25 to 54 with Large Frames

Height					Percentile			
in	cm	5	10	15	50	85	90	95
58	147							
59	150				45			
60	152				44			
61	155		29	33	41	62	74	
62	157	26	28	31	44	56	63	72
63	160	27	30	32	43	60	65	77
64	163	26	28	29	39	50	55	63
65	165	27	28	29	39	56	59	67
66	168	23	24	27	35	49	53	69
67	170	25	28	30	37	50	53	55
68	173		28	30	38	51	54	
69	175			27	35	49		
70	178				37			

Heights are without shoe heels. Values were derived from the revised AMA equations
Adapted from: Am. J. Clin. Nutr. 40:808 1984

TABLE 54: Bone-Free Arm Muscle Area (cm²) in US Men Aged 55 to 74 with Small Frames

Height					Percentile			
in	cm	5	10	15	50	85	90	95
62	157			38	46	52		
63	160		34	35	43	54	55	
64	163	26	30	31	44	53	54	56
65	165	26	30	34	48	57	60	62
66	168	25	31	35	45	54	58	64
67	170	30	36	37	45	53	55	59
68	173		35	35	43	55	60	
69	175			38	47	62		
70	178				48			
71	180				43			
72	183							
73	185							
74	188							

Heights are without shoe heels. Values were derived from the revised AMA equations. Adapted from: Am. J. Clin. Nutr. 40:808 1984

TABLE 55: Bone-Free Arm Muscle Area (cm²) in US Women Aged 55 to 74 with Small Frames

Height		Percentile						
in	cm	5	10	15	50	85	90	95
58	147		22	23	29	40	42	
59	150	22	23	24	30	39	40	44
60	152	20	22	23	30	37	41	44
61	155	18	21	23	28	36	40	42
62	157	20	23	24	30	37	40	43
63	160		19	20	27	35	36	
64	163		21	21	28	37	42	
65	165				28			
66	168				33			
67	170							
68	173							
69	175							
70	178							

Heights are without shoe heels. Values were derived from the revised AMA equations.
Adapted from: Am. J. Clin. Nutr. 40:808 1984

TABLE 56: Bone-Free Arm Muscle Area (cm²) in US Men Aged 55 to 74 with Medium Frames

Height		Percentile						
in	cm	5	10	15	50	85	90	95
62	157			39	48	61		
63	160		36	38	50	60	63	
64	163	35	39	40	51	64	66	71
65	165	35	38	41	52	63	65	72
66	168	34	39	42	51	60	62	67
67	170	35	39	42	52	65	67	70
68	173	37	40	42	52	65	67	70
69	175	31	36	40	51	62	65	72
70	178	36	41	44	53	63	65	68
71	180	36	42	44	56	65	67	71
72	183		27	39	50	67	59	
73	185			43	56			
74	188				56			

Heights are without shoe heels. Values were derived from the revised AMA equations. Adapted from: Am. J. Clin. Nutr. 40:808 1984

TABLE 57: Bone-Free Arm Muscle Area (cm²) in US Women Aged 55 to 74 with Medium Frames

Height		Percentile						
in	cm	5	10	15	50	85	90	95
58	147	21	23	25	32	46	47	51
59	150	24	26	27	35	44	48	48
60	152	21	24	26	35	45	49	57
61	155	22	24	26	34	44	49	52
62	157	24	25	26	35	45	47	54
63	160	24	26	27	35	44	45	51
64	163	21	24	26	33	44	46	49
65	165	24	25	27	34	44	45	50
66	168	24	26	27	33	41	43	49
67	170		27	28	32	41	43	
68	173				36			
69	175							
70	178							

Heights are without shoe heels. Values were derived from the revised AMA equations. Adapted from: Am. J. Clin. Nutr. 40:808 1984.

TABLE 58: Bone-Free Arm Muscle Area (cm²) in US Men Aged 55 to 74 with Large Frames

Height		Percentile						
in	cm	5	10	15	50	85	90	95
62	157							
63	160				57			
64	163				44			
65	165			44	59	66		
66	168		43	47	56	67	72	
67	170	41	43	44	56	71	73	79
68	173	41	43	46	57	69	70	74
69	175	40	45	45	58	70	72	79
70	178	43	48	50	59	70	71	87
71	180		46	47	54	70	75	
72	183		47	48	59	73	78	
73	185				59			
74	188				54			

Heights are without shoe heels. Values were derived from the revised AMA equations.
Adapted from: Am. J. Clin. Nutr. 40:808 1984.

TABLE 59: Bone-Free Arm Muscle Area (cm²) in US Women Aged 55 to 74 with Large Frames

| Height | | Percentile | | | | | | |
in	cm	5	10	15	50	85	90	95
58	147				50			
59	150				49			
60	152		28	33	41	58	60	
61	155	31	32	34	44	59	61	71
62	157	28	29	34	43	59	63	76
63	160	27	32	33	41	56	62	67
64	163	28	29	32	41	54	60	78
65	165	29	32	32	42	53	57	65
66	168		31	31	40	57	58	
67	170			30	40	58		
68	173				48			
69	175							
70	178							

Heights are without shoe heels. Values were derived from the revised AMA equations
Adapted from: Am. J. Clin. Nutr. 40:808 1984.

Chumlea has published percentiles for midarm muscle area (AMA) in individuals 65 - 90 years of age. They are derived from triceps skinfold and arm circumference measurements from 269 ambulatory, free-living Caucasian men and women in southwest Ohio. The corrected AMA formulas of Heymsfield discussed above were not used because they had not been tested in the elderly.

TABLE 60: Midarm Muscle Area in Men and Women Aged 65 to 90

| | Percentiles | | | | | |
Age	5	50	95	5	50	95
65	43.2	59.4	77.1	33.5	44.5	66.4
70	41.4	57.7	75.3	33.0	44.1	65.9
75	39.6	55.9	73.5	32.6	43.6	65.5
80	37.8	54.1	71.7	32.2	43.2	65.1
85	36.0	52.3	69.9	31.8	42.8	64.7
90	34.3	50.5	68.2	31.3	42.4	64.2

Adapted from: Chumlea, W.: J. Geront. 41:36, 1986.

Falciglia et al have published percentiles for triceps skinfold, arm circumference, arm muscle circumference and mid-arm muscle area from a larger sample of 746 noninstitutionalized, ambulatory Caucasian elderly 60-89 years of age living in the Cincinnati area. (See end of Chapter for source).

SPECIAL CONSIDERATIONS

Extremes of Body Size

Subjects at the extremes of body composition (i.e. less than the 5th percentile or greater than the 95th) are at increased risk for nutritional compromise and or disease. They may need further evaluation or at least more frequent monitoring. Possible reasons for exceeding the 95th percentile include a tall stature, obesity, or edema. Reasons for being less than the 5th percentile include short stature, malnutrition, dehydration, osteoporosis.

Which Side to Measure

Some anthropometric measures are larger on the dominant side of the body, especially those on the arm. In some cases, the differences are statistically significant (i.e, triceps skinfold, wrist circumference, and arm circumference). The side of the body used for anthropometric measures varies with the survey and the investigator. NHANES data was obtained on the right side. Data from surveys in Europe and developing countries is generally obtained on the left side. While international agreement on which side to use is desirable, the side used makes little difference as the differences between sides are less than measurement errors.

Children and Infants

Measurement errors are more likely in children due to their difficulty maintaining a standardized position. Measurements can be done either recumbent or with the infant help in a lap. In newborns, skinfold measurements should not be done the first 24 hours after birth because of early water shifts in the tissues. The smaller Lange skinfold calipers may be preferred for the very young due to their smaller size. A number of investigators release the calipers for a longer period of time (15 to 60 seconds) before taking a reading, or else wait until the reading has stabilized. This is because of the greater water content in the fat tissue of newborns.

Handicapped Subjects

Recumbent methods can be used on young, handicapped subjects although standards have not yet been established. No systematic differences between recumbent and ambulatory measurements have been shown, however. Subjects who are confined to wheelchairs should be measured supine because the results will be more accurate.

Elderly Subjects

Reference data for recumbent measures are available for the elderly aged 65 to 90. Recumbent measures have not been found to differ significantly from values reported by the National Center for Health Statistics on elderly, ambulatory subjects. It is not known, however if the same data can be used for elderly blacks as well as whites.

Obese Subjects

Reliable measurements are more difficult in the obese for several reasons. Finding the bony landmarks for precise location of measurement sites is more difficult. Secondly, the sides of the skinfold may not be parallel, and the skinfolds may be thicker than the caliper opening. Formulas for predicting total body fat have not been proved valid in obese subjects. Circumference measurements are preferred in the obese as they are more accessible and less variable. A minimum of two measures are recommended, either skinfolds or circumferences. Measurements which evaluate both peripheral and central body compartments should be included. Central measures include subscapular skinfold, supra-iliac skinfold, waist circumference, and hip circumference. Peripheral measures include triceps skinfold, biceps skinfold, arm circumference and calf circumference.

For further information on assessing body compositon consult Anthropometric Standards for the Assessment of Growth and Nutritional Status by A.R. Frisancho, University of Michigan Press, Ann Arbor, MI, 1990.

References

- Lohman T et al: Anthropometric Standardization Reference Manual. Champaign: Human Kinetics Books, 1988.

- Gray, D et al: Accuracy of recumbent height measurement. JPEN 9: 712, 1985.

- Stewart, A et al: The reliability and validity of self-reported weight and height. J Chron Dis 35:295, 1982.

- Robinson, L and Wright, B: Comparison of stated and measured patient heights and weights. Am J. Hosp. Pharm. 39:822, 1982.

- Harris, J et al: The Measurement of Man. Minneapolis: University of Minnesota Press, 1930.

- Dequeker, J et al: The significance of stature as a clinical measurement of aging. J. Am. Ger. Soc. 17:169, 1969.

- Mitchell, C and Lipschitz, D: Arm length measurement as an alternative to height in nutritional assessment of the elderly. JPEN 6:226, 1982.

- Chumlea, W et al: Estimating stature from knee height for persons 60 to 90 years of age. J Am Geriat Soc 33:116, 1985.

- Chumlea, W et al: Prediction of stature from knee height for black and white adults and children with application to mobility-impaired or handicapped persons. J. Am. Diet. Assn.94:1385, 1994.

- Chumlea, W and Guo, S: Supplement: Equations for predicting stature in white and black elderly individuals. J. Geront. 47:M197, 1992.

- Frisancho, R and Flegel, P: Elbow breadth as a measure of frame size for US males and females. Am. J. Clin. Nutr. 37:311, 1983.

- Grant, J: Handbook of Total Parenteral Nutrition. Philadelphia: WB Sanders, 1980.

- Seltzer, M: Dietetic Currents 10:17, 1983. Ross Laboratories.

- Robinett-Weiss, N et al: The Metropolitan height-weight tables: perspectives for use. J. Am. Diet. Assn. 84:1480, 1984.

- Frisancho, R: New standards of weight body and composition by frame size and height for assessment of nutritional status of adults and the elderly. Am. J. Clin. Nutr. 40:808, 1984.

- Master, A and Lasser, R: Tables of average weight and height of Americans aged 65 to 94 years. J. Am. Med. Assoc.172:658, 1960.

- National Institutes of Health, Consensus Development Conference Statement: Volume 5, Number 9, 1985.

- Bray, G: Obesity. Disease a Month, July 1989, p456.

- Manson, J et al: Body weight and longevity, J. Am. Med. Assn. 257:353, 1987.

- Clouse, R: Practical use of body weight in nutritional therapy. Clin Consult , Vol 3, No 4, 1983.

- Chumlea, W et al: Some anthropometric indices of body composition for elderly adults. J Geront. 41:36, 1986.

- Heymsfield, S et al: Anthropometric measurement of muscle mass: revised equations for calculating bone-free muscle area. Am. J. Clin. Nutr. 36:680, 1982.

- Chumlea, W et al: Nutritional anthropometric assessment in elderly persons 65 to 90 years of age. J. Nutr. for the Elderly. 4:39, 1985.

- Falciglia, G et al: Upper arm anthropometric norms in elderly white subjects. J. Am. Diet. Assoc. 88:569, 1988.

- Heymsfield, S, and Casper, K: Anthropometric assessment of the adult hospitalized patient. J.P.E.N. 11:36S, 1987.

- Himes, J et al: Parent-specific adjustments for evaluation of recumbent length and stature of children. Ped. 75:304, 1985.

- Interdepartmental Committee on Nutrition for National Defense: Manual for Nutrition Surveys. 2nd ed. Washington, 1963.

- Churchill, E et al: Anthropometry of women of the US Army 1977 (Report No. 2 - The basic univariate statistics. (AD-A044-806) Natick/TR-77/024. Natick: US Army, 1977.

- White, R and Churchill, E: The body size of soldiers. (TR72-51-CE). Natick: US Army Natick Laboratories, 1975.

- Osterkamp, L: Current perspective on assessment of human body proportions of relevance to amputees. J. Am. Diet. Assn. 95:215, 1995.

- Frisancho, AR: Anthropometric Standards for the Assessment of Growth and Nutritional Status. University of Michigan Press: Ann Arbor, MI, 1990.

- NHANES III Anthropometric Procedures Video. National Center for Health Statistics. (301) 436-8500.

CLINICAL ASSESSMENT

The focus of clinical assessment is on the physical examination and medical history and looks for signs of nutrient deficiency. Some physical abnormalities are diagnostic of nutrient deficiency, but most are mild and nonspecific. In fact, many signs can result from a lack of several nutrients as well as from non-nutritional causes. In spite of these shortcomings, their observation can be a useful index of nutritional status. Any positive findings should be further investigated or confirmed with anthropometric measurements, dietary evaluation or biochemical tests.

PHYSICAL SIGNS IN NUTRITION ASSESSMENT

Physical findings can be divided into three classes and are presented this way in the tables that follow:

- Those which are important in nutritional assessment.

- Those which are suggestive of poor nutrition and require further evaluation.

- Those due to non-nutritional causes.

In the NHANES survey the major deficiency signs were assigned to one of three risk categories (high, moderate, low) based on their specificity for a particular deficiency. Signs in the high risk category are considered highly sensitive and specific. A person presenting with one of these signs would be considered at high risk of either having or developing the deficiency.

Physical Signs Of Value In Nutrition Assessment	Physical Signs Needing Further Evaluation	Physical Signs Unrelated To Nutrient Deficiency
HAIR		**Alopecia.** Baldness.
Lackluster. Dull, dry, brittle and wire-like. Compare to local normal standards. Consider environmental causes. Protein deficiency: low risk if single finding.		**Artificial Discoloration.** Chemical or environmental.
Thinness, Sparseness. Fine and silky with wider gaps between hairs. Associated with protein deficiency.		
Straightness. Straight in cultural groups with normally curly hair. Other changes usually present. Protein deficiency: medium risk.		
Dyspigmented. Lightening of normal hair color or depigmentation. Black hair becomes grayish or reddish. Most evident distally. Rare in adults. Do not confuse with bleached or dyed hair. Protein deficiency: medium risk if two or more signs present.		
Flag Sign. Alternating bands of light and dark along the length of the hair in young children. Depigmented bands are usually of a different texture. Shows periods of better and poorer nutrition. Uncommon. Associated with protein deficiency.		
Easy Pluckability. Small clump can be pulled out with moderate force and no pain, especially on side of head. Generally occurs with other hair changes. Inspect comb or brush for excess shedding. Protein deficiency: low risk, medium if two or more signs present.		

Physical Signs Of Value In Nutrition Assessment	**Physical Signs Needing Further Evaluation**	**Physical Signs Unrelated To Nutrient Deficiency**

FACE

Diffuse Depigmentation. General lightening of skin color. In protein calorie malnutrition this is most obvious on the face.

Nasolabial Seborrhea. Scaling with dry, greasy, gray or yellowish thread-like material around nasolabial folds. Also on bridge of nose, eyebrows and backs of ears. Sebaceous gland ducts become plugged. May also be due to poor hygiene. Riboflavin deficiency: medium risk. Also associated with niacin and pyridoxine deficiency.

Moon-Face. Rounded prominence of cheeks, making mouth look "pursed in." Generally in preschool children with kwashiorkor.

Malar and Supraorbital Pigmentation. Darkened or brown pigmentation over cheeks and under eyes. Do not confuse with chloasma, Addison's disease or vitiligo. Associated with niacin deficiency.

Acne Vulgaris. Common acne. Chronic inflammation of sebaceous glands which produce small pink elevations generally on face, chest and back.

Chloasma. Yellowish-brown discoloration of face. Usually related to pregnancy oral contraceptives or sun exposure.

Acne Rosacea. Chronic condition of skin of nose, forehead and cheeks. Flushing and red coloration due to dilated capillaries plus acne-like elevations.

EYES

Night Blindness. Eyes do not adjust to darkness readily. Early sign of vitamin A deficiency.

Pale Conjunctiva. Eyelid lining and whites of eyes are pale as are bucchal mucosa (inner surface of cheeks). Mainly a symptom of anemia. Associated with iron, folate and vitamin B_{12} deficiency.

Conjunctival Xerosis. Inner lids and whites of eye appear dull, dry, roughened and pigmented. Hold lid open and rotate eyes to better identify. May look wrinkled with increased vascularity and pigmentation. Do not confuse with chemical or environmental irritation or pterygium or pinguecula. Vitamin A deficiency: high risk. Early sign.

Corneal Xerosis. Cornea becomes dull, milky, hazy or opaque, especially the lower, central area. Associated with vitamin A deficiency.

Bitot's Spots. Dry, grayish, yellow or white foamy spots on the whites of the eye (generally lateral). Usually bilateral. Most common in children. Don't confuse with pterygium. Vitamin A deficiency: high risk.

Corneal Vascularization. Tiny capillary blood vessels in colored part of eye. Nonspecific. Can occur in any inflammation or irritation of the cornea.

Corneal Opacities and Scars. Scars in the cornea. Associated with protein and vitamin A deficiency. May also result from past malnutrition, trauma or infection.

Conjunctival and Scleral Pigmentation. Unusual brownish coloring of the whites of the eyes. Common in dark skinned people but non-nutritional. May also be pigmented ring around cornea.

Ocular Fundus. Abnormalities of back of eyes, visible through opthalmoscope.

Pterygium. Wing-shaped tissue extending from the corner of the eye to the cornea.

Pannus. Virus-caused infection of colored part of the eye. Cornea becomes invaded by blood vessels and appears opaque, especially on upper part.

Pingueculae. Bilateral or unilateral yellowish accumulation of fatty material on the lateral side of the sclera near the corneal margin.

Physical Signs Of Value In Nutrition Assessment	Physical Signs Needing Further Evaluation	Physical Signs Unrelated To Nutrient Deficiency
Keratomalacia. Softening of part or all of the cornea, usually bilateral. Eyes become white or yellow gelatinous mass. No pain or discharge. Vitamin A deficiency: high risk.	**Conjunctival Injection.** Increased vascularity of the eye in the absence of infection. Riboflavin deficiency: low risk.	
Angular Palpebritis (Blepharitis). Corners of eyes become cracked and red. Often associated with angular stomatitis of lips (see below). Eyelids are inflamed. Riboflavin: medium risk. Also associated with niacin deficiency.	**Circumcorneal Injection.** Fine blood vesseling of colored part of eye. Bilateral. Best seen with ophthalmoscope. Riboflavin deficiency: low risk.	

LIPS

Bilateral Angular Stomatitis. Cracks, redness and flaking at corners of the mouth. Important only if bilateral. Also results from poor dentures, herpes and syphilis. Riboflavin deficiency: high risk. Also associated with niacin, iron and pyridoxine deficiency.	**Chronic Depigmentation.** Usually in the center of lower lip. May be healed cheilosis.	**Chapping.** Exposure to harsh climate.
Bilateral Angular Scars. White or pink scars at corners of the mouth from healed stomatitis. Riboflavin: high risk.		
Cheilosis. Vertical cracks of lips, usually the center of the lower lip. Lips are red, swollen and inner mucosa appears to extend out onto the lip. May be ulcerated. May also occur with environmental exposure. Riboflavin deficiency: medium risk. Also associated with niacin deficiency.		

TONGUE

Edema. Tooth pressure makes indentations along edges of tongue. Niacin deficiency: low risk.	**Hyperaemic and Hypertrophic Papillae.** Taste buds are large and red or pink. Tongue looks granular, pebbly or "berry-like." Consider dietary irritants. Niacin deficiency: medium risk.	**Aphthous Ulcer.** "Canker sore."
Magenta Tongue. Purplish red and swollen. Usually sore. Pale if anemia is due to folate deficiency. Other changes usually absent. Niacin deficiency: high risk.	**Geographic Tongue.** Irregular patches with no taste buds. Non-tender.	**Leukoplakia.** Thickened white patches on mucous membranes of mouth.
Atrophic Papillae. Taste buds have disappeared. Tongue appears smooth, pale and slick (even when slightly scraped). Can be central or marginal. May occur in non-nutritional anemia. Niacin deficiency: high risk. Also associated with folate, riboflavin, iron and vitamin B_{12} deficiency.		

Physical Signs Of Value In Nutrition Assessment	Physical Signs Needing Further Evaluation	Physical Signs Unrelated To Nutrient Deficiency
Glossitis. Tongue is beefy red, painful and taste buds are atrophied. Usually hypersensitive, with burning and even taste changes. Oral mucosa may also be red and swollen. Niacin deficiency: high risk if other signs (dementia, dermatitis, diarrhea) present. Also associated with folate, riboflavin, iron, vitamin B12, pyridoxine and tryptophan deficiencies. **Fissures.** Cracks on tongue surfaces with no taste buds on sides or bottom of cracks. Definite break in epithelium. Niacin deficiency: high risk.	**Pigmented Tongue.** Patchy areas of blue-black pigmentation, sometimes also on gums. No known significance.	
TEETH		
Mottled Enamel. White or brownish patches in tooth enamel. May also be pitting of enamel. Most obvious in upper front teeth. If mild, paper-white spots are seen on tips and edges of teeth with gradual fading into normal coloration. If severe, there will be pitting or brown staining. Do not confuse with enamel or staining from tetracycline taken during tooth development. Associated with fluorine excess.	**Caries.** Dental decay. May indicate high intake of sugar and sticky carbohydrate. Also lack of fluoride. **Attrition.** Cutting edges of teeth are worn and flattened. Related to toughness and hardness of diet. **Enamel Hypoplasia.** Defective tooth enamel. Usually generalized over tooth surface. **Enamel Erosion.** Areas around gum line where tooth enamel has eroded.	**Malocclusion.** Faulty meeting of teeth or jaws.
GUMS		
Spongy, Bleeding. Purplish or red, spongy and swollen. Usually bleed easily with slight pressure. Teeth must be present to occur. May also be caused by chronic use of hydantoinates (Dilantin, etc), poor hygiene and lymphoma. Vitamin C deficiency: medium risk.	**Recession of Gums.** Roots of teeth are exposed. Usually secondary to pyorrhea (gum inflammation).	**Pyorrhea.** Chronic gum inflammation around teeth, with gums receeding. Red and bleed easily. Generally not swollen.
GLANDS		
Enlarged Thyroid (Goiter). May be visible or felt. More visible with head tipped back. Also caused by cysts, tumors and hyperthyroidism. Iodine deficiency: medium to high risk.	**Gynecomastia.** Bilateral breast enlargement in males.	**Thyroid or Parotid Enlargement.** Secondary to allergic or inflammatory causes.

Physical Signs Of Value In Nutrition Assessment	Physical Signs Needing Further Evaluation	Physical Signs Unrelated To Nutrient Deficiency

Enlarged Parotid. Glands just below earlobes visible. Chronic, non-tender enlargement. Significant only if bilateral. Protein deficiency: medium risk.

SKIN

Xerosis. General dryness with fine lines, flaking and shedding of bran-like scales. Usually starts on nasolabial folds and eyebrows, spreading across neck and face. Consider environmental and hygiene factors, aging, hypothyroidism, uremia, ichthyosis. Vitamin A and/or essential fatty acid deficiency: low risk. Medium risk of vitamin A deficiency if occurs with hyperfolliculosis of arms.

Follicular Kyperkeratosis. Spine-like plaques around mouths of hair follicles, especially on arms, thighs, buttocks, shoulders, elbows and knees. Skin feels like sandpaper and looks like "gooseflesh." Doesn't disappear with rubbing. Also occurs with fungus infection and syphilis. Vitamin A and/or essential fatty acid deficiency: medium risk if on arms, low if on back.

Perifollicular Petechiae. Small, red or purple spots around hair follicles due to extravasation of blood. Hair may also have a corkscrew character. If areas other than hair follicles are affected probably due to other causes. Vitamin C deficiency: medium risk. Early sign.

Ecchymoses. Small red, purple, black or blue hemorrhagic spots on skin or mucous membranes. Usually at pressure points (backs of arms, buttocks, around joints). Also occurs in hematological disorders, trauma, liver disease and anticoagulant overdose. Vitamin C deficiency: medium risk. High risk if occurs with follicular hyperkeratosis. An early sign of deficiency.

Hyperpigmentation. On palms of the hands. Associated with folate and vitamin B_{12} deficiency.

Thickening and Pigmentation of Pressure Points. Widespread thickening of skin at knees, elbows, ankles and possibly knuckles. Skin may also be wrinkled and cracked. Usually non-nutritional if only on knees and elbows. Also consider occupational trauma. Associated with niacin deficiency.

Intertriginous Lesions. Raw, red areas in folds such as groin, buttocks and underarms. May become infected.

Mosaic Dermatitis. Large plaques of skin, adhering at center, peeling at edges. Bilateral on both shins.

Ichthyosis. Dry, rough, scaly skin due to hypertrophy of outer layer. Affects entire skin.

Acneiform Eruptions. Skin eruptions resembling acne.

Miliaria. Sweat retention by inner skin layers. Produces small, pale or red lesions in the skin. Heat rash or prickly heat.

Epidermophytoses. Fungal infection.

Sunburn.

Onchocercal Dermatosis. Parasitic worms dwelling in tumors in subcutaneous connective tissue.

Physical Signs Of Value In Nutrition Assessment	Physical Signs Needing Further Evaluation	Physical Signs Unrelated To Nutrient Deficiency

Pellagrous Dermatitis. Hyperpigmented areas bilaterally on body parts exposed to sunlight (cheeks, forearms, neck, etc.). Symmetrical with sharp edges. Acute: red, swollen with itching, cracking, burning and exudative. Chronic: dry, rough, thickened and scaly with brown pigmentation. Consider thermal, sun or chemical burns and Addison's disease. Niacin: high risk, especially if dementia or diarrhea. Also associated with tryptophan deficiency.

Scrotal or Vulval Dermatosis. Often itchy, peeling lesions of skin of scrotum and vulva. May be secondary infection. Consider fungus infection. Associated with riboflavin deficiency.

Flaky-Paint Dermatosis. Extensive hyperpigmented patches which peel off to leave hypopigmented skin or superficial ulcers. Especially on buttocks and backs of thighs. Often bilateral.

NAILS

Koilonychia. Bilateral thin, flat or concave spoon-shaped nails in older children and adults. Consider Plummer-Vinson syndrome (koilonychia, dysphagia, glossitis, angular stomatitis, anemia) and clubbing from cardiopulmonary disease. Associated with iron deficiency, protein-calorie malnutrition and long term insulin deficiency.

Brittle, Ridged Nails. Crosswise ridges or grooves in nails. Important only if nails of more than one extremity are affected.

Brittle, Longitudinally Ridged Nails. Nonspecific.

Striate Leuconychia. Crosswise stripes of depigmentation on nails. Associated with selenium deficiency. Occasionally seen in patients maintained on intravenous feeding.

SUBCUTANEOUS TISSUE

Edema. Bilateral swelling, usually of ankles and feet first. Press down on tissue for 3 seconds. Edematous tissue will pit. Occurs in conditions of sodium and water retention, pregnancy, protein-losing enteropathy, varicose veins and stasis. Associated with thiamine and protein deficiency (i.e. serum albumin < 2.5 g/dl).

Physical Signs Of Value In Nutrition Assessment	Physical Signs Needing Further Evaluation	Physical Signs Unrelated To Nutrient Deficiency
Subcutaneous Fat. Measure with skinfold calipers. Decreased in protein-calorie malnutrition.		

MUSCULOSKELETAL SYSTEM

Muscle Wasting. Evaluated with upper arm muscle measurements. Prominence of body skeleton. Excess folding of skin under buttocks in protein-calorie malnutrition.	**Winged Scapulae.** Shoulder blades protrude.	**Funnel Chest.** Funnel-shaped deformity of front of chest wall. Generally familial.

Craniotabes. Softening of the skull across the back and sides of the head under one year of age. Skull depresses and returns with the feeling of pressing on a tennis ball. Associated with active vitamin D deficiency or rickets.

Frontal and Parietal Bossing. Round swelling or thickening of front and sides of head in infants. Head may be larger than normal. Generally bilateral. Vitamin D: medium risk. Associated with past vitamin D deficiency.

Epiphyseal Enlargement. Ends of long bones enlarge, especially at wrist, knees and ankles. May be painless or tender. Consider trauma, congenital deformity, renal disease and malabsorption. Vitamin D: high risk if wrists involved. Associated with active D deficiency if painless, vitamin C deficiency if painful.

Beading of Ribs (Rachitic Rosary). Small lumps on sides of chest wall on ribs. In scorbutic rosary (associated with vitamin C deficiency) costochrondal junctions (rib and cartilage junctions) are sharp. In rachitic rosary they are smooth. Consider renal rickets and malabsorption as causes. Vitamin D: high risk. Associated with active vitamin D and calcium deficiency.

Persistently Open Anterior Fontanel. Soft spot on baby's head doesn't harden at proper time (18 months of age). May also indicate hydrocephalus. Associated with active vitamin D deficiency.

Physical Signs Of Value In Nutrition Assessment	Physical Signs Needing Further Evaluation	Physical Signs Unrelated To Nutrient Deficiency

Knock-Knees or Bowed Legs. Curve outward at knees. Legs are bowed outward. Consider congenital deformity. Vitamin D: medium risk. Associated with past vitamin D and calcium deficiency.

Pithed Frog Position. Legs flex at knees and hips and rotate out due to pain on movement. Due to hemorrhage under fibrous membranes covering the bones. Associated with vitamin C deficiency.

Diffuse or Local Skeletal Deformities. Osteomalacia in adults (adult rickets). Bones may be tender.

Deformities of the Thorax. Harrison's sulcus (a horizontal depression along the lower border of the chest). Associated with rickets.

Musculoskeletal Hemorrhages. Bleeding into the muscle. Can only be confirmed by special tests and clinical examination. Associated with vitamin C deficiency.

GASTROINTESTINAL SYSTEM

Hepatomegaly. Enlarged liver. Liver edge palpable more than 2 cms below costal margin. Feel abdomen with knees bent. Occurs with numerous conditions. Protein deficiency: medium risk.

Splenomegaly. Enlarged spleen. Usually non-nutritional causes.

NERVOUS SYSTEM

Psychomotor Change. Listless, apathetic. Protein deficiency: medium risk.

Mental Confusion. Confusion and hyperirritability. Protein deficiency: medium risk.

Sensory Loss. Associated with thiamin deficiency.

Motor Weakness. Inability to squat and then stand 3 - 4 times in a row. Associated with thiamin deficiency.

Loss of Position Sense. Associated with thiamin deficiency.

Physical Signs Of Value In Nutrition Assessment	Physical Signs Needing Further Evaluation	Physical Signs Unrelated To Nutrient Deficiency
Loss of Vibratory Sense. Tested with tuning fork. Significant only if bilateral. Consider peripheral neuropathy or other causes. Associated with thiamin and B_{12} deficiency.		
Loss of Ankle and Knee Jerks. Significant only if absolute and bilateral. Consider peripheral neuropathy of other causes. Thiamin: medium risk. Also associated with B_{12} deficiency.		
Calf Tenderness. Squeeze calf muscle firmly between thumb and forefinger. Significant only if bilateral. Consider deep vein thrombosis and peripheral neuropathy of other causes. Associated with thiamin deficiency.		
CARDIOVASCULAR SYSTEM		
Cardiac Enlargement. Enlarged heart. Generally non-nutritional. May occur in anemia and beriberi. Associated with thiamin deficiency.	**Blood Pressure Elevation.**	
Tachycardia. Rapid heart rate (above 100). May occur in anemia or beriberi. Associated with thiamin deficiency.		

PHYSICAL SIGNS OF NUTRIENT DEFICIENCY AND TOXICITY

Most clinical signs are nonspecific, thus they are best interpreted as part of a group of symptoms which are common to a particular nutrient deficiency. The greater the number of signs in a group that are present, the greater the likelihood of a true nutrient deficiency. For example, angular stomatitis may have several causes, but if it occurs with other symptoms of riboflavin deficiency, then the likelihood of a riboflavin deficiency is increased. The charts below contain many of the symptoms associated with both nutrient deficiency and excess.

Vitamin	Deficiency Symptoms	Toxicity Symptoms
VITAMIN A	• Night blindness • Dry scaly skin (xerosis) • Follicular hyperkeratosis • Decreased taste and smell • Increased infections • Retarded growth • Dry mucus membranes • Keratomalacia	**Acute** • Abdominal pain • Headache • Hypercalcemia • Irritability • Nausea • Vomiting • Skin desquamation **Chronic** • Alopecia • Anorexia, • Bone pain • High CSF pressure • Headache • Irritability • Joint pain • Nausea • Vomiting • Skin desquamation • Splenomegaly Toxicity is rare with chronic intakes of less than 9000 µg RE/d (30,000 IU). Intakes of 25,000-50,000 IU/d for several months are associated with adverse effects. Birth defects are reported with intakes of 25,000 IU/d. Acute toxicity can occur with > 500,000 IU/d (100 times RDA). Infants are susceptible with toxicity symptoms at 2100 IU/100 calories (3 - 8 times RDA).
VITAMIN D	**Rickets** (infants, children) • Bone pain • Muscle tenderness • Hypocalcemia • Tetany • Delayed tooth eruption • Delayed closure of the fontanel	• Anorexia • Bone demineralization • Constipation • Hypercalcemic symtoms (muscular weakness, pain, nausea, vomiting, polyuria, calcinosis, renal calculi)

Vitamin	Deficiency Symptoms	Toxicity Symptoms
	• Enlargement of joints of long bones • Bowed legs or knock knees (older children). Osteomalacia • Muscular weakness • Bone tenderness (especially in the spine, shoulder, ribs or pelvis) • Low bone density • Pseudo-fractures	Single doses of 50 times the RDA are reported to be toxic. Children are especially sensitive.
VITAMIN E	• Muscle weakness • Hemolytic anemia • Irritability • Edema	• Mild GI distress • Nausea • Coagulopathy in patients receiving anticonvulsants • Generally nontoxic Doses of 100 times recommended levels are tolerated without adverse effects.
VITAMIN K	• Prolonged bleeding time • Elevated prothrombin time • Hemorrhage • Anemia	Toxicity is primarily associated with pharmacological doses of the synthetic provitamin menadione. Symptoms include hepatic damage, hyperbilirubinemia and hemolytic anemia..
VITAMIN C	• Anorexia • Swollen, painful joints • Impaired wound healing • Increased susceptibility to infection • Swollen bleeding gums • Loose teeth • Ecchymoses, petechiae	• GI distress • Diarrhea • Oxaluria Diarrhea and GI distress are reported at levels 20-80 times the RDA. Levels of 100-1000 times the RDA appear safe. Deficiency symptoms with discontinuation of chronic high doses.
THIAMIN	• Anorexia • Muscular weakness • Depression Dry Beriberi • Peripheral neurititis • Atrophy of the legs	Generally nontoxic when taken orally. Parenteral doses of 100-200 times the RDA are reported to cause headache, muscle weakness, paralysis, cardiac arrhythmia's and allergic reactions.

Vitamin	Deficiency Symptoms	Toxicity Symptoms
	Wet Beriberi • Cardiac hypertrophy • Edema • Heart failure Infantile Beriberi • Anorexia • Vomiting • Diarrhea • Cyanosis • Tachycardia • Convulsions Wernicke-Korsakoff • Ophthalmoplegia • Ataxia • Psychosis • Confabulation • Impaired memory and cognitive function	
RIBOFLAVIN	• Cheilosis • Angular stomatitis • Glossitis • Nasolabial seborrheic dermatitis • Scrotal and vulval dermatitis • Peripheral neuropathy (hyperesthesia, coldness, pain, decreased sensitivity to touch, temperature, vibration and position).	Nontoxic. Because of poor absorption high oral doses are well tolerated.
NIACIN	• Anxiety • Nausea • Vomiting • Headache • Dizziness • Irritability • Angular stomatitis • Cheilosis • Glossitis • Diarrhea • Anemia • Pellagrous dermatitis (cracking, desquamation, hyperpigmentation of face, neck, backs of hands and forearms, parts exposed to sunlight)	• Blood vessel dilation • Itching skin, rash • Liver damage • Cardiac arrhythmia High doses of nicotinic acid (2-4 g/d) can cause side effects. Nicotinamide at 50 - 100 times the RDA does not.

Vitamin	Deficiency Symptoms	Toxicity Symptoms
PYRIDOXINE	• Peripheral neuropathies • Cheilosis • Glossitis • Stomatitis • Seizures • Irritability	Generally nontoxic. Doses of 500 mg/d have been used for several months without significant bad effects but larger doses have caused reversible neuropathies with chronic use. Deficiency symptoms occur with discontinuance of high doses. Intakes of 100 times the RDA appear safe.
FOLATE	• Nuclear hypersegmentation of circulating polymorphonuclear leukocytes • Megaloblastic anemia • Weakness • Depression • Polyneuropathy	Nontoxic. Other than a few reports of allergic reactions, current information indicates doses 2000 times the RDA are safe.
VITAMIN B$_{12}$	• Megaloblastic anemia • Peripheral neuropathy	Nontoxic. Other than a few reports of allergic reactions, current information indicates doses 1000 times the RDA are safe.
PANTOTHENIC ACID	• Fatigue • Insomnia • Vomiting	Nontoxic.
BIOTIN	• Dermatitis • Glossitis • Anorexia • Nausea • Depression • Hypercholesterolemia	Nontoxic.

Mineral	Deficiency Symptoms	Toxicity Symptoms
CHROMIUM	• Hyperglycemia • Excess insulin requirements • Weight loss • Hyperlipidemia • Metabolic encephalopathy • Peripheral neuropathy	• Dermatitis • Hepatitis • Gastrointestinal disorders • Lung cancer (chronic exposure) Toxic reactions to IV chromium are not expected.
COPPER	• Hypochromic, microcytic anemia • Neutropenia • Seborrheic dermatosis • Apathy • Hypothermia • Swollen joints • CNS changes • Skin and hair depigmentation • Pallor • Hypotonia • Psychomotor retardation • Decreased visual acuity	• Wilson's disease • Hemolytic anemia • Hepatic necrosis
FLOURIDE	• Dental caries • Osteoporosis	• Dental fluorosis • Skeletal fluorosis Dental fluorosis occurs during tooth development at levels greater than 2 ppm. Skeletal fluorosis occurs with intakes greater than 10 g/d for 10 years or more. Oral doses of 5 to 10 gm are lethal.
IODINE	• Goiter • Weight gain • Somnolence • Cold intolerance • Bradycardia • Dry skin • Constipation • Hyporeflexia • Increased blood pressure • Weakness • Mental changes	• Supression of thyroid activity. Can result from excess exposure to drugs (amiodarone), contrast media and topical iodine.

Mineral	Deficiency Symptoms	Toxicity Symptoms
IRON	• Anemia • Fatigue • Dypsnea on exertion • Headache • Glossitis • Burning sensation of the tongue • Pallor • Tachycardia • Paresthesias	• Hemosiderosis • Hemachromatosis with hyperpigmentation, hepatic cirrhosis, diabetes mellitus. About 25% of subjects has a systemic reaction (fever, hypotension, vomiting, headache, convulsions) to higher doses of parenteral iron (2.5 to 10 times the currently approved single-dose allowance).
SELENIUM	• Dilated cardiomyopathy (Keshan's disease) • Myalgia • Muscle weakness • Myositis • Pancreatic • Degeneration • Increased platelet aggregation • Increased red cell fragility	• Garlic breath odor • Headache • Nausea • Vomiting • Chronic dermatitis • Loss of hair, nails • Excess fatigue • Dizziness • Pulmonary edema No signs of abnormality at intakes of 100 - 600 µg/d but 1500 µg is toxic.
ZINC	• Delayed wound healing • Night blindness • Photophobia • Decreased sense of smell • Decreased sense of taste • Glucose intolerance • Diarrhea • Alopecia • Skin lesions • Growth retardation (children) • Delayed sexual maturity (children)	• Decreased serum copper • Copper deficiency • Hyperamylasemia • Immunosupression • Testicular atrophy IV doses of 50 - 100 mg/d are tolerated if infused slowly.

References

• Jeliffe, D: The Assessment of the Nutritional Status of the Community. World Health Organization Monograph, Ser. No. 53, Geneva, 1966.

• Interdepartmental Committee on Nutrition for National Defense: Manual for Nutritional Surveys, 2nd ed. Washington, 1963.

• Sandstead, H, Carter, J and Darby, W: How to diagnose nutritional disorders in daily practice. Nutrition Today 4:20, 1969.

• Preliminary Findings of the First Health and Nutrition Examination Survey, United States, 1971-72, Anthropometric and Clinical Findings. DHEW Publication No. (HRA) 75-1229, Public Health Service, Rockville, Md. April, 1975.

• McClaren, D: A Colour Atlas and Text of Diet-Related Disorders, 2nd ed. Mosby-Yearbook Europe Limited, 1992.

• Coombs, G: The vitamins: fundamental aspects in nutrition and health. Academic Press, Inc. San Diego, 1992.

• Deglin, J and Vallerand, A: Davis's Drug Guide for Nurses, 5th ed. F.A. Davis Company, Philadelphia, 1997.

• Baumgartner, T: Clinical Guide to Parenteral Micronutrition, 2nd ed. Fujisawa, USA, Inc., 1991

BIOCHEMICAL ASSESSMENT

Numerous laboratory tests can be useful in assessing nutritional status. Serum albumin can be an index of protein status. Urinary urea nitrogen can be used to estimate nitrogen balance. Prealbumin can be used to guage the adequacy of nutrition support. Caution is necessary when interpreting test results. Some lab tests are inappropriate for some subjects in some situations. Creatinine excretion cannot be used to estimate muscle mass in those with renal failure because this test assumes normal renal function. Extended prothrombin times may not indicate vitamin K deficiency in those with coagulation defects. Some tests of protein status underestimate nutrition status in conditions of stress. Some tests of vitamin and mineral status are imprecise with limited standards available for comparison.

The results of a single laboratory test should be interpreted carefully. A lab test done serially will give more accurate information. Lab findings can be used with more confidence when supportive information is available, e.g., diet history, clinical symptoms, other lab results etc. When ordering laboratory tests, consider whether the outcome will change the nutrition care plan and whether or not the test is cost-effective.

Suggested normal or age-appropriate values are included here. It should be remembered that normal values vary somewhat with each laboratory and standardized or normal values for the individual laboratory should be used when interpreting test results. SI units, the abbreviation for Systeme International dUnites, are included with each test, where appropriate. The SI is a uniform system of reporting numerical values permitting interchangeability of information between health care providers of different nations. This system presents hematological and clinical chemistry values in molar concentrations with the liter as the reference volume, e.g., mol/L.

TESTS OF PROTEIN STATUS

Over 500 plasma proteins have been identified. They perform a wide variety of functions although sometimes the function is not well defined. Mostly they stay in the circulation but can leave the capillaries by an active transport system or else leak through the junctions between cells. Most are synthesized by the liver. Plasma levels reflect the balance between synthesis and degradation. Each protein is regulated independently of the others. Protein levels can be altered by disease, physiological characteristics (age, sex, race, pregnancy), and by congenital and acquired abnormalities.

Acute phase reactants (APRs) are proteins whose plasma levels change in response to inflammatory states (infection, postsurgery, trauma, post-myocardial infarction, malignancy, and tissue necrosis). This is referred to as the acute phase response. Some are positive reactants (their levels increase with stress) and others are negative reactants (their levels decrease). Most reach their maximum response in 2 - 5 days. Those with liver disease, malnutrition, or protein-losing syndromes often show a blunted acute phase response.

A primary goal of nutritional therapy is to maintain or replete the body's protein compartment. To do this requires some method of monitoring. The ideal protein should have a short half-life, a small body pool, a rapid synthetic rate, a constant catabolic rate, and be sensitive to changes in protein and calorie intake. Currently no one protein meets all of these conditions. The table below reports information relevant to the use of some visceral protein markers used to assess protein status.

Test	Clinical Significance

TOTAL PROTEIN

Normal Values
- Adult/elderly
  6.4 - 8.3 g/dl
  64 - 83 g/L
- Child
  6.2 - 8 g/dl
- Infant
  6.0 - 6.7 g/dl
- Newborn
  4.6 - 7.4 g/dl
- Premature infant
  4.2 - 7.6 g/dl

Increased
- Vomiting
- Diarrhea
- Excess sweating
- Salt-losing syndromes
- Diuresis (drugs, hyperosmolar states)
- Steroids (including oral contraceptives)
- Increased gamma-globulin synthesis

Decreased
- Volume expansion (dextran, IV fluids, pregnancy, salt-retention)
- Malnutrition
- Chronic liver disease
- Nephrotic syndrome
- Inflammatory bowel disease
- Burns
- Exudative losses

Total serum protein is about 60% albumin and 40% globulin's. Both provide oncotic pressure which helps maintain water in the circulation. Albumin is responsible for 80% of this. Severely depressed levels result in edema.

Total protein levels can be affected by changes in fluid balance, synthesis, catabolism, and protein losses. Levels can be 10% lower in recumbent subjects. Exercise transiently increases levels.

Levels increase with dehydration from inadequate fluid intake or increased fluid loss. Excess loss can occur via the kidney, GI tract, and skin. Levels can decrease with volume expansion. Changes in the actual amount of protein result from changes in synthesis and/or catabolism and losses. Steroids (including oral contraceptives) increase protein synthesis. Increased total protein levels, when hydration is normal, are usually the result of increased gamma globulin synthesis.

A decrease in one protein may be offset by changes in another. For example, increased synthesis of acute phase proteins may be offset by decreased albumin synthesis. An albumin to globulin ratio (A:G ratio) may be helpful in determining the cause of the change.

ALBUMIN

Normal Values
- Adult/elderly
  3.5 - 5.0 g/dl
  35 - 50 g/L
- Child
  4.0 - 5.9 g/dl
- Infant
  4.4 - 5.4 g/dl
- Newborn
  3.5 - 5.4 g/dl

Albumin is the most abundant protein in plasma. It has a large body pool (about 60% of total serum protein), and a long half life (about 20 days). Its main function is to maintain colloidal osmotic pressure, keeping fluid within the circulation. It also transports blood components such as drugs, hormones, enzymes, metals, ions, fatty acids, amino acids, bilirubin, and other metabolites. Forty percent of albumin is extravascular, mainly in the skin. Albumin is exchanged between extravascular and intravascular spaces. Albumin is synthesized by the liver and is a measure of liver function. Ten to 20% of functioning hepatocytes will maintain a normal albumin. In a steady-state 200 mg/kg/d (4% of pool) is synthesized and degraded each day.

Test	Clinical Significance

Test

- Premature infant
  3.0-4.2 g/dl

Increased
- Dehydration

Decreased
- Liver disease
- Protein-losing enteropathy (mucosal ulceration)
- Protein-losing nephropathy (nephrotic syndrome, glomerulonephritis)
- Third-space losses (ascites, burns, effusions)
- Malnutrition
- Dilution (excess IV fluids)
- Increased capillary permeability (collagen vascular diseases e.g. lupus)
- Stress (trauma, infection, surgery, infection)
- Malignancy
- Tuberculosis

GLOBULIN

Normal Value
- Adult/elderly
  2.3 - 3.4 g/dl

Increased
- Immunologic tumors (e.g. multiple myeloma)
- Collagen vascular disease (e.g. SLE)

Decreased
- Malnutrition
- Immune deficiency

ALBUMIN GLOBULIN RATIO (A:G Ratio)
Normally greater than 1.0

Clinical Significance

Albumin synthesis decreases within 24 hours of fasting (due to lack of substrate) and returns to normal with refeeding. With extended fasting albumin levels decrease slowly due to the large pool, slow turnover, and intravascular transfer. Decreased levels may be seen only after long periods of malnutrition. Hypoalbuminemia also results from impaired synthesis (liver disease), and increased catabolism. The stress response from injury, infection, and inflammation results in decreased synthesis, increased degradation, and increased intravascular loss from increased vascular permeability ("third-spacing"). Albumin levels don't increase in stressed patients until the stress response abates. Albumin can also be lost via organs (gut, kidneys) and damaged tissues. Severe losses of albumin can result in edema and reduced substance transport. A change from standing to recumbent position with bedrest as well as rapid infusion of large volumes of IV fluids can also contribute to a drop in albumin. Hyperalbuminemia is usually due to dehydration.

Low levels are associated with increased morbidity and mortality, length of stay, infection rate, and development of decubitus ulcers in institutionalized patients. Levels less than 2.8 are associated with development of edema.

Albumin is not a good index of short term protein energy deficit but it is a good index of chronic protein deficiency.

Globulins make up 40% of total proteins. They are the key building blocks of antibodies and they also contribute to oncotic pressure, although albumin is responsible for 80%. They also function as transport proteins. High levels of total protein without dehydration usually indicates increased synthesis of gamma globulins.

Changes in total protein may result from changes in albumin, globulins, or both. A change in one can be offset by a change in the other, thus leaving total protein unchanged. Sometimes it is useful to determine the albumin globulin ratio to help determine the cause of an abnormal total protein level. Elevated globulin or low albumin can be the cause of a low ratio.

If globulin value is not available it can be calculated from albumin and total protein as follows.

A:G Ratio = albumin ÷ total protein - albumin

Test	Clinical Significance

PREALBUMIN
(Transthyretin)
(Thyroxin-binding prealbumin)

Normal Values
- Adult
  19 - 43 mg/dl
  190 - 430 mg/L

Increased
- Renal failure
- Steroids
- Pregnancy

Decreased
- Acute catabolic states (stress, infection, trauma, surgery, burns)
- Liver disease (cirrhosis, hepatitis)
- Nephrotic syndrome
- Malnutrition
- Hemorrhage

Prealbumin is a transport protein for some thyroxin (thyroid hormone) and, together with retinol-binding protein, for vitamin A. Prealbumin combines in a 1:1 ratio with the vitamin A carrier protein retinol-binding protein (RBP). This prevents urinary loss of the vitamin. The prealbumin plasma pool is small and the half-life is two days. Levels are significantly reduced with liver disease due to impaired synthesis, so the protein can be an index of synthetic ability in a nonstressed subject.

Prealbumin responds rapidly to changes in protein and energy intake. As such it can be used as basis for assessing malnutrition and following changing nutrition status. Levels of less than 17 mg/dl have been suggested as indicated for nutrition intervention. Levels less than 11 indicate significant protein-energy malnutrition. Increased mortality is associated with levels less than five. Levels decrease with stress as protein synthetic priorities change. Levels can drop 5 to 9 mg/dl in first week post-op.

Prealbumin will increase when 55 to 60% of calorie and protein needs are met. Levels can double or increase five to nine mg/dl in one week with adequate nutrition support. Less than a two mg/dl increase in a week is inadequate and should prompt a review of feeding mode, and amount and type of nutrients. A doubling of plasma levels or a level of 18 is reported to correspond with positive nitrogen balance.

Levels may be slightly elevated in pregnancy and renal disease due to reduced catabolism by the kidney and by steroid therapy but trends can still reflect response to nutritional therapy. Levels are not affected as early or as much as other proteins in liver disease. Levels remain low in burn patients, even with nutrition support, until grafts are placed. Prealbumin is not significantly affected by hydration or albumin infusions. Levels may be altered by infusion of blood products. Prealbumin can increase with steroid intake, pregnancy, and chronic renal failure.

TRANSFERRIN
(Siderophilin)

Normal Values
- Adult
  200 - 400 mg/dl
- Child
  203 - 360 mg/dl
- Newborn
  130 - 275 mg/dl
Degree of depletion
  > 200 adequate
  150 - 200 mild
  100 - 150 moderate
  < 100 severe
Transferrin levels can be estimated by multiplying 0.7

Most transferrin is synthesized by the liver. The body pool is smaller than albumin and the half-life shorter (8 - 10 days) Transferrin's main function is the transport of iron from its absorption site in the intestine to the bone marrow, liver, or spleen for storage. Almost all of plasma iron is bound by transferrin. Plasma levels of free iron are normally very low. This reduces urinary iron loss and avoids the toxic effects of high levels of free iron, making it unavailable to bacteria during an infection, for example. Synthesis is regulated by iron stores. When iron levels are low, transferrin rises in proportion to the deficiency. Each molecule has 2 iron-binding sites. Transferrin is normally only 33% saturated. Transferrin can be measured directly or estimated from total iron-binding capacity (TIBC).

Depressed levels occur in liver disease, protein-losing disorders (nephrotic syndrome, protein-losing enteropathy) and malnutrition. Because it is an negative acute phase reactant, low levels are seen in chronic or acute inflammatory states and in malignancy. It may also be altered by nonnutrition causes (see left).

Test	Clinical Significance

times total iron-binding capacity (TIBC)

Increased
- Pregnancy
- Oral contraceptives
- Iron deficiency
- Acute hepatitis

Decreased
- Severe liver disease
- Protein calorie malnutrition
- Nephrotic syndrome
- Anemia
- Neoplasia
- Protein-losing enteropathy

Levels are reported to decrease in severe protein-calorie malnutrition but transferrin is not sensitive to moderate changes in nutrition status. It is also not a good tool to assess response to nutrition support because of its longer half-life.

Antibiotics that may decrease levels include aminoglycosides, tetracycline, and some cephalosporins.

RETINOL-BINDING PROTEIN (RBP)

Normal Values
- 3.0 - 6.0 mg/dl
- 30 - 60 mg/L

Increased
- Renal disease

Decreased
- Liver disease
- Vitamin A deficiency
- Stress states
- Hyperthyroidism
- Zinc deficiency
- Cystic fibrosis

RBP transports vitamin A in the plasma. The RBP-vitamin A complex is carried bound to prealbumin in a 1:1 ratio. It responds quickly to protein and energy depletion due to a small body pool and short half life (12-24 hours).

Levels parallel those of prealbumin except in acute renal failure. Here levels are significantly higher due to reduced renal catabolism and excretion of the retinol-free form of RBP. In stable renal failure trends can be followed to evaluate adequacy of nutrition therapy.

Decreased levels in liver disease are attributed to decreased rate of protein synthesis. Increased levels may occur for awhile in hepatitis due to release of stored RBP by an injured liver.

SOMATAMEDIN-C (SMC) (Insulin-like growth factor-1) (IGF-1)

Normal Values
0.10 - 0.40 mg/L

SMC is important in the stimulation of growth. Serum concentrations are regulated by both growth hormone and nutritional intake. Most is produced in the liver and circulates protein-bound. The half-life is 2 to 4 hours.

Levels drease with fasting and increase rapidly with nutritional support and are not altered by the stress response. Lab procedures must separate SMC from binding proteins for accurate results.

SMC appears to be useful in assessing basal nutritional status and response to nutrition support. Malnourished patients, especially those with protein deficiency, have lower basal levels than normals. Values increase rapidly with nutrition support, more so than RBP, prealbumin, transferrin, or albumin. They also fall quickly when nutrition support stopped.

SMC correlates well with nitrogen balance. A 100% increase in IGF-1 correlates with positive nitrogen balance. Can be useful when nitrogen balance is unreliable (i.e. renal failure, GI disease, burns, or questionable urine collections).

Test	Clinical Significance

FIBRONECTIN

Normal Values
- 220 - 400 mg/dl

Decreased
- Malnutrition
- Stress states

Fibronectin is the primary protein controlling phagocytosis. It also has roles in wound healing and maintenance of vascular integrity. Low levels are associated with poor would healing. The half-life is about 15 hours.

Fibronectin may decrease with stress (infection, shock, burn) or at least not increase. It responds rapidly to changes in intake. It has value in nutrition panels because it is not exclusively synthesized in the liver and may be useful without normal hepatic function. The test is not readily available and more research is needed regarding response to nutrition support.

C-REACTIVE PROTEIN (CRP)

Normal Values
< 0.8 mg/dl

Increased
- Infections (viral, bacterial, parasitic, fungal)
- Myocardial infarction
- Surgery
- Ulcerative colitis
- Crohn's disease
- Rheumatic diseases (except SLE)
- Renal transplant rejection
- Graft Vs host disease

CRP is an acute phase protein which increases in conditions of tissue injury or inflammation. Most is synthesized in the liver and small amounts are normally found in the plasma. It seems to function as an immunomodulator during an immune response. Levels rise before other acute phase proteins (within 4 - 6 hours). Serial measurements may give an index of disease activity and response to therapy.

Measurement of C-reactive protein is useful in following those with inflammatory disorders. It may detect occult infections post op, monitor disease activity in rheumatic disease and inflammatory bowel disease, and detect transplant rejection. CRP is the first acute phase reactant to increase and its increases are greater. Levels begin to decrease when hypermetabolism begins to abate. Then other short half-life proteins become more useful as nutritional markers.

3-METHYLHISTIDINE (3-ME)

3-Methylhistidine has been studied for potential use in estimating somatic protein mass. During muscle catabolism 3-methylhistidine is released from muscle and excreted in the urine. Like creatinine, 3-ME excretion is proportional to muscle mass and determination of 3-ME excreted in a 24 hour urine collection reflects muscle catabolism during that time. Age, sex, starvation, trauma, infection, meat consumption, and the completeness of the urine collection all affect the validity of the test. At the present time, 3-ME is is used primarily for research purposes.

CREATININE-HEIGHT INDEX (CHI)

Average creatinine excretion
- Males: 23 mg/kg/d
- Females: 18 mg/kg/d

Increased
- Stress (sepsis, fever, trauma)
- Strenuous exercise
- Second half of menstrual cycle

Almost all of the body's creatine content is in muscle. Creatine is converted to creatinine which then diffuses out of muscle into the blood for filtration and elimination by the kidney. This occurs at a fairly constant rate. Creatinine excretion can provide a reasonable estimate of muscle mass if its limitations are kept in mind and subjects selected appropriately.

Expressing creatinine excretion in relation to height rather than weight is considered more reliable because of variations in body weight from fat tissue and fluid imbalance. To estimate CHI the excretion rate of an individual is compared to the expected excretion rate for an individual of similar height and sex using this formula:

Test	Clinical Significance

Decreased
- Protein-free diet
- Elderly
- Emotional stress

CHI = actual 24 hr creatinine x 100 ÷ expected 24 hr creatinine

example:

A 188 cm male of medium frame has a 24 hour urinary creatinine excretion of 1500 mgs. The expected creatinine excretion for a man this size is 1846 mgs.

CHI = 1500 x 100 ÷ 1846 = 81%

Expected creatinine excretion rates are found in Tables 1 and 2. Values should be 90 - 110% of expected.

Aside from the estimated 4 - 8% normal daily variation in excretion, other factors can alter results. Excretion is increased in the early states of injury (fever, infection, trauma), by strenuous exercise, and in the second half of the menstrual cycle. Excretion is reduced by renal failure as GFR falls and with aging due to reduced muscle mass. Urinary creatinine is also altered by diet, primarily meat intake.

For the best results urine collections should not be done during periods of emotional stress, vigorous exercise, early phase of major injury, infection, or fever or in severe renal failure. The diet can provide up to 20% of the creatinine. Dietary intake should also be similar during collection periods. While standard excretion rates were derived on a diet free of creatine and creatinine (i.e. meat-free), those with moderate to severe depletion of lean body mass will not be missed even with dietary protein intake. A reduction of 20% in the obtained value is recommended if the diet contains a source of creatinine.

Heymsfield found good correlation between urinary creatinine excretion and arm muscle area (calculated from mid-arm circumference and triceps skinfold thickness).

NITROGEN BALANCE
Positive nitrogen balance
- Pregnancy
- Growth
- Athletic training

Negative nitrogen balance
- Increased catabolism (trauma, surgery, infection)
- Poor quality protein
- Inadequate protein intake

The main product of protein catabolism is urea formed in the liver from amino groups when amino acids are catabolized. Urea is excreted by the kidney. Nitrogen balance is the difference between nitrogen intake and nitrogen excretion as urea. In healthy people it approximates zero. Estimation requires a 24 hour urine collection for urinary urea nitrogen (UUN) or total urinary nitrogen (TUN). Best results require a steady state, consistent nutrition support, normal renal function, and accurate urine collections, not always available in a clinical situation. A 24 hour collection is recommended over shorter collections. Calculation is as follows:

NB = (protein ÷ 6.25) - (UUN + 4)

Protein intake includes that from IV amino acids or enteral feeding. Protein is divided by 6.25 to convert grams of protein or animo acids to grams of nitrogen. A factor of four is added to cover nonurea nitrogen losses (skin, hair, nails, stool, and other nitrogen-containing compounds in the urine). An additional factor proportional to the size of the burn is

Test	Clinical Significance
	included for burned subjects. The goal for anabolism is plus 4 to 6 grams of nitrogen.

In an unstressed patient a UUN x 1.25 closely approximates TUN. When a TUN is used a factor of only two is added to cover nonurinary losses.

In an unstressed patient urea makes up about 80% of the TUN. As hypercatabolism increases the proportion of the TUN that is urea decreases to as low as 25%.

Results becomes less reliable in liver disease when urea synthesis is compromised and in renal disease when urea excretion is compromised. In the latter case urea kinetics should be used instead (see below).

PROTEIN CATABOLIC RATE (PCR)

Nitrogen balance is unreliable with renal dysfunction (i.e., creatinine clearance < 50 ml/min) due to altered fluid and urea excretion.

Creatinine clearance = (140 - age) (kg) ÷ (72) (serum creatinine)

For women, multiple above result by 0.8.

Urea kinetics can be used in place of nitrogen balance to calculate protein catabolic rate (PCR) in those with renal failure, renal dysfunction, or changing renal function. PCR is the amount of protein catabolized in a specified time interval. The results are usually expressed in g/d. PCR correlates well with nitrogen balance and can be compared to protein intake for an estimation of nitrogen balance. If protein intake is greater than PCR, nitrogen balance is positive and the patient is assumed to be anabolic. If intake is less, nitrogen balance is negative and the patient is assumed to be catabolic.

PCR (g/d) = 9.35 GUN + 11

PCR is calculated from the urea generation rate (GUN). Urea generation parallels protein catabolism and urea diffuses freely throughout body water. Urea generation rate is calculated from changes in BUN, volume of body water urea is dissolved in, and residual urinary urea excretion. Results are expressed in mg/min. The method of calculation will vary somewhat depending on whether a patient is being dialyzed and whether there is residual renal function. The 11 represents the grams of obligatory nitrogen loss via stool, skin, and other nonurea nitrogenous compounds. This can be adjusted for body size by using the following formula.

PCR (g/d) = 9.35 GUN + 0.294 V_1

V_1 = volume of total body water at dry weight (ml)

Total body water is estimated by multiplying dry weight in kilograms by 0.58 (lean male) or .55 (lean female) and multiplying the result by 1000. Results are in milliters.

Definitions of terms used in urea kinetics and samples of calculations are shown on next page.

Test	Clinical Significance

KrUN = residual urea clearance in ml/min

GUN = urea nitrogen generation in mg/min

UUN = urinary urea nitrogen concentration in mg/ml

U = urine volume in ml

BUN = serum urea nitrogen in mg/ml

BUN_1 = first BUN measured

BUN_2 = second BUN measured

mean BUN = BUN_1 + $BUN_2 \div 2$

V_1 = estimated volume of body water (ml) urea is dissolved in based on dry weight

V_2 = V_1 + ml body water gained between dialyses

t = minutes in urine collection

ø = minutes between BUN_1 and BUN_2

example

PCR in a stable, predialysis patient with a relatively constant BUN, a creatinine clearance < 50, and some residual renal function is calculated as follows. Residual urea clearance (KrUN) is calculated first.

1. KrUN (ml/min) = (UUN ÷ mean BUN) (U ÷ t)

2. GUN (mg/min) = (BUN) (KrUN)

3. PCR (g/d) = 9.35 GUN + 11

UUN = 7 g = 7000 mg/1800 ml = 3.8 mg/ml

BUN = 50 mg/dl = 0.50 mg/ml

U = 1800 ml

t = 24° = 1440 min

1. KrU = (3.8 ÷ 0.5) (1800 ÷ 1440) = (7.6) (1.25) = 9.5 ml/min

2. GUN = (0.5) (9.5) = 4.75 mg/min

3. PCR = (9.35) (4.75) + 11 = 55 g/d

example

PCR in a nondialyzed, unstable/catabolic male patient with a creatinine clearance of < 50 and increasing BUN is calculated as follows. The accumulation of urea in body water is combined with the quantity of urea excreted in urine.

1. KrUN (ml/ml) = (UUN ÷ mean BUN) (U ÷ t)

2. GUN mg/min) = (BUN_2 - BUN_1) (V) ÷ ø + (KrUN x mean BUN)

3. PCR (g/d) = 9.35 GUN + 11

Test	Clinical Significance

$U = 600$ ml

UUN $= 2.4$ g $= 0.4$ mg/ml urine

$BUN_1 = 50$ mg/dl $= 0.5$ mg/ml

$BUN_2 = 70$ mg/dl $= 0.7$ mg/ml

$t = 24° = 1440$ min

dry weight $= 65$ kg

$V = 65$ kg x .58 x 1000 $= 37700$ ml

$\emptyset = 1440$ min

1. KrUN $= (0.4 \div 0.6) (600 \div 1440) = (0.66) (0.42) = 0.28$ ml/min

2. GUN $= (0.7 - 0.5) (37700) \div 1440 + (0.28) (0.6)$

   $= (0.2) (37700) \div 1440 + (0.17)$

   $= 7540 \div 1440 + 0.17$

   $= 5.2$ mg/ml

3. PCR $= (9.35) (5.4) + 11 = 60$ g/d

example

PCR in a dialyzed female patient with minimal residual renal function is calculated as follows. PCR is determined between dialyses to avoid adjusting for urea losses in dialysate.

1. GUN (mg/min) $= (V_2 \times BUN_2) - (V_1 \times BUN_1) \div \emptyset$

2. PCR (g/d) $= 9.35$ GUN $+ 11$

dry weight $= 62$ kg

predialysis weight $= 65$ kg

$V_1 = 62$ kg x .58 $= 35.96$L x 1000 $= 35960$ ml

$V_2 = 35960 + 3000$ ml $= 38960$

$BUN_1 = 30$ mg/dl $= 0.3$ mg/ml

$BUN_2 = 45$ mg/dl $= 0.45$ mg/ml

$\emptyset = 1560$

1. GUN $= (38960 \times 0.45) - (35960 \times 0.3) \div 1560$

   $= (17532) - (10788) \div 1560$

   $= 4.32$ mg/min

2. PCR $= (9.35) (4.32) + 11 = 51$ g/d

Test	Clinical Significance

example

PCR in a dialyzed patient with urinary urea loss is calculated as follows. Urea accumulating in body water between dialyses is combined with urea excreted in urine.

1. KrUN (ml/min) = (UUN ÷ mean BUN) (U ÷ t)

2. GUN (mg/min) = (V_2 x BUN_2) - (V_1 x BUN_1) ÷ ø + (KrUN x mean BUN)

3. PCR = 9.35 GUN + 11

UUN = 2.6 g nitrogen or 4 mg/ml

BUN_1 = 25 g/dl or .25 mg/ml

BUN_2 = 32 g/dl or .32 mg/ml

U = 650 ml

t = 2880 min

ø = 2700 min

dry weight = 60 kg

predialysis weight = 67 kg

V_1 = 60 x .55 = 33 L x 1000 = 33000 ml

V_2 = 33000 + 5000 = 3800

1. KrUN = (4 ÷ 0.285) (650 ÷ 2880) = (14) (0.225)

   = 3.15 ml/min

2. GUN = (38000 x 0.32) - (33000 x 0.25) ÷ 2700 + (3.15 x. 0.285)

   = (12160 - 8250) ÷ 2700 + 0.9

   = 3910 ÷ 2700 + 0.9

   = 1.45 + 0.9

   = 2.35 mg/min

3. PCR = (9.35) (2.35) + 11

   = 33 g/d

TABLE 1: Expected 24 Hour Urinary Creatinine Excretion for Men

Height		Small Frame		Medium Frame		Large Frame	
in	cm	kgs	mgs	kgs	mgs	kgs	mgs
61	155	52.7	1212	56.1	1290	60.7	1396
62	158	54.1	1244	57.7	1327	62.0	1426
63	160	55.4	1274	59.1	1359	63.6	1463
64	163	56.8	1306	60.4	1389	65.2	1500
65	165	58.4	1343	62.0	1426	66.8	1536
66	168	60.2	1385	63.9	1470	68.9	1585
67	170	62.0	1426	65.9	1516	71.1	1635
68	173	63.9	1470	67.7	1557	72.9	1677
69	175	65.9	1516	69.5	1598	74.8	1720
70	178	67.7	1557	71.6	1647	76.8	1766
71	180	69.5	1599	73.6	1693	79.1	1819
72	183	71.4	1642	75.7	1741	81.1	1865
73	185	73.4	1688	77.7	1787	83.4	1918
74	188	75.2	1730	80.0	1846	85.7	1971
75	191	77.0	1771	82.3	1893	87.7	2017

Table 1 lists the expected daily creatinine excretion for men based on height, and frame size. These values are the product of the average creatinine excretion rate and the ideal body weight for the appropriate height and frame size. The average excretion rate for men is 23 mg/kg/day. Ideal body weights are based on the 1959 Metropolitan Insurance Company tables.

TABLE 2: Expected 24 Hour Urinary Creatinine Excretion for Women

Height		Small Frame		Medium Frame		Large Frame	
in	cm	kgs	mgs	kgs	mgs	kgs	mgs
56	142	43.2	778	46.1	830	50.7	913
57	145	44.3	797	47.3	851	51.8	932
58	147	45.4	817	48.6	875	53.2	958
59	150	46.8	842	50.0	900	54.5	981
60	152	48.2	868	51.4	925	55.9	1006
61	155	49.5	891	52.7	949	57.3	1031
62	158	50.9	916	54.3	977	58.9	1060
63	160	52.3	941	55.9	1006	60.6	1091
64	163	53.9	970	57.9	1042	62.5	1125
65	165	55.7	1003	59.8	1076	64.3	1157
66	168	57.5	1035	61.6	1109	66.1	1190
67	170	59.3	1067	63.4	1141	67.9	1222
68	173	61.4	1105	65.2	1174	70.0	1260
69	175	63.2	1138	67	1206	72.0	1296
70	178	65.0	1170	68.9	1240	74.1	1334

Table 2 lists the expected daily creatinine excretion for women based on height, and frame size. These values are the product of the average creatinine excretion rate and the ideal body weight for the appropriate height and frame size. The average excretion rate for women is 18 mg/kg/day. Ideal body weights are based on the 1959 Metropolitan Insurance Company tables.

TESTS OF HYDRATION STATUS

About 60% of body weight is water, depending on gender, age, and body fat. Water provides the medium where the body's metabolic processes occur. Water balance or hydration is determined by water intake versus water output.

Sources of water include food, fluids, and metabolic water (water released when food is oxidized). Food varies widely in water content from 0 % for fats to 95% for some fruits and vegetables. Water is lost through the lungs, skin, urine, and stool. Below is a typical fluid intake and output.

Intake (cc)		Output (cc)	
Food	750	Urine	1200
Liquids	1150	Stool	150
Metabolic water	350	Insensible loss	900
Total	2250	Total	2250

Normal water loss through the skin is about 500 ml/d and 400 ml through the lungs. This loss makes up the "insensible losses." Water loss via stool is about 150 ml/d. Urine output is variable. The minimum obligatory urine output is about 700 ml/d. load. Renal solute load determines the volume of water necessary to form urine. Renal solute load can be calculated by allowing one milliliter of water for each milliequivalent of sodium, potassium, and chloride and 5.7 per gram of protein. The presence of catabolism or anabolism may alter the final value. Healthy kidneys can concentrate urine to 1200 to 1400 mOsm/L. Additional water is needed to excrete more solute. For example, if an individual can concentrate urine to 1200 mOsm/L and the renal solute load is 1400 mOsm, then 1166 ml will be needed to excrete this solute load. Kidneys function better when urine output is 1.5 to 2 times the renal solute.

Several guidelines exist for estimating fluid needs. They are:
- One ml per calorie
- 1500 ml/square meter body surface area
- ml/kg based on age and weight

Age	mg / kg / d*	
Average Adults (25 - 55)	35	
Active Adults (16 - 30)	40	
Older Patients (55 - 65)	30	
Elderly (> 65)	25	*Ideal body weight

Fluid needs may be elevated by the presence of infection, vomiting, diarrhea, fever, diuretic therapy, high protein feedings, burns, nasogastric suction, fistulas, and drain output. Conditions where fluid may need to be restricted include congestive heart failure, renal failure, liver failure, or head trauma.

Tube fed patients will usually need additional water. Most enteral formulas contain between 70 and 95% water. Additional water can be given by diluting the feeding, giving water boluses every few hours, or giving additional water with medications.

When output consistently exceeds intake dehydration results. Hypertonic dehydration occurs when water loss exceeds sodium loss, (e.g. fever, air-fluidized beds, hyperglycemia, diabetes insipidus, post obstructive diuresis, diuretics, laxatives, sweating, hyperventilation, hypercalcemia, and high protein tube feedings). Isotonic dehydration results from loss of equal amounts of water and sodium, (e.g. nasogastric suction, or diarrhea). Hypotonic dehydration results from sodium loss in excess of water loss as with diuretics or a low-sodium diet.

Total body water content decreases with age. The elderly are at increased risk of dehydration and they have significant morbidity and mortality as a result, especially when dehydration is accompanied by infection. Factors associated with aging increase their risk. Their thirst perception is altered, their kidneys lose concentrating ability, and antidiuretic hormone (ADH) may be less effective. Some choose to reduce their fluid intake due to incontinence. They are also frequent users of drugs that increase fluid loss (diuretics and laxatives). In warm weather they are less able to regulate their body temperature. Some need to rely on others for their fluid needs (decreased mobility, dementia). The elderly also suffer more adverse effects from dehydration than do younger persons e.g. constipation, impaction, skin breakdown, falls from dizziness, or organ damage from already compromised blood flow.

Physical symptoms of dehydration include weight loss, loss of skin turgor, confusion, lethargy, headache, anorexia, vomiting, weakness, orthostatic hypotension, decreased urine output, concentrated urine, and occasionally, convulsions. More than a 5% weight loss is significant and suggestive of dehydration.

Lab findings which help to evaluate hydration include serum electrolytes, hematocrit, hemoglobin, creatinine, blood urea nitrogen (BUN), BUN to creatinine ratio, serum and urine osmolality, urine specific gravity, and intake and output records.

Test	Clinical Significance
SERUM SODIUM • 135 - 145 meq/L	Often reflects changes in water balance more than sodium balance. If a patient has not received a large sodium load, elevated values suggest dehydration. Levels of of 148 meq/L or more are seen with fluid deficit.
HEMATOCRIT • Male 42 - 52% • Female 37 - 47% • Child 31 - 43%	Elevated levels may indicate hemoconcentration and dehydration.
BUN:CREATININE RATIO • 12 - 20 (usually 12 - 16)	The ratio is better than BUN alone where elevated values may indicate impaired renal function. Values of 25 or greater suggest dehydration due to fluid deficit.
SERUM OSMOLALITY • Adult/elderly 285 - 295 mOsm/kg • Child 275 - 290 mOsm/L	Measures the concentration of particles in the serum and urine. Values vary with hydration. Osmolality is more useful than hematocrit and BUN in evaluating hydration. Above normal values are associated with hypertonic dehydration, normal with isotonic dehydration. Serum osmolality can be estimated: osmolarity (mOsm) = serum Na^+ x 2 + serum glucose ÷ 18 + BUN ÷ 2.8
URINE SPECIFIC GRAVITY • Adult 1.010 - 1.025 Decreases with age • < 2 years 1.001-1.018	Measures the concentration of particles in the urine and the kidney's ability to concentrate and dilute urine. It is less accurate than urine osmolality but values roughly correlate. May be elevated when dehydration due to fluid deficit. Low urine volume would also be expected.
URINE OSMOLALITY usually 350 - 400 mOsm/L	

A variety of fluids can be used for oral rehydration: water, broth, carbonated beverages, fruit juices, and sports drinks. When choosing fluids, take into account the electrolyte content, and the osmolality. Sodium and potassium content should be compatible with dietary allowances. Fluids with a lower osmolality will cause less GI distress and be absorbed faster. Many clinicians use sports drinks (Gatorade or Exceed) for rehydration because they provide electrolytes along with fluid. If dehydration is severe, rehydration may need to be done intravenously or by feeding tube.

Clinical symptoms and history are more important in assessing overhydration than electrolytes. Symptoms include pitting edema, weight increase, hypertension (especially systolic), rapid breathing, distended neck veins, and fast pulse. The primary cause is renal dysfunction, but positive fluid balance may also be due to cardiac and liver dysfunction, hypoproteinemia, excess IV saline, and steroid therapy. Treatment usually includes diuretics and sodium and fluid restrictions.

TESTS OF HEMATOLOGICAL STATUS

Anemia is not a disease but a defect of an underlying process. The medical history, physical exam, and laboratory data all help in the diagnosis. Questions regarding blood loss, medications, diet, family history, presence of fever, and weight loss may suggest a cause. Physical signs (e.g. hepatomegaly, splenomegaly) provide more clues. A complete blood count (CBC) provides information about red blood cells, white blood cells, and platelets. A white blood cell differential may also be included. The hemoglobin and hematocrit quantify the degree of deficiency of anemia and the red cell indices help classify the type. Evaluation of a peripheral blood sample provides further diagnostic information about red cells, white cells, and platelets. A deficient blood component suggests a bone marrow production or peripheral destruction. An elevated blood component indicates a normal marrow response or a malignant proliferation. Potential causes of anemia include acute or chronic blood loss, impaired red cell production, sideroblastic anemia, anemia of chronic disease, or impaired DNA synthesis. The CBC can also be used to evaluate the response to treatment of hematological disease.

Blood Loss

Acute Blood Loss: A blood loss of up to 20% can be tolerated in healthy people without clinical manifestations. Hematocrit and hemoglobin remain normal initially. As extravascular fluid and albumin are transferred to the intravascular space hematocrit falls to a maximum about 3 days later. The anemia will be a normochromic, normocytic one initially. Increased RBC production is then stimulated by the release of erythropoietin. Evidence of red cell regeneration will normally be seen in 3 to 5 days when the reticulocyte count increases. White cells and platelets increase also. Anemia and increased reticulocyte count without signs of external bleeding suggests internal bleeding or hemolytic anemia. If elevated bilirubin and other characteristic cell abnormalities are not present, the bleeding is likely to be internal.

Chronic Blood Loss: Chronic blood loss (malignancy, ulcers) produces anemia when iron stores are depleted or when red cell production cannot keep pace with loss.

Impaired Red Blood Cell Production

Impaired red cell generation may result from a lack of precursors. Hemoglobin synthesis requires adequate iron and the proteins protophorphrin and globin. Pyridoxine is a cofactor in the synthesis of protophorphrin. Without adequate supplies of these precursors, inadequate hemoglobin production results in hypochromic (pale), microcytic (small) red cells. A pyridoxine deficiency or reduced activation of pyridoxine (alcoholics) retards hemoglobin synthesis. Iron deficiency, or a block in iron utilization, leads to incorporation of zinc into the protoporphrin ring. The ratio of zinc protoporphrin to hemoglobin is a sensitive test of iron deficiency.

Iron deficiency is the prime cause of anemia usually resulting from inadequate intake or depletion of stores. Dietary inadequacy is mainly a problem during periods of increased need (growth, pregnancy, lactation). Iron malabsorption may occur with achlorhydria (partial or total gastrectomy), enteritis (celiac disease) or pica (the ingestion of clay or starch). Depletion of stores through chronic blood loss (GI bleeding in men and postmenopausal women, and menstrual loss in premenopausal women) is the more common cause in the US.

Symptoms of iron deficiency anemia include: abnormal nails (brittle, spoon shaped, ridged), glossitis (sore, burning tongue with flattened papillae), angular stomatitis (cracks and ulcers at corners of the mouth), and esophageal webs or strictures.

Laboratory data may include reduced serum ferritin, reduced serum iron, increased transferrin, decreased transferrin saturation and reduced MCV and MCHC. The peripheral smear shows microcytic, hypochromic red cells.

After the cause is found, iron stores are best repleted with oral ferrous sulfate. Response can be followed with the reticulocyte count which should approach maximum in 7 - 10 days. Hemoglobin should be normal in about 8 weeks.

Sideroblastic Anemia

Sideroblastic anemias (hereditary or acquired) result from impaired iron utilization resulting in reduced heme synthesis despite adequate iron. Excess iron is deposited in the developing red cell creating an easily identified characteristic appearance (ringed sideroblasts). Hypochromic, microcytic red cells are seen. Iron absorption continues to be stimulated resulting in increased serum iron, saturated transferrin, and reduced transferrin synthesis. Iron begins to overflow storage areas and deposits in organs (heart, pancreas, liver) producing organ dysfunction (diabetes, cirrhosis, cardiomyopathy). Some of the hereditary forms respond to large doses of pyridoxine even though the body is not deficient. Acquired forms may result from unknown causes, drugs (antituberculosis drugs, alcohol, chemotherapy) or are associated with other disorders (multiple myeloma, lymphoma, megaloblastic anemia, collagen vascular disorders, and myxedema). They are unresponsive to blood forming agents.

Anemia of Chronic Disease

The second most common type of anemia behind iron deficiency is anemia of chronic disease. It is often seen with chronic nonhematological diseases and results from impaired iron utilization. Findings include decreased serum iron and transferrin, decreased transferrin saturation, and adequate or increased iron stores. Iron from destroyed RBCs is trapped in storage sites and not recycled to produce new RBCs The life span of RBCs is also reduced and the bone marrow is unable to adequately compensate. These factors seem related to the continued release of interleukin-1 (IL-1) found in chronic inflammation or neoplasia. This anemia usually develops one to two months after the onset of a chronic disease. Generally the RBC are normocytic and normochronic. The reticulocyte count is normal or low and marrow iron stores are adequate or increased. A common finding is sideroblasts less than 20% of normal.

Megaloblastic Anemia

Megaloblastic anemias are characterized by reduced DNA synthetic rate. Vitamin B_{12} and folate deficiency are the most common causes. Symptoms of vitamin B_{12} deficiency include weakness, sore tongue, and paresthesias (numbness, tingling, loss of vibration, and position sense), an unsteady gait, and gastrointestinal complaints (heartburn, anorexia, diarrhea). Folate deficiency produces the same symptoms but without the neurological changes. Both produce the same peripheral blood and bone marrow findings. Red cells are macrocytic. MCV and MCH are elevated but MCHC is normal. The reticulocyte count is normal or low (marrow is unable to produce red cells). A peripheral smear shows hypersegmented neutrophils and other characteristic cell changes. If B_{12} and folate are normal, other causes should be sought. Therapy is repletion of folate and vitamin B_{12} stores. Parenteral or IM vitamin B_{12} is needed with pernicious anemia due to malabsorption of the vitamin. Folic acid can be given orally or IV. Within three to five days reticulocyte count will rise, and serum iron will fall.

Aplastic Anemia

Aplastic anemia is generally an acquired defect in stem cell production by the bone marrow. Causes can be from chemical or drug induced injury, radiation exposure, or infection. The remaining causes are unknown.

Iron Overload

Normal daily losses of 1 to 2 milligrams of iron are offset by absorption of ingested iron. Any excess iron administration or increased absorption cannot be matched by excretion and leads to the gradual accumulation of excess iron in tissues outside the reticuloendothelial system storage sites in body organs (liver, heart, pancreas) producing cirrhosis, cardiomyopathy or cardiac arrhythmias, and glucose intolerance. Deposition in the skin produces a bronzed appearance. Arthritis may also occur.

Primary hemochromatosis results from an inborn error of metabolism affecting mainly males and leading to absorption of an additional 2 to 3 more milligrams per day of iron, much of which is deposited in organ tissue, especially the liver. Iron stores in the reticuloendothelial system (spleen, bone marrow) may be normal despite the excess in tissue. Laboratory findings include transferrin saturation greater than 80% and serum ferritin levels above 500 µg/L. Liver biopsy confirms the diagnosis.

Secondary hemachromatosis is usually the result of ineffective red cell formation. When normal reticuloendothelial storage sites become saturated iron then becomes deposited in organ tissues. Treatment of the accompanying anemia with transfusion further adds to the iron overload.

Test	Clinical Significance

RED BLOOD CELLS (RBC)
Normal Values
Adult/Elderly
• Male
  4.7 - 6.1 million/µl
• Female
  4.2 - 5.4 million/µl
• Infant/child
  3.8 - 5.5 million/µl
• Newborn
  4.8 - 7.1 million/µl
 	
Increased
 	
• Dehydration
• High altitude living
• Cardiovascular disease
• Pulmonary disease
• Polycythemia vera
 	
Decreased
 	
• Overhydration
• Hemorrhage
• Hemolysis
• Inadequate diet
• Pregnancy (hemodilution)
• Leukemia
• Anemia
• Renal disease
• Multiple myeloma
• Pernicious anemia
• Rheumatic fever
• Pregnancy
• Hodgkin's disease
	An RBC count is a routine part of a complete blood count (CBC). It measures the number of RBCs in a cubic millimeter of blood and provides a basis for calculating hematocrit, MCH, and MCHC.
	
	Normal values vary with age and gender. Over and under hydration may obscure true values. Values less than 90% of normal indicate anemia.
	
	High values are associated with the need for increased oxygen transport capacity (e.g., high altitude, heart and lung disease) or increased production from bone marrow disorders (e.g. polycythemia vera).
	
	The normal lifespan for a RBC is 120 days. At the end of that time the cell is removed from circulation and hemolyzed. Shorter life spans result from peripheral vascular disease and artificial heart valves. An enlarged spleen may also destroy normal RBCs.
	
	The drugs gentamycin, and methyldopa may increase red cell count. Drugs which decrease red cell count include chloramphenicol, quinidine, and hydantoin.

Test	Clinical Significance

• Lymphoma
• Chemotherapy
• Thalassemia

HEMATOCRIT (HCT)
(Packed Cell Volume)
Normal Values
• Male
  42 - 52%
  0.42 - 0.52 volume fraction
• Female
  37 - 47%
  0.37 - 0.43 volume fraction
• Pregnancy
  > 33%
• Child
  31 - 43%
• Infant
  30 - 40%
• Newborn
  44 - 64%
Values in the elderly may be
  slightly lower

Increased
• High altitude living
• Dehydration
• Polycythemia vera
• Shock, trauma, surgery, burns
• Eclampsia

Decreased
• Anemia
• Malnutrition
• Hyperthyroidism
• Hemolysis, hemorrhage
• Organ disease
  (cirrhosis, renal, liver)
• Leukemia
• Overhydration
• Bone marrow failure
• Hodgkin's disease
• Pregnancy
• Rheumatoid arthritis
• Multiple myeloma

Hematocrit is a routine part of a CBC and measures the percent of RBCs in the total blood volume. Results closely reflect hemoglobin and RBC values. Hematocrit (in %) is usually three times hemoglobin (in g/dl) when RBCs are of normal size with normal amounts of hemoglobin. Hematocrit is calculated from the RBC count and the MCV and thus a less accurate index of anemia than direct measurement of hemoglobin.

Values vary with age and gender with a tendency toward lower values after age 60. Values may not be reliable immediately after hemorrhage, transfusions, or burns. A very high white blood cell may alter values as does over and under hydration. Abnormal values are associated with the same conditions as abnormal RBC and hemoglobin levels.

Drugs which may decrease hematocrit include chloramphenicol and penicillin.

Test	Clinical Significance

HEMOGLOBIN (Hb)

Normal Values

- Male
  14 - 18 g/dl
  8.7 - 11.2 mmol/L
- Female
  12 - 16 g/dl
  7.4 - 9.9 mmol/L
- Pregnancy
  > 11g/dl
- Child
  11 - 16 g/dl
- Infant
  10 - 15 g/dl
- Newborn
  14 - 24 g/dl

Increased

- High altitude living
- Dehydration
- Polycythemia vera
- Chronic obstructive pulmonary
  disease (COPD)
- Congestive heart failure
- Congenital heart disease
- Severe burns

Decreased

- Overhydration
- Anemia
- Malnutrition
- Hemolysis, hemorrhage
- Leukemia
- Lymphoma
- Hodgkins disease
- Cancer
- Systemic lupus erythematous
- Sarcoidosis
- Renal disease
- Splenomegaly
- Sickle cell anemia

Hemoglobin measurement is a routine part of a CBC. It measures the total amount of hemoglobin in peripheral blood. Hemoglobin is the part of the RBC that carries oxygen and carbon dioxide and makes up about 90% of the red cell. Decreases in hemoglobin are called anemia. Increases are called polycythemia.

Normal values vary with age, gender, and ethnicity. Levels tend to be lower after age 60. Slightly lower levels are found in blacks and premature infants. Lower values in pregnancy reflect increased blood volume despite an increased number of RBCs.

The drugs gentamycin and methyldopa may increase hemoglobin. Antibiotics, aspirin, indomethacin, rifampin, sulfonamides, and anti-cancer drugs may decrease it.

MEAN CORPUSCULAR VOLUME (MCV)

Normal Values

- Adult/elderly/child
  80 - 95 fl

MCV is one of the red blood cell indices (MCV, MCH, MCHC). It measures of the average size of a RBC and is useful in classifying anemias. Normal values vary by age and gender. Cells may be abnormally small (microcytic), abnormally large (macrocytic) or normal in size (normocytic). Values can be falsely elevated by an increased reticulocyte count.

Test	Clinical Significance

• Newborn
96 - 108 fl

Increased

• Liver disease
• Folate deficiency
• Vitamin B$_{12}$ deficiency
• Alcoholism
• Antimetabolite therapy

Decreased

• Iron deficiency
• Thalassemia

MEAN CORPUSCULAR HEMOGLOBIN (MCH)

Normal Values

• Adults/elderly/child
27 - 31 pg
• Newborn
32 - 34 pg

Increased

• Macrocytic anemia

Decreased

• Microcytic anemia

MCH is a measure of the average weight of hemoglobin in a RBC. Causes of abnormal values parallel those for MCV. Values can be falsely elevated by hyperlipidemia. WBC counts greater than 50,000, and high heparin concentrations. Clinical usefulness is limited but MCHC can be used for laboratory quality control.

MEAN CORPUSCULAR HEMOGLOBIN CONCENTRATION (MCHC)

Normal Values

• Adult/elderly/child
32 - 36 g/dl
32 - 36%
320 - 360 g/L
• Newborns
32 - 33 g/dl
32 - 33%

Increased

• Spherocytosis
• Infants, newborns

Decreased

• Iron deficiency anemia
• Macrocytic anemias
• Thalassemia
• Chronic blood loss
• B$_6$ responsive anemia

MCHC measures the average concentration of hemoglobin per total red cell volume. It is derived from hemoglobin and hematocrit.

Low values indicate the cell has a deficiency of hemoglobin and is hypochromic. Normal values indicate cells are normocytic. Values are falsely elevated by lipidemia and high heparin concentrations.

Clinical use is limited but MCHC can be used for laboratory quality control.

Test	Clinical Significance
RED CELL DISTRIBUTION WIDTH (RDW)	RDW is a measure of the degree of size variation (or anisocytosis) among red blood cells. It can be useful in the classification of anemias.

RED CELL DISTRIBUTION WIDTH (RDW)

Normal Values

• Adult
  11 - 14.5%

Increased

• Dietary deficiency
  (iron, B_{12}, folate)
• Abnormal hemoglobin
• Immune hemolytic anemia

Decreased

• Hemorrhage

RETICULOCYTE COUNT
(Retic. count)

Normal Values

• Adult/elderly/child
  0.5 - 2% of total RBCs
• Infant
  0.5 - 3.1%
• Newborn
  2.5 - 6.5%

Increased

• Sickle cell anemia
• 3 - 4 days after hemorrhage
• Post splenectomy
• Pregnancy
• Leukemia
• Treatment of anemia
• Hemolytic anemia
• Anemia therapy

Decreased

• Iron deficiency
• Aplastic anemia
• Pernicious anemia
• Chronic infection
• Radiation therapy
• Marrow failure
• Myelodysplasia
• Folate, B_{12}, or iron deficiency
• Liver cirrhosis
• Post transfusion

Reticulocytes are immature RBCs with a life span of three to four days. They are normally seen in small amounts in a peripheral blood smear. A reticulocyte count is an index of red cell production by the bone marrow. A normal or decreased count together with significant anemia suggests lack of bone marrow response as in iron, folate, or vitamin B_{12} deficiency or else bone marrow infiltration. An increased count suggest rapid cell turnover (e.g. acute blood loss or hemolysis).

A reticulocyte count can also be used to follow response to treatment of anemia. A high count is expected with anemia and indicates increased RBC production. A normal or low count indicates inadequate marrow production and possibly the cause of the anemia.

A reticulocyte index can be calculated to determine if the increased count indicates an adequate bone marrow response.

retic. index = % reticulocytes x (patient hct ÷ normal hct)

Values less than 1.0 indicate inadequate compensation by the bone marrow as in iron, folate, B_{12} deficiency, or marrow failure.

Test	Clinical Significance

FERRITIN

Normal Values

- Male
  12 - 300 ng/ml or µg/L
- Female
  10 - 150 ng/ml or µg/L
- 6 mo - 15 yr
  7 - 142 ng/ml
- 2 - 5 mo
  50 - 200 ng/ml
- 0 - 2 months
  200 - 600 ng/ml
- Newborn
  25 - 200 ng/ml

Increased

- Hemochromatosis
- Hemosiderosis
- Megaloblastic anemia
- Hemolytic anemia
- Thalassemia
- Liver disease
- Inflammatory disease
- Hodgkin's disease
- Lymphoma
- Leukemia
- Breast cancer
- Recent transfusion or high iron meal
- Iron preparations

Decreased

- Iron deficiency anemia
- Severe protein depletion
- Hemodialysis

Ferritin is the major iron storage protein and normally present in concentrations proportional to stored iron. It provides an index of iron stores in iron deficiency and iron overload. Normally one ng/L corresponds to eight mg stored iron. Used in conjunction with total iron binding capacity and iron levels, it can help classify the type of anemia.

Levels are significantly higher in men and postmenopausal women Low levels are associated with iron or protein depletion. High levels are associated with iron excess. Since ferritin is an acute phase protein it may not be reliable in inflammatory conditions, neoplasia, or liver disease.

IRON (Fe)

Normal Values

- 60 - 190 µg/dl
- 13 - 31 µmol/L

Increased

- Multiple transfusions
- Hemosiderosis
- Hemochromatosis
- Hemolytic anemia (thalassemia)
- Hepatitis, hepatic necrosis
- Acute leukemia

Iron absorbed into the circulation is bound to transferrin and transported to the bone marrow for incorporation into hemoglobin. After removal of the iron, transferrin is released back into circulation. When red cells are destroyed the iron is stored in the reticuloendothelial system of the spleen, marrow, and liver. Serum iron measures the quantity of iron that is bound to transferrin. Normally one-third of transferrin's iron binding sites are saturated. Very little free iron normally exists in the plasma. Iron levels may vary significantly throughout the day, therefore its best to draw levels in the morning after a 12 hour fast and before any blood transfusions.

Iron deficiency can be caused by inadequate intake, malabsorption (achlorhydria, gastrectomy, pica, enteritis), increased needs (growth, pregnancy), and blood loss (GI bleeding, menstruation). A deficiency will reduce hemoglobin producing small, pale RBCs.

Test	Clinical Significance

• Nephrosis
• Drugs

Decreased

• Inadequate intake/absorption
• Chronic blood loss
• Pregnancy (late)
• Chronic disease (lupus, rheumatoid arthritis, chronic infection)
• Hypothyroidism
• Chronic GI loss
• Neoplasms
• Drugs

Drugs which may elevate iron levels include chloramphenical, dextran, estrogen, ethanol, iron preparations, methyldopa, and oral contraceptives. Drugs which reduce iron levels include deferoxamine, methicillin, testosterone, ACTH, cholestyramine, chloramphenicol, and colchicine.

TOTAL IRON-BINDING CAPACITY (TIBC)

Normal Values

• 25 - 420 µg/dl
  45 - 73 µmol/L

Increased

• Iron deficiency anemia
• Pregnancy (late)
• Polycythemia vera

Decreased

• Hypoproteinemia
• Hemolytic anemia
• Pernicious anemia
• Sickle cell anemia
• Liver cirrhosis
• Inflammatory disease

Transferrin saturation:
normally 30 - 40%

Increased

• Hemochromatosis
• Increased iron intake
• Thalassemia
• Pyridoxine deficiency
• Aplastic anemia
• Hemosiderosis

Decreased

• Iron deficiency anemia
• Malignancy
• Anemia of chronic disease

The protein transferrin carries absorbed iron to the bone marrow for incorporation into hemoglobin. Transferrin synthesis is regulated by iron stores. When iron stores are low transferrin levels increase proportional to the deficiency. This is an early index of iron deficiency and the last index to return to normal when the deficiency is corrected. TIBC is a measure of transferrin, but labs more often measure transferrin directly. Transferrin can be estimated by multiplying TIBC by 0.7.

Serum iron measures the quantity of iron bound to transferrin. Ninety-nine percent of iron is bound to about one-third of the transferrin. Transferrin saturation is useful in determining the cause of abnormal iron and TIBC. Transferrin is normally 30 to 40% saturated. Transferrin saturation can be calculated as follows:

% transferrin saturation = iron x 100 ÷ TIBC

Transferrin is a protein synthesized by the liver and as such is not always reflective of iron metabolism. Levels decrease with stress states and inflammatory conditions.

Drugs which may increase TIBC include fluorides, oral contraceptives, chloramphenicol, and estrogen. Drugs that may decrease TIBC include ACTH and chloramphenicol.

Test	Clinical Significance

PROTHROMBIN TIME (PT)

Normal Values
- 11 - 12.5 seconds
  85 - 100% of control
  Anticoagulant therapy
- 1.5 to 2 times control
  20 - 30% of control

Increased
- Vitamin K deficiency
- Liver disease
- Anticoagulant therapy
- Biliary obstruction
- Salicylate intoxication
- Disseminated intravascular clotting (DIC)
- Excess alcohol intake
- Hypervitaminosis A
- Dehydration
- Zollinger-Ellison syndrome
- Systemic lupus erythematosis

Decreased
- Ileitis, enteritis
- Dehydration

Prothrombin time measures the clotting ability of prothrombin and other clotting factors synthesized by the liver. Several are vitamin K-dependent. When factor production or vitamin K is deficient, PT is prolonged.

With severe liver disease (cirrhosis, hepatitis, tumor) production of clotting factors is reduced and PT elevated. In obstructive biliary disease (stones, tumors, cholestasis) vitamin K-dependent clotting factors are not adequately synthesized due to vitamin K malabsorption. Giving vitamin K will differentiate between the two causes. If PT returns to normal this indicates biliary obstruction and vitamin K malabsorption. If not, liver disease and the inability to synthesize clotting factors is indicated.

Another reporting method for PT is the INR (International Normalized Ratio), developed to standardize reporting results regardless of lab reagents or method used. In anticoagulation therapy a prolonged PT (or INR) is desired to treat or prevent blood clots. Anticoagulants delay clotting by interfering with the action of the vitamin K-dependent clotting factors. Adequacy of anticoagulation therapy can be followed by regular PT or INR determinations.

Drugs which may elevate PT include anticoagulants, aspirin, allopurinol, antibiotics, barbiturates, chloral hydrate, chlorpromazine, clofibrate, cholestyramine, chloramphenicol, cimetidine, colestipol, heparin, methyldopa, neomycin, quinine, quinidine, and sulfonamides.

Drugs which may decrease PT include anabolic steroids, barbiturates, chloral hydrate, digitalis, diphenhydramine, estrogen, griseofulvin, oral contraceptives, and vitamin K.

FOLATE

Normal Values

Serum Folate
- 5 - 20 µg/ml
  14 - 34 mmol/L
- Red Cell Folate
  160 - 800 ng/ml

Increased
- Vegetarians
- Hemolyzed blood sample
- Transfusions
- Pernicious anemia
- Blind Loop Syndrome

Decreased
- Inadequate intake
- Malabsorption (Crohn's, celiac disease, ulcerative colitis)
- Malignancy

Serum folate is measured to help diagnose the cause of megaloblastic anemia. It is usually measured in conjunction with vitamin B12. Levels of folate are sensitive to short term variation in intake and therefore should be measured before consumption of a good quality diet or nutrition supplements. For this reason red cell folate is a better index of long term deficiency. Levels should be checked before transfusions are given.

The prime causes of deficiency are inadequate intake (lack of fresh foods), malabsorption (drugs, small bowel disease), inadequate utilization (drugs, vitamin B12 deficiency, alcoholism, vitamin C deficiency, inborn errors), increased needs (parasites, pregnancy, lactation, growth, tumors), and increased excretion (dialysis, exfoliative dermatitis).

Drugs which may reduce folate levels include alcohol, aminopterin, aminosalicylic acid, ampicillin, antimalarials, chloramphenicol, erythromycin, estrogens, methotrexate, oral contraceptives, penicillin, phenobarbital, phenytoin, tetracyclines, trimethoprim, and triamterene.

Test	Clinical Significance

- Lymphoma, leukemia
- Myelofibrosis
- Pregnancy
- Sickle cell anemia
- Thalassemia
- Small cell cancer
- Hypothyroidism
- Exfoliative dermatitis

VITAMIN B$_{12}$

Normal Values
- Adult
  100 - 700 pg/ml
  74 - 517 pmol/L
- Newborn
  160 - 1300 pg/ml

Increased
- Polycythemia vera
- Congestive heart failure

Decreased
- Pernicious anemia
- Gastrectomy
- Inflammatory bowel disease
- Blind loop
- Vegetarian diet
- Alcoholism
- Folate deficiency
- Liver disease (hepatitis, cirrhosis, tumors)
- Iron deficiency
- Fish tapeworm
- Hyperthyroidism

Vitamin B$_{12}$ levels are used to help diagnose the cause of megaloblastic anemia. They are usually measured in conjunction with folate as diagnosis generally requires both values. Levels should be checked before any vitamin B$_{12}$ injections are given. When a deficiency is established the cause of the deficiency must then be determined.

Causes of a deficiency include inadequate intake, usually strict vegetarians and alcoholics. Malabsorption of the vitamin can result from lack of intrinsic factor (pernicious anemia), pancreatic insufficiency (maldigestion), competition from bacteria (blind loop), and ileal disease (resection or disease). Congenital lack of enzymes or drug antagonists can produce inadequate utilization. Vitamin needs are increased by hyperthyroidism, growth, pregnancy, lactation, and parasites. Increased losses occur with liver disease (reduced storage) and high doses of ascorbic acid (vitamin destruction).

Drugs that may reduce B$_{12}$ levels include para-aminosalicylic acid, oral hypoglycemics, neomycin, cholestyramine, colchicine, and cimetidine.

TABLE 3: Classification of Some Anemias

Test	B12 Deficiency	Folate Deficiency	Iron Deficiency	Anemia Of Chronic Disease
RBC count	D	D	D	D
Hemoglobin	D	D	D	slight D
Hematocrit	D	D	D	D
MCV	I	I	D	N
MCH	I	I	D	N
MCHC	N	N	D	N
Reticulocyte count	N or D	N or D	N or D	N or D
RDW	N or I	N or I	I	N
Serum ferritin	I	I	D	N or I
TIBC	N	N	N or I	N or D
Transferrin	N	N	N or I	N or D
Transferrin saturation (%)	N	N	D	N or D
Serum iron	N	N	D	D
Serum folate	N or I	D	N	N
Red cell folate	D	D	N	N
Vitamin B$_{12}$	D	N	N	N
Red cells	normochromic, macrocytic	normochromic, macrocytic	hypochromic, microcytic	hypochromic, microcytic (both mild)
Other	hypersegmented neutrophils, macroovalocytes	hypersegmented neutrophils, macroovalocytes	anisocytosis	poikilocytosis (slight), anisocytosis (moderate)

I = Increased, N = Normal, D = Decreased

TABLE 4: Laboratory Findings in the Development of Folate Deficient Anemia

Test	Normal	Negative Folate Balance	Folate Depletion	Folate Deficienct Erythropoiesis	Folate Deficiency Anemia
Serum folate (ng/ml)	> 5	< 3	< 3	< 3	< 3
RBC folate (ng/ml)	> 200	> 200	< 160	< 120	< 100
Lobe average	< 3.5	< 3.5	< 3.5	> 3.5	> 3.5
RBCs	Normal	Normal	Normal	Normal	Macroovalocytic
MCV	Normal	Normal	Normal	Normal	Elevated
Hemoglobin (g/dl)	> 12	> 12	> 12	> 12	< 12

TABLE 5: Laboratory Findings in the Development of Vitamin B$_{12}$ Deficient Anemia.

Test	Normal	Negative B$_{12}$ Balance	B$_{12}$ Depletion	B$_{12}$ Deficient Erythro-poiesis	B$_{12}$ Deficient Anemia
Hypersegmentation*	No	No	No	Yes	Yes
RBC folate (ng/dl)	> 160	> 160	> 160	< 140	< 140
RBCs	Normal	Normal	Normal	Normal	Macroovalocytic
MCV	Normal	Normal	Normal	Normal	Elevated
Hemoglobin	Normal	Normal	Normal	Normal	Low

Increased number of lobes in granulocytic nuclei.

TABLE 6: Laboratory Findings in the Development of Iron Deficient Anemia

Test	Normal	Iron Depletion	Iron Deficient Blood	Iron Deficiency Anemia
TIBC (µmol/L)	54 - 64	64	70	73
Serum ferritin (µg/L)	40 - 160	20	10	< 10
Serum iron (µmol/L)	12 - 30	21	< 11	< 7
Transferrin saturation*	20 - 50	30	< 15	< 10
Zinc protoporphyrin to heme ratio (µmol/mol)	< 80	↑	↑↑	↑↑↑
RDW (%)	14.5	high	high	high
RBCs	normal	normal	normal	microcytic hypochromic

Serum iron divided by total iron-binding capacity x 100

TESTS OF IMMUNE STATUS

Nutritional deficiency significantly impacts the immune system and immunocompetence is a sensitive indicator of nutritional status. Infection is the most important complication of nutritional deficiency. Studies in developing countries with a high incidence of malnutrition show that immune incompetence precedes the presence of an overt infection.

Test	Clinical Significance

TOTAL LYMPHOCYTE COUNT (TLC)
Normal Values
  1000 - 4000 per cubic millimeter
  20 - 40% of total white cell count
Increased (> 4000)
• Leukemia
• Infectious mononucleosis
• Some bacterial infections (TB, brucellosis, pertussis)
• Viral infections (CMV, measles, mumps, chickenpox, infectious hepatitis, toxoplasmosis)
• Crohn's disease, ulcerative colitis
• Serum sickness, drug hypersensitivity
• Hypoadrenalism
• Multiple myeloma
• Hypothyroidism (Grave's disease)
Decreased
• Malnutrition
• Steroid therapy
• Immunosupressive therapy
• Chemotherapy
• Radiation therapy
• Aplastic anemia
• Hodgkin's disease, other malignancies
• Immune disorders (inherited, AIDS)
• Congestive heart failure
• Renal failure
• Obstruction of lymph system (tumor, Whipple's disease, intestinal lymphectasia)
	TLC = % lymphocytes x WBC ÷ 100
	
	Levels < 1500 are reported to be associated with increased mortality and indicative of nutrient deficits. TLC is also subject to alteration by other factors: sepsis, hypercatabolism, cancer, steroid therapy, radiation therapy, chemotherapy, and immune deficiency disorders.

Test	Clinical Significance
DELAYED CUTANEOUS HYPERSENSITIVITY (DCH) **Decreased** • Malnutrition • Infection • Lymphoma • Sarcoidosis • Chemotherapy • Radiation therapy • Metabolic stress • Steroid therapy • Chronic disease (renal, liver)	DCH measures skin response to both new and recall (those previously exposed to) antigens. It is a reliable index of cell-mediated immunity. An induration at the injection site of 2 millimeters or greater is considered a positive response. Responses between 1 and 2 mm can be difficult to judge. Lack of a response is anergy, the inability to adequately respond to and destroy foreign antigens. Anergy correlates with increased infections and mortality. The degree and size of the skin response also correlates well with visceral protein status as judged by serum albumin. Skin response decreases with overall malnutrition as well as individual nutrient deficiencies of zinc, iron, folate, pyridoxine, and essential fatty acids. Skin response is also reduced by factors other than malnutrition (see left).

TESTS OF MINERAL STATUS

There are six major electrolytes in blood. Three, potassium, magnesium, and phosphorus, are in greatest concentration within the cells. Sodium and chloride are the major extracellular electrolytes. The flow of calcium into and out of cells is important to muscular contractions. Healthy bodies are able to maintain normal fluid and electrolyte composition but a number of disorders cause abnormal electrolyte and fluid balance which requires monitoring. Administration of intravenous fluids also requires periodic assessment of serum electrolytes.

Test

Clinical Significance

SODIUM (NA⁺)

Normal Values
- Adult/elderly
  136 - 145 mEq/L
  136 - 145 mmol/L
- Child
  136 - 145 mEq/L
- Infant
  134 - 150 mEq/L
- Newborn
  134 - 144 mEq/L

Increased
- Excess sodium intake (oral, IV)
- Decreased sodium loss (Cushing's disease, hyperaldosteronism)
- Excess free water loss (sweat, burns, diabetes insipidus, osmotic diuresis)

Decreased
- Decreased sodium intake (oral, IV)
- Increased sodium loss (Addison's, diarrhea, vomiting, nasogastric suction, diuretics, chronic renal insufficiency)
- Excess water intake (oral, IV)
- Congestive heart failure
- SIADH
- Third-space sodium loss
- Ascites
- Peripheral edema
- Pleural effusions
- Loss into the bowel (ileus, obstruction)
- Osmotic dilution

Sodium is the primary cation in the extracellular space. Its prime function is maintenance of plasma osmolality and fluid balance. Typical intake is 90 - 250 mEq/d. Maximum tolerance is 400 mEq/d. (Three liters of normal saline in 24 hours would provide 465 mEq.) The major route of excretion is the kidneys which can excrete up to 300 mEq/d. Some sodium is also lost through the skin (sweat) and GI fluids.

Serum sodium levels are a balance between intake and excretion by the kidney. As free water intake increases, sodium concentration decreases causing the kidney to conserve sodium and excrete water. As free water decreases, sodium concentration increases leading to water conservation by the kidney. Other factors (ADH, aldosterone, natriuretic factor) are also involved. Urine sodium is a more sensitive index of sodium balance. High lipid, protein, or glucose levels and mannitol will cause falsely low levels of sodium due to displacement of sodium in the blood sample.

Hyponatremia can be classified on the basis of plasma osmolality. Hypoosmolar hyponatremia results from depletion of effective circulating volume (ECV), that is, the portion of extracellular fluid that perfuses the cells. The body can "perceive" a decrease in ECV with either excess total body water (congestive heart failure, cirrhosis, nephrotic syndrome) or with total body water depletion (diarrhea, vomiting, skin loss). This leads to ADH (antidiuretic hormone) secretion, and thirst. The increased fluid intake and decreased water excretion results in hypoosmolarity and hyponatremia.

Causes include severe renal failure, diuretic therapy, mineralocorticoid deficiency and salt losing syndromes, and water intake beyond excretion ability. Hypothyroidism and hypocorticolism are also associated with reduced ECV and water retention. The syndrome of inappropriate ADH secretion (SIADH) is another cause. This can result from tumors, pulmonary disorders, and central nervous system disease. Some drugs (chlorpropamide, carbamazepine, tolbutamide) produce an SIADH-like syndrome by enhancing the effects of ADH.

Hyperosmolar hyponatremia can be produced by hyperglycemia and mannitol, both of which draw water out of the cells producing hyponatremia.

Pseudohyponatremia occurs when plasma contains large amounts of lipid or proteins which replace sodium in the test sample. Osmolality is not affected.

Test	Clinical Significance

Urine osmolality helps assess renal water excretion. Hyponatremia with low urine osmolality or specific gravity suggests appropriately supressed ADH secretion. Elevated urine osmolality sugests impaired renal water excretion. Urinary sodium is useful in assessing those with hyponatremia and impaired water excretion. If low, this suggest hypovolemia due to sodium and water loss or decreased effective circulating volume. If high, renal disease is indicated as the cause of the hyponatremia.

Some clinical symptoms of hyponatremia (weakness, confusion, lethargy, seizures, coma, and death) are related to water entering the brain in the body's attempt to correct hypoosmolality by moving water into body cells. Other symptoms include anorexia, fatigue, cramps, diarrhea, hypotension and oliguria. Drugs that may reduce sodium levels include diuretics, sulfates, laxatives, sulfonylureas, triamterene, carbamazepine, and vasopressin.

Hypernatremia is always associated with increased osmolality. It results from loss of water in excess of solute or else a gain in sodium. The normal response to hypernatremia is increased ADH secretion, thirst, and retention of water. Hypernatremia generally occurs in those without access to water (comatose, infants) or with hypothalmic disorders that alter thirst response (tumors, sarcoidosis, granulomatous disease, vascular disorders) or osmoreceptor function (hyperaldosteronism, Cushing's). Hypernatremia may also result from CNS disorders (anoxic brain damage, trauma, infections, neurosurgery). Other causes include excess sodium intake from hypertonic solutions or formulas. Another cause is defective ADH secretion (diabetes insipidus or impaired renal response to ADH (nephrogenic diabetes insipidus). Renal failure, hypokalemia, hypercalcemia, drugs, pregnancy, sickle cell anemia, osmotic diuresis or congenital causes may cause the latter.

Drugs which may increase sodium include anabolic steroids, corticosteroids, antibiotics, cough medicines, clonidine, methyldopa, NSAIDS, oral contrceptives, calcium, fluoride, and iron.

Symptoms of hypernatremia include dry mucous membranes, thirst, agitation, hyperreflexia, mania, and convulsions.

POTASSIUM (K⁺)

Normal Values

- Adult/elderly
  3.5 - 5.0 mEq/L
  3.5 - 5.0 mmol/L
- Child
  3.4 - 4.7 mEq/L
- Infant
  4.1 - 5.3 mEq/L
- Newborn
  3.9 - 5.9 mEq/L

Potassium is the major cation within the cell. It has roles in muscle function, nerve conduction, acid-base balance, maintenance of osmotic pressure, and cardiac function. Daily needs are between 45 and 145 mEq/d. Body content varies with age, sex, weight, and muscle mass. The serum content is small and minor changes have significant results. Several factors affect levels. Increased aldosterone secretion increases renal excretion of potassium as sodium and chloride are resorbed. Changes in blood pH cause potassium to move in and out of cells. Serum levels vary inversely with serum pH as potassium enters and leaves the cells. A 0.1 change in pH can change plasma potassium by 0.4 to 0.6 mEq/L (the higher the pH, the lower the potassium). The kidney doesn't conserve potassium. Even with no intake 40 - 50 mEq/d are excreted daily

Test	Clinical Significance

Increased

- Increased intake (oral, IV)
- Decreased loss (renal failure, Addison's disease)
- Hypoaldosteronism
- Potassium wasting diuretics
- Extracellular shift (acidosis, infection, crush injury)
- Hemolysis

Decreased

- Decreased intake (oral, IV)
- Excess GI loss,
- Hyperaldosteronism
- Cushing's syndrome
- Renal tubular acidosis
- Excess licorice (natural)
- Intracellular shift (alkalosis; glucose, insulin, or calcium administration)

potentially causing a deficiency. Levels should be followed closely with renal failure, acidosis, and those taking potassium-sparing diuretics and digoxin (toxicity is increased by hypokalemia).

Hypokalemia results from inadequate intake (TPN, starvation), increased GI losses (diarrhea, fistulas, vomiting, nasogastric suction) and increased excretion (renal tubular disorders, hypoaldosteronism, Cushing's syndrome). Drugs which may increase GI losses include laxatives and enemas. Drugs which increase urinary excretion include potassium-wasting diuretics, insulin, lithium carbonate, penicillin antibiotics (carbenicillin, ticarcillin, nafcillin, ampicillin), aminoglycoside antibiotics, amphotericin B, and aspirin. Symptoms of hypokalemia include weakness, paralysis, ileus, increased sensitivity to digoxin, cardiac arrhythmias, and electrocardiogram changes. Clinical situations requiring treatment usually occur at levels < 3 mEq/L.

Hyperkalemia results from excess intake (IVs, TPN, oral) especially with impaired renal excretion (renal disease, hypoaldosteronism), extracellular shift (acidosis), and insulin deficiency (insulin promotes entry of glucose and potassium into the cell). Tissue breakdown (rhabdomyolysis, trauma, hemolysis, and tumor lysis after chemotherapy) increases plasma levels. Drugs which may increase levels include penicillin antibiotics, cancer drugs, ACE inhibitors, heparin, potassium penicillin, isoniazid, lithium, potassium-sparing diuretics (spironolactone, triamterene), and potassium supplements. Symptoms of hyperkalemia include nausea, vomiting, diarrhea, irritability, electrocardiogram changes and, on occasion, cardiac arrest. Potassium supplementation should be given cautiously in those on potassium-sparing diuretics, ACE inhibitors and digitalis, and those with impaired renal function.

CHLORIDE (CL⁻)

Normal Values

- Adult/elderly
  90 - 110 mEq/l
  98 - 106 mmol/l
- Child
  90 - 110 mEq/l
- Newborn
  96 - 106 mEq/l

Increased

- Dehydration
- Renal tubular acidosis
- Excess saline infusion
- Cushing's syndrome
- Eclampsia
- Multiple myeloma
- Kidney dysfunction
- Metabolic acidosis

Chloride is the major extracellular anion. It exists in combination as sodium chloride or as hydrochloric acid. It influences water balance, serum osmolality, and acid-base balance. When carbon dioxide increases and blood becomes more acid, bicarbonate moves out of cells into the blood. Chloride will then shift into the cell to maintain electrical neutrality. Chloride deficiency and excess rarely occur alone and levels follow those of sodium.

Signs of hypochloremia include hyperexcitability of nerves and muscles, shallow breathing, hypotension, and tetany. Drugs which may decrease serum levels include aldosterone, bicarbonates, corticosteroids, loop diuretics, thiazide diuretics, and triamterene.

Signs of hyperchloremia include lethargy, weakness, and deep breathing. Drugs which may increase plasma levels include acetazolamide, ammonium chloride, androgens, chlorothiazide, cortisone, estrogens, guanethidine, hydrochlorothiazide, methyldopa, and nonsteroidal antiinflammatory drugs (NSAIDS).

Test	**Clinical Significance**

• Hyperventilation
• Anemia

Decreased

• Overhydration
• Congestive heart failure
• Syndrome of inappropriate antidiuretic hormone (SIADH)
• Vomiting
• Gastric suction
• Chronic respiratory
• Acidosis
• Salt-losing nephritis
• Addison's disease
• Burns
• Metabolic alkalosis
• Diuretic therapy
• Hypokalemia

CALCIUM (CA^{++})

Normal Values

Total calcium
• Adult
  9 - 10.5 mg/dl
  2.25 - 2.75 mmol/L
• Child
  8.8 - 10.8 mg/dl
  2.2 - 2.7 mmol/L
• Newborn
  9 - 10.6 mg/dl
  2.3 - 2.65 mmol/L
• Slightly lower values in the elderly
Ionized calcium
• Adult
  4.5 - 5.6 mg/dl
  1.05 - 1.30 mmol/L

Increased

• Excess vitamin D
• Milk-alkali syndrome (excess milk and antacid intake)
• Malignant tumors (especially breast, renal, lung)
• Hyperparathyroidism
• Hyperthyroidism
• Granulomatous disease (sarcoidosis, TB)
• Addison's disease

Calcium has roles in muscle contraction, cardiac function, nerve conduction, and blood clotting. A typical calcium intake is one gram per day, about 75% from dairy products. Absorption in the duodenum and proximal jejunum is about 20-30%. Approximately 98% of calcium is stored in the bones and teeth. They act as calcium reserves for maintaining blood levels. Three hormones help regulate calcium. Parathyroid hormone (PTH) affects bone and the kidney to increase blood calcium. Vitamin D in its active form increases calcium and phosphate absorption and enhances the effects of PTH. Calcitonin inhibits bone breakdown and the influence of PTH and vitamin D.

Calcium exists in the blood in two forms. About 45% is free (ionized) and the rest is bound to albumin. Total calcium measures both. Because a number of factors influence ionized calcium it cannot be reliably estimated from total calcium. When serum albumin is low, total calcium is low due to decreased binding. As a rule, calcium decreases 0.8 mg for every one gram decrease in albumin. A normal total calcium with a low albumin means hypercalcemia. Ionized calcium is not affected by albumin and thus is considered by many to be more sensitive and reliable.

The most common causes of hypocalcemia include use of citrated blood products during surgery, renal disease, parathyroid insufficiency, pancreatitis, vitamin D deficiency, and magnesium deficiency (due to decreased secretion of PTH). In renal disease hyperparathyroidism often compensates for the low calcium that results from binding by excess phosphate or hypocalcemia caused by insufficient activation of vitamin D by the kidney. Decreased ionized calcium can cause cardiovascular disorders (cardiac insufficiency, arrhythmias) and neuromuscular irritability (irregular muscle spasms or tetany). A chronic deficiency may lead to depression and psychosis. For better absorption oral calcium supplements are best taken 1 to 1 1/2 hours after meals in divided doses and used cautiously in those with low gastric acidity (e.g. elderly, AIDS).

Test	Clinical Significance

- Paget's disease of bone
- Cancer (lung, renal)
- Acromegaly
- Prolonged immobilization, bone fractures
- Hodgkins, lymphoma, leukemia
- Multiple
- Sarcoidosis
- Renal transplant
- Drugs

Decreased
- Hypoparathyroidism
- Renal failure
- Renal transplant
- Rickets, osteomalacia
- Hyperphosphatemia
- Vitamin D deficiency
- Fat malabsorption (fatty acids bind calcium)
- Acute pancreatitis
- Alcoholism, cirrhosis
- Hypoalbuminemia
- Hypomagnesemia
- Hemodilution
- Drugs

Hyperparathyroidism, malignancies, and granulomatous diseases are the prime causes of elevated levels. Other causes include excessive calcium or vitamin D intake, immobilization, and drugs. Malignancies may affect bone directly by increasing breakdown, or by secreting PTH-like substances. Symptoms of hypercalcemia include constipation, anorexia, nausea, vomiting, abdominal pain, polyuria, and renal stones. Calcium should be used cautiously in patients receiving digitalis or who have calcium deposition in soft tissue (e.g. renal calculi). Excess vitamin D in hyperparathyroidism may cause hypercalcemia.

Drugs that may increase calcium levels include calcium supplements, hydralazine, lithium, thiazide diuretics, and vitamin D.

Drugs that may decrease calcium levels include acetazolamide, anticonvulsants, aspirin, calcitonin, cisplatin, corticosteroids, heparin, laxatives, loop diuretics, magnesium salts, and oral contraceptives.

MAGNESIUM (MG^{++})
Normal Values
- Adult
  1.2 - 2.0 mEq/L
  0.6 - 1.0 mmol/L
- Child
  1.4 - 1.7 mEq/L
  0.71 - 0.78 mmol/L
- Newborn
  1.2 - 1.8 mEq/L
  0.6 - 0.9 mmol/L

Increased
- Uncontrolled diabetes
- Renal insufficiency
- Addison's disease
- Hypothyroidism
- Excess intake (magnesium-containing antacids, laxatives, enemas salts, TPN)
- Dehydration

Magnesium is important for muscle contraction, nerve conduction, and is a cofactor in over 300 enzymes. Good sources are green vegetables, meat, grains, and seafood. About 20 to 60% is absorbed in the small intestine, depending on need. Fat malabsorption reduces absorption by forming insoluble soaps with magnesium. Ninety-nine percent of magnesium is split between bone and soft tissue. Body content is primarily regulated by the kidney. Calcium, magnesium, and phosphorus are all intracellular electrolytes and regulated by vitamin D and PTH. A depletion of one is associated with depletion of the others.

Causes of magnesium depletion include inadequate intake, malabsorption (diarrhea, fistula, malabsorption syndromes), and increased excretion (alcoholism, chronic renal disease). Hypomagnesemia is common in diabetics and is associated with decreased PTH, altered vitamin D metabolism, and insulin deficiency or resistance. Adequate dietary intake is important. In alcoholics hypomagnesemia is from a combination of poor intake, vomiting, diarrhea, increased excretion, and hyperaldosteronism. Requirements increase in pregnancy and premature labor and preeclampsia/eclampsia are associated with a deficiency. Those with Paget's disease of the bone have more active disease with hypomagnesemia, probably from increased mineral uptake by bone. Elevated intake is recommended. Levels can drop acutely from

Test	Clinical Significance

- Adrenalectomy
- Hemolysis

Decreased

- Diabetic acidosis
- Hemodialysis
- Pancreatitis
- Hemodialysis
- Hyperaldosteronism
- Diuretic abuse
- Inadequate intake
- Malabsorption syndromes
- Chronic renal disease
- Hypoparathyroidism
- Hyperthyroidism
- Acoholism,
- Toxemia of pregnancy

PHOSPHATE
(P, Phosphate, PO₄)

Normal Values

- Adult
  3.0 - 4.5 mg/L
  0.97 - 1.45 mmol/L
- Child
  4.5 - 6.5 mg/dl
  1.45 - 2.10 mmol/L
- Newborn
  4.3 - 9.3 mg/dl
  1.4 - 3.0 mmol/L
- Slightly lower values in the elderly

Increased

- Excess intake (IV, oral, laxatives, enemas)
- Excess vitamin D
- Hypoparathyroidism
- Renal failure
- Acromegaly
- Bone metastases
- Hypocalcemia
- Addison's disease
- Sarcoidosis
- Liver disease, cirrhosis
- Hemolysis

Decreased

- Inadequate intake

intracellular shifts with the administration of glucose or amimo acids, especially following starvation or insulin therapy for hyperglycemia. Protein loading may increase urinary excretion. Several drugs (diuretics, aminoglycoside antibiotics, cisplatin, and cyclosporine) increase renal loss of magnesiuim.

Symptoms of deficiency include anorexia, nausea, vomiting, weakness, lethargy, muscle tremors, tetany, hypocalcemia, and cardiac dysfunction (coronary vasospasm, arrhythmias, acute infarct, sudden death).

Hypermagnesemia is uncommon and most cases result from magnesium-containing drugs (antacids, laxatives, enemas, salts), excess in TPN solutions, or renal failure. Symptoms include hypotension, lethargy, and respiratory depression. Magnesium should be given cautiously in renal dysfunction. Adequate protein intake is needed for best magnesium retention. At least two mEq are needed per gram of nitrogen for anabolism.

Phosphorus has roles in bone formation, acid-base balance, and energy transfer. Phosphate is widespread in foods and dietary deficiency is uncommon. Good sources include high protein foods (meat, beans), and bran. Carbonated beverages can also be a significant source. Intake is reported to be one to two grams per day. Absorption is very efficient (70 to 90%) but is reduced by antacids and vitamin D deficiency. The kidney excretes excess phosphate under the influence of PTH which inhibits renal reabsorption. Most is combined in the skeleton with calcium as hydroxyapatite. Fifteen percent is in the blood as a phosphate salt. Most phosphate is intracellular.

Blood levels are regulated by PTH, vitamin D, and growth hormone. PTH increases both phosphate absorption and excretion (by inhibiting renal reabsorption). Vitamin D increases both intestinal absorption and renal reabsorption. Growth hormone also plays a role in controlling blood levels by decreasing renal excretion of phosphate. Calcium and phosphorus have an inverse relationship. A decrease in one increases the other.

Causes of hypophosphatemia include infusion of glucose (TPN, treatment of diabetic ketoacidosis) as phosphate enters the cells with glucose. Intracellular shifts of phosphate also occur with alkalosis (hyperventilation), refeeding of starved persons, and recovery from burns. Vitamin D deficiency, and binding by antacids (aluminum hydroxide, magnesium hydroxide, aluminum carbonate) reduce absorption. Excretion is increased by diuretics and hyperparathyroidism. Mannitol may also reduce serum levels. Hypophosphatemia is seen with excess antacid use.

Symptoms include cardiopulmonary dysfunction, neuromuscular dysfunction (weakness), glucose intolerance, impaired phagocytosis, red cell dysfunction (impaired release of oxygen by hemoglobin), CNS dysfunction (confusion, seizures), and with chronic deficiency rickets in children and osteomalacia in adults. Severe deficiency leads to decreased

Test	Clinical Significance

- Chronic antacid use
- Chronic diuretic use
- Hyperparathyroidism
- Hypercalcemia
- Chronic alcoholism
- Vitamin D deficiency
- Osteomalacia/rickets
- Continuous IV glucose
- Hyperinsulinemia
- Diabetic acidosis

phosphate-containing compounds like ATP, which in turn is the cause of most symptoms, ie. muscle weakness, respiratory and myocardial insufficiency, and liver damage.

The most frequent cause of hyperphosphatemia is decreased renal excretion by diseased kidneys. Other potential causes include excess intake (enemas, laxatives, IV solutions), excess vitamin D, or increased cell breakdown with infection, extreme exercise, rhabdomyolysis, or treatment of neoplastic disease (tumor lysis syndrome). Neonates may also have elevated levels because of an immature regulating system. Drugs that may increase phosphate levels include methicillin, and excess vitamin D.

Symptoms include paralysis, confusion, weakness, hypertension, arrhythmias, and calcium phosphate deposition in soft tissues, especially when hypercalcemia also present.

Infusion of TPN solutions should provide adequate phosphate, especially in the malnourished and those with chronic diuretic or antacid use. Several recommendations for supplementation have been made (e.g., 0.14 mmol/k/d or 30 - 60 mEq/d for adults). Two mEq phosphate approximately equals one mmol or 31 mg. Lipids are also a source of phosphate (7.5 mmol/500 cc). The retention of one gram of nitrogen is associated with retention of 809 mg (0.8g) of phosphate.

BICARBONATE

Bicarbonate is the main extracellular buffer. Along with the lungs, kidneys, and other buffer systems it helps maintain the pH of the extracellular fluid. Bicarbonate is in equilibrium with carbon dioxide and carbonic acid (dissolved carbon dioxide) and is interconverted depending upon blood pH, respiratory and kidney function. Plasma bicarbonate levels and pH are controlled by lung ventilation and renal excretion. See acid-base balance elsewhere in this chapter.

TESTS OF TRACE ELEMENT STATUS

Trace elements are those that are present in the body in very small amounts (less than 100 mgs). When deficient they can have significant effects on body function. About 20 are believed essential. Four (zinc, iron, iodine, selenium) have Recommended Daily Allowances. Five others (chromium, copper, fluoride, manganese, molybdenum) have Estimated Safe and Adequate Daily Dietary Intakes established. Only 10 have been added to TPN solutions. The American Medical association has established guidelines for administration of only four (zinc, copper, chromium, and manganese). Below is some of what is currently known about some of these trace elements.

Test	Clinical Significance
ZINC (Zn) **Reference Range** • Plasma 　10.7 - 18.4 µmol/L 　70 - 120 µg/dl • Serum values 　5 - 15% higher than plasma • Fasting values < 10.7 mol/L 　suggests marginal intake • Urine 　2.3 - 15.3 µmol/d 　0.15 - 1.0 mg/d **Increased** • Zinc therapy (Wilson's disease) • Contaminated food/beverage (galvanized container storage) • Excess intake (supplements) • Excess inhalation (metal fumes) • Hemolysis • Tissue necrosis **Decreased** • Inadequate intake (alcoholics, vegetarians, anorexia nervosa) • TPN without zinc supplement • Stress states (infection, inflammation) • Steroids • Pregnancy/estrogen • Hypoalbuminemia (reduced binding) • Alcoholism, cirrhosis • Sickle cell anemia, thalassemia • Penicillamine therapy (Wilson's disease) • Burns	Zinc in a cofactor in over 300 enzymes which are important to cell growth and replication, sexual maturation and reproduction, collagen synthesis, wound healing, taste acuity, night vision, and immune function. Good sources are meat, liver, eggs, seafood (especially oysters). Absorption is normally about 30% and reduced by dietary phytate and fiber (although more of a problem worldwide than in the U.S.). Zinc competes with copper for absorption. Zinc is transported in the blood mainly by albumin. About 55% of zinc is loosely bound to protein and available for metabolic use. About 40 % is tightly bound and is not. In alcoholic cirrhosis serum albumin has a decreased affinity for zinc. Most excretion is via intestinal secretions, especially pancreatic secretions. Only a small amount is lost via urine (500 µg/d), although urinary loss may be elevated with cirrhosis, high alcohol intake, sickle cell anemia, and post surgical status. Minor losses occur through hair, skin, and sweat. A variety of tests (serum, saliva, urine, and red cell zinc, enzyme function, and taste acuity) have been used to evaluate zinc status. To date there is no one defining test of a deficiency. Levels may also be difficult to interpret. When albumin levels are down (in stress and malnutrition) zinc levels will be low despite adequate stores. Steroid therapy, exogenous estrogen, and pregnancy decrease zinc levels. Inflammation and infection produce an acute redistribution of zinc to the liver and tissues. Levels may fall by half. Alkaline phosphatase can be a good index of zinc deficiency as below normal levels are associated with zinc deficiency. Plasma levels are elevated by short term fasting, hemolysis, and tissue necrosis. A deficiency is usually due to poor intake associated with increased loss. It is prevalent in pregnancy and lactation due to increased urinary or lactation loss. Decreased absorption is associated with small bowel disease. Deficiency symptoms include skin lesions, behavioral changes, diarrhea, depression, impaired taste acuity, impaired wound healing, alopecia, night blindness, and growth retardation. Diarrhea continues even without enteral feeding if due to zinc deficiency. Deficiency is treated with zinc sulfate to provide 25 - 50 mg/d elemental zinc. Excess zinc can be toxic although 50 - 100 mg/d can be tolerated if infused steadily over 24 hours. Zinc should be monitored frequently in TPN patients. Positive zinc balance is important to nitrogen retention and anabolism in nutritionally

Test	Clinical Significance

• Small bowel disease (Crohn's, short bowel, jejunoileal bypass)

depleted patients. TPN patients maintained in positive zinc balance show improved nitrogen retention and insulin secretion.

The AMA Expert panel recommended 2.5 - 4 mg/d. An additional 2 mg is recommended in acute catabolic states. Larger doses will be needed with a deficiency or if there are large losses of intestinal fluid (diarrhea or ileostomy output), Twelve to 17 mg/L of small bowel fluid is recommended. For tumor-bearing adults on TPN 70 - 80 μg/kg/d is suggested.

COPPER (Cu)
Reference Range
• Male
 70 - 140 μg/dl
 11 - 22 μmol/L
• Female
 80 - 155 μg/dl
 12.6 - 24.4 μmol/L
• Pregnancy
 120 - 300 μg/dl
 18.9 - 47.2 μmol/L
• Ages 6 - 12 yr
 12.6 - 29.9 μmol/L
 80 - 190 μg/dl
• Infants
 3.1 - 11 μmol/L
 20 - 70 μg/dl
• Diurnal variation (highest values in the AM)

Increased
• Wilson's disease
• Excess intake (copper salts)
• Contaminated water or dialysis fluid
• Oral contraceptives
• Pregnancy
• Infection
• Smoking
• Malignancy
• Inflammation

Decreased
• Hypochromic anemia unresponsive to iron
• Steroids
• Penicillamine therapy
• Burns, stress

Copper is a component of many enzymes and involved in red and white blood cell formation, bone mineralization, elastin and collagen synthesis, and antioxidant protection. Good sources are organ meats, seafood, nuts, and seeds.

Forty to 50% is absorbed in the stomach and duodenum. Copper competes for absorption with iron and zinc, and absorption is reduced by excess fiber intake. Excretion is mainly through bile. The liver is the prime storage site. Ninety five percent of plasma copper is bound to ceruloplasmin. Transportation to the tissues may be limited by protein depletion due to inadequate synthesis of ceruloplasmin.

Higher levels are found in women (due to higher ceruloplasmin levels stimulated by estrogen in pregnancy and oral contraceptive use), smokers, cirrhosis, malignancy, and in inflammatory states (infection, surgery).

A deficiency is suggested by neutropenia, a microcytic and hypochromic anemia, low reticulocyte count, adequate iron status, and low copper and ceruloplasmin levels. Increased loss is associated with stress, burns, biliary fistula, and GI suction. Severe deficiency is rare. The main abnormalities reported in TPN-induced deficiency are microcytosis and neutropenia. Other symptoms include skin pallor, and hair depigmentation. A deficiency is rapidly corrected with 1 mg/d but maintenance levels will also correct abnormalities. The chelating drug penicillamine and amino acids in the TPN may increase renal excretion.

Diagnosis of overload may be difficult due to factors that increase serum levels. Toxicity is mainly from excess intake, IV or oral. Administration of copper in gram amounts acutely produces hemolytic anemia, and hepatic necrosis. Chronic excess may result in liver accumulation and damage.

Copper should be routinely supplemented in TPN. An intake of 0.5 to 1.5 mg/d is recommended by the AMA expert panel, although this recommendation may be too high as balance is reported with 0.25 mg/d and repletion has been demonstrated with 0.4 to 1.0 mg/d. Supplementation should be used cautiously in conditions of overload (Wilson's disease), biliary obstruction, intrahepatic cholestasis (primary biliary cirrhosis), and liver disease (cirrhosis).

Test	Clinical Significance

- Biliary fistula
- Excess zinc intake

CHROMIUM (Cr)
Reference Values
- Plasma
  0.3 µg/L
- Serum
  0.03 - 18 ng/ml

Chromium is a component of glucose tolerance factor (GTF) which promotes the action of insulin at tissue level. Chromium may also have a role in lipoprotein metabolism. The bioavailability of chromium in cheese, calf liver, and wheat germ is relatively high. The best assurance of an adequate intake is with a varied diet.

Average intake is 60 - 90 µg/d and 0.5 - 2% is absorbed, with greater absorption at the lower intakes. Absorption is reduced by excess fiber and phytates. After absorption chromium is incorporated into glucose tolerance factor (GTF) in the liver. Carbohydrate intake promotes the release of GTF along with insulin. During its presence in the circulation chromium is filtered by the kidney, the prime route of excretion. This normally follows a cyclic pattern with increased excretion following meals. TPN may promote continuous release and excretion of chromium and make documentation of a deficiency difficult.

Assessment of status is difficult. Expected serum levels are 0.038 µg/L or greater. Low serum and hair levels are associated with aging, increased parity, juvenile diabetes, and coronary artery disease.

Deficiency is generally a result of inadequate supplementation in association with excess glucose (e.g. TPN). Symptoms include glucose intolerance unresponsive to insulin, weight loss, excessive insulin needs, peripheral neuropathy, metabolic encephalopathy, and hyperlipidemia. Diagnosis is best confirmed with improved glucose tolerance after supplementation. This may be done with glucose tolerance testing. Blood sugar should be monitored during supplementation as insulin needs may decrease.

The toxicity of chromium III is very low. Chromium IV (industrial contact) is more toxic. Excess exposure is associated with dermatitis, hepatitis, GI disorders, organ deposition, and with chronic exposure, lung cancer.

Daily supplementation is recommended in TPN, especially if needed for an extended time. The AMA expert committee recommends 10 - 15 µg/d for stable adults.

FLUORIDE (Fl)
Reference Values
- Plasma
  10 - 200 µg/L
  0.5 - 10.5 µmol/L
- Blood
  50 - 500 µg/L

The only known role of fluoride is its presence in bones and teeth, reducing the incidence of dental caries (when present during tooth formation) and osteoporosis. It is widespread in food, but the main source is fluoridated water. Fluoride-containing dental products can also be a significant source.

Average intake is 0.5 to 5 mg/d with about 80% absorbed from the stomach and intestines. About 20% of intake is retained and most of this (95%) is deposited as fluoroapatite in bones and teeth. About 50% of

Test	Clinical Significance

2.6 - 26.3 µmol/L
- Urine
  0.2 - 3.2 mg/L
  0.01 - 17 mmol/L
- Levels increase with age
  200 - 300 µg/dl associated
  with fatality

fluoride is excreted through urine over the next 24 hours. Acidification of urine increases resorption by the kidney, alkalinization reduces it.

There are no symptoms associated with a deficiency except for increased dental caries and osteoporosis.

Supplemental fluoride may not be appropriate for those in geographical areas with high fluoride levels. Pregnant women and infants should be supplemented cautiously due to limited capacity for the fetus and infants to excrete the mineral. Excess intake during tooth formation produces fluorosis (mottling, enamel hypoplasia). Hypermineralization of bone indicates skeletal fluorosis and can be crippling. Five to ten grams is fatal. The acidity of gastric contents produces hydrofluoric acid which is corrosive to mucous membranes.

Parenteral fluoride requirements are not available. The AMA expert panel did not make recommendations but others have suggested 1 - 2 mg/day for adults. Supplementation is recommended for growing children or adolescents and patients with osteoporosis during long term TPN. Fluoride toxicity has not been associated with TPN. Fluoride status is rarely measured in TPN patients. Unknown quantities are received as a contaminant in the water used to prepare the solutions. It is prudent to periodically assess for toxicity in those suspectedof having a high body content or who show massive bone loss or demineralization. Whole blood or urine levels can be used.

IRON (Fe)

Normal Values
- Male
  75 - 175 µg/dl
- Female
  65 - 165 µg/dl
- Children
  50 - 120 µg/dl
- Newborn
  100 - 250 µg/dl

Increased
- Alcoholism
- Hemolytic anemia (thalassemia)
- Hemochromatosis (excess absorption)
- Acute hepatitis or necrosis
- Lead poisoning
- Excess intake (oral, IV, iron cooking pots, transfusions)

Decreased
- Chronic blood loss
- Late pregnancy

Iron has a prime role in oxygen and carbon dioxide transport as a component of red cell hemoglobin. Good sources include, meat, eggs, vegetables, and fortified cereal products.

Average intake is 15 mg/d (10 in the elderly). Men need 1 mg/d, women 2 mg/d, and pregnant women 4 mg/d. Absorption is regulated by the intestine in response to need and reserves. Absorption is increased by a low pH, ascorbic acid, and the presence of amino acids. Absorption is reduced by excess fiber, tannins, oxalates, carbonates, phosphates, and divalent cations (copper, zinc, calcium, magnesium). Iron is recycled and potential for elimination is limited, primarily through desquamation of skin and intestinal cells.

Normal levels are > 60 µg/dl. With infection iron is redistributed to the liver so it is unavailable to bacteria which have high iron needs. Ferritin levels, a good index of iron stores, are elevated with inflammation, giving misleading results.

A deficiency is the primary cause of anemia and results from decreased intake, decreased absorption (e.g. post-gastrectomy), and excess loss (menstruation, gastrointestinal bleeding). Common symptoms include shortness of breath with exertion, pallor, and tachycardia.

Iron toxicity results in the deposition of excess iron in body organs. This can be from excess intake (frequently associated with excess alcohol and ascorbic acid), multiple transfusions, or excess accumulation from disease (thalassemia, hemochromatosis).

Test	Clinical Significance
• Insufficient intake • Excess loss (menstruation) • Inadequate absorption (gastrectomy)	The AMA expert committee made no recommendations for adding iron to TPN. Others have suggested 0.5 to 5 mg as maintenance levels. It is usually omitted from TPN short term, relying on iron stores. It is recommended in long term TPN and possibly with pregnancy. Other nutrients important to red cell formation (folate, pyridoxine, vitamin B$_{12}$, copper, and protein) should also be adequate. Subjects should be monitored for iron deficiency as well as iron overload during supplementation.

MANGANESE (Mn)
Reference Values
• Serum/plasma
  7.0 - 20 nmol/L
  0.4 - 1.1 ng/ml
  0.38 - 1.04 µg/L
• Whole blood
  140 - 220 nmol/L
  7.7 - 12.1 ng/ml
• Urine
  0 - 0.3 µg/dl
 	
Increased
• Hepatitis
• Postnecrotic cirrhosis
• Cholestasis
• Industrial exposure
	Manganese is involved with formation of connective tissue, growth, reproduction, and carbohydrate and lipid metabolism. It is widespread throughout the food supply.
	
	Average intake is 3.5 mg/d. Absorption is about 50% and is reduced by phytates, iron, calcium, and phosphate. Storage is concentrated in the liver. Most loss occurs via biliary, and to some extent, intestinal secretions.
	
	Currently there are no readily available, reliable tests.
	
	One deficiency has been reported in humans. Symptoms included impaired growth, skeletal abnormalities, decreased reproductive function, and ataxia.
	
	Higher serum levels are found with in hepatitis, postnecrotic cirrhosis, cholestasis, and chronic (industrial) exposure.
	
	Unsupplemented TPN is associated with negative manganese balance but there is minimal evidence for TPN-induced deficiency. Recommended maintenance levels are 0.15 to 0.8 mg/d but should be less for patients with cholestasis or biliary disease.

MOLYBDENUM (Mb)
Reference Range
• Plasma
  0.1 - 3 µg/L
  1.0 - 31.3 nmol/L
• Whole blood
  0.8 - 3.3 µg/L
  8.3 - 34.4 nmol/L
 	
Increased
• Excess intake (supplements, tungsten exposure)
 	
Decreased
• Sulfite oxidase deficiency (inborn error of metabolism)
• Prolonged TPN without supplementation
	Molybdenum acts as a cofactor for several oxidation-reduction enzymes. Xanthine oxidase catabolizes the oxidation of xanthine to uric acid. The metabolism of sulfur-containing amino acids methionine and cystine are dependent on sulfite oxidase. Purines are detoxified by aldehyde oxidase. Thus manganese is considered essential to man.
	
	Average intake is 200 - 500 µg/d with wide variations by geographical area. It is rapidly and well absorbed in the upper GI tract. The largest amount is stored in the liver. Most loss is via the urine with small amounts eliminated in bile. A low protein intake seems to impair the liver's ability to store the element. High levels of molybdenum promote hepatic copper retention.
	
	Monitoring status is difficult with few interpretive guidelines and test methodology available. Plasma levels vary widely with geographical area. If a deficiency or toxicity is suspected, levels of purines, sulfate, and copper should be measured.
	
	Dietary deficiencies are not reported. Excess losses occur with active Crohn's disease. A reported deficiency in a Crohn's patient with short

Test	Clinical Significance

bowel syndrome was associated with symptoms of increased heart and respiratory rates, headaches, nausea, vomiting, night blindness, lethargy, and edema. Biochemical changes included low plasma uric acid levels and high methionine and sulfate levels.

High dietary intakes are associated with a high incidence of hyperuricemic gout, and high levels of molybdenum, uric acid, and xanthine oxidase. Molybdenum has a low toxicity but it does cause significant urinary copper losses and a chronic daily intake of more than 0.5 mg should not be exceeded. A high copper and low molybdenum intake can adversely affect iron status.

The element is not widely added to TPN. Supplementation recommendations were not made by the AMA's Expert Panel but others recommend 100 - 200 µg/d. Use caution with supplementing pregnant subjects and neonates due to decreased capacity to excrete excess. Levels should be adjusted for renal dysfunction and biliary obstruction. Molybdenum should not be included unless copper is present as it can aggravate a copper deficiency.

SELENIUM (Se)
Reference Range
- Serum/plasma
  0.58 - 1.82 µmol/L
  46 - 143 ng/ml
- Whole blood
  74 - 2.97 µmol/L
  58 - 234 ng/ml
- Urine
  0.1 - 2 µmol/L
  7 - 160 µg/L
- Hair
  2.5 - 17.8 nmol/g
  0.2 - 1.4 µg/g
- Lower levels in newborns

Increased
- Increased intake (supplements)
- Keshan's disease/juvenile cardiomyopathy (high soil content)
- Industrial exposure
- Reticuloendothelial neoplasia

Decreased
- Inadequate intake (low soil content)
- TPN without supplementation
- Pregnancy
- Gastrointestinal cancer

Selenium is a component of the enzyme glutathione peroxidase, a free radical scavenger and important antioxidant. Average intake is 83 - 129 µg/d. Estimated safe and adequate dietary intakes is 50 - 200 µg/d for adults. Absorption is 50 - 75%. Excretion is mainly via urine. Best sources are cereals, seafood, and organ meats.

Plasma levels are a better index of status as they are more sensitive to changes in intake and disease. They vary with geographical area. Erythrocyte glutathione peroxidase assay is useful to detect a deficiency as selenium is a component.

A deficiency has been seen in very malnourished children and unsupplemented TPN patients. At risk are premature infants, growing children, and those with low intake (mainly foods from selenium-poor soil). Decreased levels are seen in critical illness due to increased loss. Symptoms include muscle weakness, myalgias, pancreatic degeneration, macrocytosis, and red cell fragility, and with chronic depletion, cardiomyopathy.

Toxicity is reported with industrial exposure (frequently lung disease) and in those living in areas of high soil concentration. Symptoms include chronic dermatitis, hair and nail loss, fatigue, pulmonary edema, and garlic odor on the breath. Short term excess exposure usually doesn't cause problems. Urine levels give a good indication of excess exposure. A maximum chronic intake should not exceed 200 µg/d. There has been no reported toxicity with TPN.

The AMA Expert panel did not make recommendations but others suggest 30 µg/d is adequate for adults receiving TPN. Use caution with renal disease, pregnancy, and infants due to limited ability to excrete excess. Need may be increased with nasogastric suction, small bowel fistulas, and inflammatory bowel disease.

Test	Clinical Significance

• Protein calorie malnutrition

IODINE (I)
Reference Range
• Plasma
  2 - 4 µg/dl
  60 ng/ml
• Levels < 0.1 µg/dl are associated with goiter
• Urinary excretion of < 40 µg/d indicates a deficiency

Iodine is involved in the synthesis and release of the thyroid hormones which are involved in growth, reproduction, cardiac function, neuromuscular function, and cellular metabolism. The best sources are seafood, eggs, meat, milk, cereal, and iodized salt.

Average intake is 500 µg/d. An intake of 1 µg/d is needed to prevent goiter. Iodine is absorbed mainly through the GI tract but also the lungs, skin, and other mucous membranes. It is concentrated in the thyroid gland as thyroid hormones. Excretion is mainly through urine. Increased metabolism (e.g. exercise, pregnancy) increases urinary excretion. Profuse sweating increases skin loss.

Essentially all iodine in the blood is present as the thyroid hormones triiodothyronine and thyroxin. Thyroxine-binding globulin, thyroxin-binding prealbumin, and albumin bind 99% of thyroid hormones.

A deficiency leads to reduced synthesis of thyroid hormones, which in turn increases thyroid stimulating hormone. The main symptom is goiter, but others include weight gain, somnolence, cold intolerance, bradycardia, hypertension, dry skin, constipation, and weakness. Urinary excretion of less than 40 µg/d indicates a deficiency. Deficiency is usually the result of inadequate intake or excess foods containing goitrogens (cabbage, cassava, rutabagas, turnips) which make iodine unavailable to the thyroid. It may also result from gland failure, or reduced thyroid-stimulating hormone (TSH) due to pituitary or hypothalmic dysfunction. Iodine needs are increased by a cold environment, stress, goitrogenic foods, and antithyroid medications.

Excess iodine intake from drugs (amiodarone), radiographic contrast media, and germicides can cause excess body stores, decreased thyroid hormone synthesis, hypothyroidism, and goiter. Oral intakes of 10 times recommended levels do not have negative effects.

Supplements are not usually needed in short-term TPN because of cutaneous absorption of iodine from iodine-containing germicides.

No adverse reactions have been reported to recommended routine supplementation in TPN. Recommended parenteral supplementation for adults on long-term TPN is 70 - 300 µg/d. Several tests of thyroid function are available to assess iodine adequacy but they are not usually done in TPN patients.

TABLE 7: Suggested Adult Daily Parenteral Intake of Trace Minerals

Nutrient	Stable	Catabolic	GI Losses
Zinc	2.5 - 4 mg	2 mg additional	12.2 mg/L small bowel fluid 17.1 mg/kg stool or ileostomy output
Copper	0.5 - 1.5 mg		
Chromium	10 - 15 μg		20 μg
Manganese	0.15 - 0.8 mg		

TABLE 8: Estimated Safe and Adequate Daily Intake of Trace Minerals

Nutrient	Amount
Chromium	10 - 200 μg
Copper	0.4 - 3 mg
Fluoride	0.1 - 4 mg
Manganese	0.3 - 5 mg
Molybdenum	15 - 250 μg

TESTS OF VITAMIN STATUS

Nutrient	Clinical Significance

VITAMIN A
(Retinol)
(Retinal)
(Retinoic Acid)

Reference Values
- Serum retinol > 2 years
  20 - 50 µg/dl
  0.7 - 1.75 µmol/L
  Higher levels in males
  Infants
  30 - 200 IU/dl
  9 - 60 µg/dl
- Serum carotene
  0.8 - 4.0 µg/ml
  1.5 - 7.4 µmol/L
  Levels > 250 µg/dl indicate carotenemia

Increased Levels
- Corticosteroids
- Oral contraceptives
- Renal disease
- Hypoparathyroidism

Decreased Levels
- Liver disease
- Stressed states (trauma, infection)
- Protein malnutrition
- Fat malabsorption (cystic fibrosis, sprue, obstructive jaundice, pancreatitis)

Vitamin A is a group of compounds with the biological activity of retinol. The vitamin is essential for vision, growth, cell differentiation, and reproduction. Preformed vitamin A is found in animal tissues. Carotenoid pigments found in plants are converted to vitamin A in the GI tract. Vitamin A activity is expressed in several ways although retinol equivalents is preferred. One retinol equivalent equals 12 µg retinol, 3.33 IU retinol, and 6 mg or 10 IU B-carotene. Good sources of vitamin A include dark green or yellow fruits and vegetables, liver, and dairy products.

Vitamin A is absorbed along with fat and transported by chylomicrons to the liver where it is linked to retinol binding protein (RBP) and stored. When needed it circulates bound to RBP which is complexed in a 1:1 ratio with another hepatic protein, prealbumin. Serum levels of RBP normally vary with the amount of vitamin A that must be carried. After delivery and release of the vitamin, RBP is returned to the kidney for degradation. Ninety percent of the body's vitamin A is stored in the liver. The liver has a huge capacity to store vitamin A but after it reaches a certain level, excess is eliminated through bile. Adequate vitamin E intake increases the ability to retain and utilize vitamin A.

A serum retinol level is the most common measure of vitamin status and reliable if the subject is not malnourished and liver and kidney function are normal. Plasma RBP levels correlate well with retinol levels and offer an alternative if plasma retinol levels are not available. Vitamin A levels are lower in stressed states (infection, trauma, surgery), liver disease, and protein malnutrition when synthesis of RBP and prealbumin are depressed. Levels are higher in renal disease due to less degradation of RBP. Corticosteroids increase vitamin A transport elevating serum levels and depleting reserves. Oral contraceptives elevate plasma vitamin A significantly, probably due to steroid-induced changes in the rate of RBP synthesis and release.

Measuring serum carotene is an indirect measurement of vitamin A status. Increased levels are found with high vegetable intake and hypothyroidism. Low levels are found with low vegetable intake and fat malabsorption. Excess carotenoid intake leads to orange-tinged skin.

Except for stressed states, serum retinol doesn't fall to low levels until liver stores are almost gone. Levels less than 0.7 µmol/L (20 µg/dl) usually indicate low intake and tissue stores. Levels < 10 µg/dl or 0.35 µmol/L indicate severe deficiency. Levels between 0.7 and 1.05 µmol/L need further investigation. Low values are associated with inadequate intake, liver disease, and fat malabsorption. Tissues most affected are rapidly proliferating ones (linings of the mouth, GI tract, respiratory tract, GU tract, cornea, and rapidly growing bone in non-adults and embryos. Initial symptoms are impaired dark adaptation and follicular hyperkeratosis. Severe deficiency is associated with follicular

Test	Clinical Significance

and corneal hyperkeratinization, impaired growth, reduced resistance to infection, and malabsorption. Some drugs alter the livers' ability to store the vitamin.

Adverse reactions are mainly due to excess administration, either IV or IM. When liver storage and retinol-binding capacity is exceeded toxicity develops. Chronic toxicity may result from intakes of 25,000 to 50,000 IU/d for a month. Symptoms include bone and joint pain, hair loss, dry lips, and hepatomegaly. Acute toxicity may result from one excess dose of 25,000 IU/kg. Symptoms include abdominal pain, nausea, vomiting, severe headaches, dizziness, lethargy, and irritability, hair loss, hepatosplenomegaly, jaundice, and leukopenia. When storage capacity is exceeded, retinyl esters are released into the plasma where they bind to cell membranes rupturing them. Serum retinyl esters greater than 10% of plasma retinol levels indicate excessive liver stores and toxicity. High levels are mainly found with vitamin supplements and in renal failure. Risk of toxicity can be reduced by giving vitamin E simultaneously.

The AMA expert panel recommendations for parenteral vitamin A are 3300 IU (1000 mg) per day for adults. Subjects initially low in vitamin A should probably get IM injections as well. Vitamin A requirements in renal disease may be reduced. Vitamin A supplementation according to the AMA expert panel guidelines maintain normal plasma levels. Multiple vitamin solutions should be diluted before IV administration, preferably in at least 500 ml fluid. Pediatric vitamins can be given in 100 ml. Much parenteral vitamin A is lost from adherence to bags and tubing and from photodegradation such that only 1/4 to 1/3 may actually be delivered to the patient. Bile flow during TPN is usually less reducing one route of excretion. Also analysis of parenteral multivitamin formulations has shown significantly higher vitamin A levels than the label indicated.

VITAMIN D
Reference Serum Values
- 25 - OH vitamin D
  25 - 40 ng/ml
Deficient
  < 25 nmol/L
  > 10 ng/ml
Toxic
  > 375 nmol/L

Increased
- Renal disease
- Excess intake

Decreased
- Inadequate intake
- Lack of UV exposure
- Fat malabsorption

Vitamin D has important roles in calcium and phosphate metabolism and bone mineralization. It promotes calcium and phosphorus absorption, stimulates removal of calcium and phosphorus from the bone to maintain serum levels, and promotes reabsorption of calcium by the kidney. Vitamin D_3 (cholecalciferol) is synthesized in the skin from 7-dehydrocholesterol after exposure to UV light. Vitamin D_2 (ergocalciferol) is produced by irradiation of ergosterol, a sterol found in plants. Good sources of vitamin D include fortified dairy products, fortified margarines, fish, and seafood.

Vitamin D is absorbed with other lipid substances in the ileum. Bile is necessary for absorption. The majority of the vitamin is stored in the liver. Excess is excreted primarily through bile and a small amount via the urine. Without oral intake biliary excretion is reduced which leads to accumulation of vitamin D. Vitamin D is activated by hydroxylation first by the liver to 25-hydroxy vitamin D and then by the kidney to 1,25-hydroxy-vitamin D. Activation requires adequate liver and kidney function.

Test	Clinical Significance

• Liver disease
• Renal disease
• Anticonvulsants

Serum 25-hydroxy vitamin D is the most useful measure of status. Because of its long circulating half-life (about 3 weeks) it represents both intake and synthesis in the skin over weeks to months.

Liver and kidney disease reduce the amount of active vitamin D synthesized. A commercial form of 1,25-OH vitamin D is available. Metabolism of vitamin D is also impaired by the drugs phenytoin, and barbiturates, thus the potential for osteomalacia or rickets with chronic use.

Vitamin D should not be given with hypercalcemia or vitamin D toxicity. Excess can lead to calcification of soft tissues. It should also be used cautiously in those with atherosclerosis or coronary artery disease and impaired renal function. Signs of overdose include hypercalcemia, weakness, headache, muscle and bone pain, hypertension, and cardiac arrhythmia's (especially with digitalis). Oral intakes of more than 5000 IU are usually needed to produce toxic symptoms.

The AMA expert panel recommended parenteral intakes of 200 IU/d for those over 11 years of age. This dose appears safe. Additional vitamin can be given IM is needed. Adequate calcium and phosphorus should also be included. Patients should be monitored for hypercalcemia, the first sign of excess. Hypercalcemia may be preceded by a decrease in alkaline phosphatase. If hypercalcemia occurs, calcium levels should be adjusted first and if necessary, vitamin D discontinued. Because of reduced oral intake and biliary stimulation vitamin D may accumulate during TPN.

VITAMIN E
(Tocopherol)
Normal Values
• Plasma tocopherol
  0.5 mg/dl or >
  12 µmol/L or >
• Tocopherol : lipid ratio
Adults
  > 0.8 mg/g lipid
Infants
  > 0.6 mg/g lipid

Increased

• Elevated serum lipids

Decreased

• Cystic fibrosis
• Celiac disease
• Sprue
• Chronic
• Pancreatitis
• Biliary ostruction
• Low serum lipids

Vitamin E is a group of tocopherols that are synthesized by plants and are widely available in foods. Vitamin E acts as a lipid antioxidant, protecting cells from oxidative damage by free radicals. Since these oxidation products can be carcinogenic, vitamin E may help prevent malignancies. Vitamin E requirements are determined by polyunsaturated fat intake. Recommended intakes are 0.4 to 0.6 mg/g polyunsaturated fatty acids. Good sources include vegetable oils, margarines, nuts, egg yolk, and liver.

Twenty-five to 85% of intake is absorbed except in premature infants with underdeveloped digestive systems. Bile is needed for incorporation into micelles prior to absorption. Fat tissue, liver, and muscle contain the most. Excess is metabolized and excreted in the urine. Vitamin E activity is expressed in a-tocopherol equivalents (TE). One mg d-tocopherol equals 1 tocopherol equivalent (TE) or 1.49 IU.

A plasma level of 0.5 mg/dl or higher is considered adequate in children and adults. Plasma levels correlate directly with total lipids, cholesterol, and LDL. If any one is elevated plasma vitamin E may be abnormally high. Conversely, low vitamin E levels may be due to low plasma lipids. Reporting vitamin E levels in relation to lipid levels has been recommended as a more reliable way of reporting status. Plasma tocopherol levels of < 0.8 mg/g lipid in adults or < 0.6 mg/g lipid in infants may indicate a deficiency.

Test	Clinical Significance

Deficiencies in man are uncommon due to its wide distribution. Causes of fat malabsorption (biliary obstruction, chronic pancreatitis, cystic fibrosis, celiac sprue) may produce a deficiency. Neurological and psychomotor symptoms result. Deficiency has also been reported in premature infants. Symptoms include edema, hemolytic anemia, thrombocytosis, and erythematous, papular skin lesions.

Toxicity is not well known but excess intakes may cause transient GI symptoms and competitively inhibit absorption of other fat soluble vitamins.

Supplementation in TPN as part of a multivitamin solution is recommended. The AMA expert panel recommended 10 IU/d in subjects > 11 years. Fat emulsions also supply the vitamin but in variable amounts. As part of a multivitamin solution, when adequately diluted in at least 500 ml of IV fluid, vitamin E is considered safe. The vitamin has also been shown to adhere to delivery bags and tubes.

VITAMIN K
Phylloquinone (Vitamin K_1)
Menaquinones (Vitamin K_2)
Menadione (Vitamin K_3)

Decreased

- Inadequate intake
- Newborns
- Fat malabsorption
- Liver disease (not responsive to vitamin K)
- Biliary insufficiency or obstruction
- Chronic aspirin use
- Mineral oil ingestion
- Broad spectrum antibiotics
- Anticoagulant therapy
- Large dose vitamin E

Vitamin K_1 is found in plants, vitamin K_2 is synthesized by bacteria (up to 50% of requirements), and vitamin K_3 is a synthetic form. The vitamins function as cofactors in the activition of several blood clotting proteins. An intake of 1.0 µg/k/d is adequate to maintain normal blood clotting. Good sources include liver and green, leafy vegetables.

All are absorbed with fat and stored in the liver. The vitamin is excreted in urine and via the GI tract. There is some regeneration or recycling of the vitamin to help conserve stores.

The most used tests of vitamin K status have been functional tests of clotting ability (e.g., prothrombin time) and the normalization of clotting activity after administration of the vitamin. If not normalized, liver dysfunction is suspected.

Deficiency is seen in newborns without active bacterial flora. Symptoms include elevated prothrombin time and possible hemorrhagic disease. It can be prevented with IM or oral vitamin K at birth. Deficiency is also seen with malabsorption, prolonged oral antibiotic therapy, renal insufficiency, anticoagulant therapy, trauma, fasting, and in TPN patients. Anticoagulants interfere with the metabolism of vitamin K thus prolonging clotting time. They also interfere with the regeneration of the vitamin. Large doses of salicylates can also interfere with vitamin K metabolism producing bleeding.

Excess vitamin, when given to subjects on anticoagulants, can promote formation of thromboemboli. Toxicity mainly results from giving excess synthetic vitamin (menadione) which can cause liver damage, hemolytic anemia, and hyperbilirubinemia.

The AMA expert panel recommended 2 - 4 mg/week for TPN patients not on anticoagulants. Some antibiotics may produce deficiency not only by altering gut synthesis but interfering in the activation/metabolism of the

Test	Clinical Significance

vitamin. The vitamin should be supplemented sufficiently to prevent excess bleeding.

VITAMIN C
(Ascorbic Acid)
Normal Values
• Plasma
  23 - 84 µmol/L
  0.4 - 1.5 mg/dl
• Leukocytes
  114 - 301 nmol/108 cells
  20 - 53 µg/108 cells
Higher levels in females
Lower levels in smokers

Ascorbic acid has roles in the synthesis of collagen (important in wound healing), folate and iron metabolism (important in preventing and treating anemia), drug metabolism, amino acid metabolism, synthesis of adrenal hormones, and immune function. Good sources include citrus fruits, berries, melons, tomatoes, green peppers, and leafy vegetables. It is easily destroyed by heat during cooking.

It is readily absorbed in the stomach and upper small intestine, although absorption is significantly reduced with high intakes. Its half-life in the body is 16 days. The average body pool is 1500 mg. About 3 - 4% of this is utilized every day. Intakes of 60 mg/d will usually maintain this body pool. As plasma levels exceed 1.4 mg/dl urinary excretion increases. With large doses ascorbic acid is excreted intact. Sulfonamide drugs, aspirin, and barbiturates also increase urinary excretion.

Plasma and leukocyte (WBC) levels of ascorbic acid are the current methods of choice for determining status. Plasma levels are more sensitive to recent intake, and WBC levels are a better measure of tissue levels and the body pool. Acceptable levels are 0.3 mg/dl or greater. Intakes of > 100 mg/d will saturate body reserves and elevate serum levels above 1.0 mg/dl. Lower plasma levels are found in men, smokers, oral contraceptive users, wound healing, severe emotional stress, chronic and acute infection, trauma, and post surgery.

Levels of less than 11 µmol/L suggest deficiency. Symptoms include swollen/bleeding gums, fatigue, arthralgias, tender and swollen legs, subcutaneous hemorrhages, impaired wound healing, and psychological disturbances. First signs occur with plasma levels of 0.13 to 0.24 mg/dl.

Large oral doses (> 1000 mg) may cause nausea, vomiting, and diarrhea due to its high osmotic effect. Chronic excessive intakes may cause uric acid, cysteine, or oxalate stones, and rebound scurvy when discontinued abruptly. Doses > 600 mg may have a diuretic effect. Large doses also acidify urine, reducing renal excretion of acidic drugs, prolonging their response. Conversely, excretion of alkaline drugs will be increased.

Ascorbic acid is present in parenteral multivitamin solutions. Solutions must be diluted before IV infusion, in at least 500 ml (100 mg for pediatric preparations). The AMA expert panel has recommended doses of 100 mg/d for subjects > 11 years receiving TPN. This level is adequate for nonstressed subjects. More will often be needed in stressed subjects (infections, post surgery). It is best added to TPN on the day of infusion due to potential for destruction by contact with copper.

Test	Clinical Significance

VITAMIN B₁
(Thiamin)

Normal Values

- Serum/plasma
  10 - 64 ng/ml
- Blood
  79 - 178 nmol/L
- Stimulation test
  0 - 15%

Increased

- Excess intake

Decreased

- Alcoholism
- Increased needs (fever, malignancy, pregnancy, dialysis, high carbohydrate intake)
- Diuretics

Thiamin functions as the coenzyme thiamin pyrophosphate in enzymatic reactions involved in energy metabolism. It also has a role in maintaining lipid integrity in the nerve myelin sheaths. Good sources include whole grain or enriched cereals, organ meats, lean pork, legumes, nuts and seeds. Thiamin antagonists present in coffee, tea, betel, and raw fish may alter availability. Recommended intakes are 0.5 mg/1000 calories. Older persons may need more due to less efficient utilization and recommended intake is 1.0 mg/d even with consumption of less than 2000 calories.

Thiamin is rapidly absorbed in the proximal small bowel and transported to the liver. It is excreted in the urine both intact and as its metabolites.

Blood levels are not a useful index of deficiency. Excretion of less than 50 µg/d is considered evidence of a deficiency. The most reliable index of status is the erythrocyte transketolase stimulation test. It measures the activity of the enzyme erythrocyte transketolase (a thiamin-dependent enzyme) in red blood cells both before and after addition of the vitamin. Activity coefficients of greater than 1.3 represent a deficiency. If the results are reported as "percentage of stimulation" or "TPP" effect, normal values are less than 25%.

Deficiencies are usually associated with poverty, disease, or alcoholism. Deficiency may also be exacerbated by increased needs (fever, malignancy, high carbohydrate intake, and TPN. Diuretics increase urinary loss. A deficiency (beriberi) takes several forms. Symptoms include peripheral neurologic symptoms (e.g. foot drop), abnormal electrocardiograms, enlarged heart, dyspnea, and congestive heart failure.

Adverse reactions are uncommon but symptoms include warmth, itching, urticaria, weakness, sweating, nausea, throat tightness, pulmonary edema, and cardiovascular collapse. Doses up to 200 times maintenance are not usually toxic.

The AMA expert panel recommended 3 mg/d in parenteral solutions for those 11 years and older and this appears adequate.

VITAMIN B₂
(Riboflavin)

Normal Values

- Urinary riboflavin excretion
  > 266 nmol/d
  > 100 µg/d
  > 66 µg/g creatinine
  > 19.8 µmol/mol creatinine
- Activity coefficient < 1.3
- Percent stimulation < 30%

Decreased

- Alcoholism
- Chronic barbiturate use

Riboflavin functions mainly as 2 coenzymes in oxidation-reduction reactions in the formation of ATP. Good sources include meat, poultry, fish, dairy products, and enriched grain products. Recommended intake is 0.6 mg/1000 calories.

Riboflavin is readily absorbed in the upper small bowel. The absorption mechanism is saturated at 25 mg. Copper, iron, niacin, ascorbic acid, caffeine, and saccharin may complex with the vitamin reducing its availability. It circulates complexed mainly to albumin. Excess is rapidly excreted in the urine.

Urinary riboflavin excretion is one of two good laboratory tests of riboflavin adequacy currently available. Excretion values of healthy adults are listed at left. Adults excreting less than 1 mg during the 4 hours after a loading dose of 5 mg are considered deficient. Urinary excretion is

Test	Clinical Significance

• Inadequate intake
• Liver disease

increased during fasting and in catabolic or inflammatory states.

A functional test of vitamin status is measurement of erythrocyte glutathione reductase (EGR-a riboflavin-dependent enzyme) activity before and after addition of the cofactor FAD (flavin adenine dinucleotide). Activity increases greater than 30-40% suggest a deficiency. Activity coefficients greater than 1.3 should be confirmed with a urinary riboflavin measurement. Low values can be seen with increased requirements (e.g. tissue repair, testosterone therapy) and with vitamin B deficiencies.

Isolated riboflavin deficiencies are rare. They usually are found with deficiencies of other B complex vitamins. Riboflavin coenzymes are involved in the activation of pyridoxine, folate, niacin, and vitamin K. Deficiency symtoms include glossitis, dermatitis, neuropathy, and a normocytic anemia. The vitamin is light sensitive and newborns treated with phototherapy for hyperbilirubinemia may develop a deficiency. A small supplement is protective.

Toxicity is low and minimal evidence of adverse reactions is seen at recommended IV doses.

The vitamin is essential for TPN solutions. The AMA expert panel recommended 3.6 mg/d for those 11 years or older. This level appears to be adequate. The vitamin may decrease significantly with exposure of the TPN solution to light.

NIACIN
(Nicotinic Acid)
(Niacinamide)
Urinary excretion
• 2-pyridone
  12 mg/d
• N-methyl nicotinamide
  12 mg/d

Decreased

• Hartnup's disease (urinary tryptophan loss)
• Isoniazid drug therapy
• Carcinoid tumors

Niacin refers to both nicotinic acid and niacinamide. They are components of 2 coenzymes involved in protein, fat, and carbohydrate metabolism. Good dietary sources of niacin are legumes, lean red meat, liver, yeast, and poultry. The amino acid tryptophan can be converted to niacin by pyridoxine. Efficiency of conversion varies with the individual. One niacin equivalent equals 60 mg tryptophan or 1 mg niacin. Recommended intake is 6.6 niacin equivalents/1000 calories. A minimum intake of 13 mg is recommended with calorie intakes of less than 2000.

Niacin is readily absorbed, transported to many tissues, and converted into its coenzyme forms, nicotinamide adenine dinucleotide (NAD) and nicotinamide adenine dinucleotide phosphate (NADP) which are required by many cell enzymes.

Blood and urine niacin levels are not considered a reliable index of status. Niacin status is usually determined by measurement of the urinary metabolites 2-pyridone and N-methyl nicotinamide. Excretions of either of less than 10 μmol/d or 1.5 - 2 mg/d indicate low intake and deficient status. Normal excretion is 12 mg/d. A ratio of 2-pyridone to N-methyl nicotinamide ofless than 1.0 is also considered evidence of deficient intake.

Niacin deficiency is known as pellagra with symptoms of diarrhea, dementia, dermatitis and death. Tuberculosis therapy with isoniazid, especially with marginal intake, may produce a deficiency. Isoniazid

Test	Clinical Significance

interferes with pyridoxine metabolism which is required for the formation of niacin from tryptophan. Drug therapy with paramycin and 5-fluorouracil may also precipitate a deficiency. With carcinoid tumors tryptophan is used by the tumor to produce large amounts of serotonin.

Niacin is generally well tolerated. Nicotinic acid (but not niacinamide) in large doses causes vasodilation and a reduction in blood cholesterol. Other side effects include arrythmias and GI distress. Taking aspirin with nicotinic acid blocks the blocks the flushing reaction. Because of the vasodilation effect of large doses, they should be used cautiously with anti-hypertensive drugs.

The recommended parenteral intake of 40 mg/d by the AMA expert panel is considered generous as the contribution of tryptophan was not accounted for.

VITAMIN B₆
(Pyridoxine)
(Pyridoxal)
(Pyridoxamine)

Reference Values
(Pyridoxal-5-phosphate)

• Men
51.8 - 59.8 pmol/ml
• Women
37.6-68.3 pmol/ml

Decreased

• Alcohol abuse
• Malignancies
• Liver disease
• Renal disease
• High protein intake
• Drug therapy (isoniazid, methotrexate, penicillamine, hydralazine, cycloserine, oral contraceptives)

Vitamin B₆ includes the substances pyridoxine, pyridoxal, and pyridoxamine. All 3 forms are phosphorylated to plasma pyridoxal 5-phosphate (PLP), the primary form in the plasma. Their main function is as cofactors for enzymes involved in amino acid, carbohydrate, and lipid metabolism and the conversion of tryptophan to niacin. Good sources include meat, yeast, seeds, and bran. The vitamin is heat sensitive and can be destroyed in cooking.

The vitamin is readily absorbed in the upper small bowel and the liver is the major storage site and responsible for activation of the vitamin. Zinc and riboflavin are also involved.

Plasma pyridoxal-5-phosphate is considered a reliable indicator of vitamin status. It measures the active form and also reflects tissue levels. When intake stops, levels begin falling. Levels less than 20 nmol/L or 5 ng/ml represent deficiency. Levels are also reduced by oral contraceptives, isoniazid, methotrexate, and excess alcohol. Levels can be inversely affected by protein intake.

Pyridoxine can also be measured by microbiological assay, chromatography, or by measuring serum aspartate aminotransferase (SAT) before and after adding vitamin B₆. The vitamin is a cofactor for SAT. A tryptophan loading test also measures vitamin status by measuring urinary xanthurenic acid, a metabolite, after giving 2 grams of tryptophan. If vitamin levels are normal, excretion will exceed 50 µmol/24 hours. This test is not practical due to the need for a timed urine collection.

An isolated deficiency is rare but symptoms include dermatitis, cheilosis, glossitis, microcytic anemia (pyridoxine-responsive), irritability, depression, and convulsions. Alcohol increases vitamin metabolism. Requirements are increased with malignancies and a high protein intake. Vitamin half-life is reduced and plasma clearance rate is increased in renal and liver disease. Several drugs are vitamin antagonists. Isoniazid increases urinary excretion, and is dose related. Penicillamine taken for Wilson's disease complexes with the vitamin. Hydralazine and the

Test	Clinical Significance

antibiotic, cycloserine, interfere with vitamin metabolism. Vitamin supplements are often used with long term intake of these drugs.

Intakes of more than 2 gm/d are reported to cause neuropathy. More than 5 mg/d should be avoided with levadopa therapy. Subjects taking levodopa alone for Parkinson's disease should avoid consuming more than 5 mg/d to avoid reversing drug effect.

Pyridoxine is added to parenteral vitamin mixtures. The recommended level for use in TPN is 4 mg/d for subjects > 11 years.

FOLATE
(Folic Acid)
(Folacin)
(Folinic Acid)

Reference Range

- Serum folate
  6 - 25 ng/ml
- RBC folate
  160 - 800 ng/ml

Decreased

- Inadequate intake (alcohol, lack of fresh foods)
- Malabsorption (celiac disease, blind loop, Crohn's)
- Inadequate utilization (antagonist drugs, vitamin B_{12} deficiency, alcohol, vitamin C deficiency)
- Increased needs (malignancy, pregnancy, growth, lactation, blood formation)
- Increased excretion (dialysis, exfoliative dermatitis)

Folate is a generic term for a group of similar compounds. Folate is important to DNA synthesis, red cell production, and amino acid metabolism. It is widely distributed in food but green leafy vegetables, fruit, and dairy products are good sources. Much can be lost in food preparation as it is heat sensitive. Body stores are limited.

About 50% of dietary folate is bioavailable. Absorption is mainly in the upper small intestine. Vitamin B_{12} is a cofactor in the conversion of folate prior to entering cells from the circulation.

Serum folate is a the most sensitive test of early folate depletion, preceding reductions in red cell folate and anemia. Levels are affected by recent folate intake. Values less than 7 nmol or 3 ng/ml indicate a low intake or negative folate balance. Red cell folate is a better index of tissue stores but misleading if the subject has received transfusions. Red cell folate levels reflect intake over several months because of the 3 month life span of red cells. Levels below 340 nmol/L or 150 ng/ml indicate tissue depletion. Because of the close link between the functions of folate and vitamin B_{12}, both folate and vitamin B_{12} should be measured together. Levels in hospital patients should be checked before initiation of a well balanced diet, nutrition supplements, or transfusions. If red cell levels are measured, vitamim B_{12} should be measured at the same time as it is a cofactor in cell folate uptake. Without adequate amounts of vitamin B_{12}, folate remains trapped in the serum.

A deficiency can result from inadequate intake, impaired absorption, increased needs, or defective metabolism. Poor intake is the most common cause. Symptoms of a deficiency include abnormal DNA synthesis (hypersegmented cells, megaloblastic bone marrow and macrocytic anemia). Alcoholics, the poor, and many elderly are especially susceptible. Malabsorption due to widespread intestinal disease (tropical sprue, gluten-sensitive enteropathy, Crohn's disease) is another common cause. Needs are increased when there is increased cell growth (in the third trimester of pregnancy, lactation, infancy) and in some hyperproliferative disorders (hemolytic anemias) and rapidly dividing tumors (leukemia, high grade lymphoma, small cell carcinoma). Inborn errors of metabolism may also occur. Supplementation is needed in dialysis patients due to dialysis loss.

Certain drugs (methotrexate, aminopterin, pyrimethamine, 5-flurouracil) are folate antagonists because of similar chemical structure. Folinic acid

Test	Clinical Significance

(the active form) or citrovorum factor is used with methotrexate to reduce drug toxicity. Folinic acid can be given with pyrimethamine to prevent bone marrow suppression. Five to 10 mg/day has been recommended to prevent drug toxicity. Anticonvulsant drugs (phenytoin, barbiturates, primidone) lead to folate deficiency with long term use. Low folate levels have also been found in subjects taking the antituberculosis drugs isoniazid and cycloserine.

The toxicity of folic acid is very low. Intakes of up to 15 mg/d are reported to have no effects. The 400 µg in parenteral vitamin solutions is adequate to meet daily needs and to replete deficits.

VITAMIN B₁₂
(Cobalamin)
Normal Values
Fasting serum level
200 - 900 pg/ml
0.2 - 1.0 ng/ml
Decreased
• Inadequate intake (vegans, alcoholics)
• Inadequate absorption (pernicious anemia, ileal resection, gastrectomy, blind loop)
• Decreased utilization (antagonists)
• Increased need (hyperthyroidismn, growth)
• Increased excretion (liver disease, dialysis)

Vitamin B₁₂ compounds function as coenzymes in the conversion of folate prior to DNA synthesis and cell division, as well as protein, carbohydrate, and lipid metabolism. Good sources include animal foods: meat, eggs, cheese, and milk.

After being released from food sources by digestion, free vitamin B₁₂ is bound to intrinsic factor (IF) produced by the stomach lining. This complex is absorbed in the terminal ileum, and then transported to the liver, the primary storage site. About 70% is absorbed with the percentage decreasing as vitamin intake increases.

Serum vitamin B₁₂ levels are the best screening test. Levels less than 111 pmol/L (150 pg/ml) are usually considered deficient. A Shilling test may then be done to determine if IF is lacking.

A deficiency can result from inadequate intake, increased needs, defective absorption, defective transport (rare), and defective enzyme activity (rare). Deficiencies are reported in pregnant and lactating women and breastfed infants of strict vegetarians. The most common cause is inadequate absorption, mainly pernicious anemia. Pernicious anemia is an acquired failure to secrete intrinsic factor by gastric parietal cells. Other causes of malabsorption include: gastrectomy, surgically produced blind loop (bacterial overgrowth with competition for the vitamin), tapeworm, celiac sprue, tropical sprue, ileal resection, and ileitis. A deficiency is usually slow in onset. With a previously adequate intake, deficiency takes 3 to 5 years to develop. Deficiency develops in 3 to 5 years after a total gastrectomy, and usually 10 to 20 years after a subtotal gastrectomy. Pancreatic insufficiency compromises release of B₁₂ from its dietary protein binders. Intestinal infestation by fish tapeworm from raw fish competes for the vitamin. Some drugs reduce vitamin absorption (para-aminosalicylic acid, oral hypoglycemic agents, neomycin, cholestyramine, potassium chloride, colchicine, cimetidine). Symptoms include weakness, sore tongue, neurological abnormalities, gastrointestinal complaints and a megaloblastic anemia.

The vitamin is nontoxic in amounts up to 10,000 times recommended intakes and excess is excreted in the urine. Vitamin B₁₂ can be given IV or IM. Allergic reactions are rare.

Test	Clinical Significance

BIOTIN
Normal Values
- Serum
  0.82 - 2.87 nmol/L
- Blood, plasma, serum
  1500 pmol/L
- Urine
  160 nmol/24 hours
  70 nmol/L

Biotin is a water-soluble B complex vitamin involved in carbohydrate, protein, lipid, and cholesterol metabolism. It is widely available in the diet, but also synthesized by intestinal bacteria although synthesis doesn't provide adequate amounts. It is thought to be absorbed in the upper small bowel.

Blood, serum, plasma, and urinary levels can indicate a deficiency although there is inconsistency as to acceptable levels. A blood, serum, or plasma level of about 1500 pmol/L or a urine level of about 160 nmol/24 hours (nmol/L) seems to indicate an adequate intake.

Deficiencies are rare and usually due to excess intake of raw egg white which contains avidin. Avidin binds with biotin preventing its absorption. Avidin is easily destroyed by heat. Alcohol use is associated with low levels. Hepatic cirrhosis may prevent normal storage and utilization. Inadequate levels are also associated with use of the epileptic drugs phenytoin, carbamazepine, and primidone. Deficiency symptoms include anorexia, nausea, vomiting, glossitis, pallor, depression, alopecia, dermatitis, and elevated serum cholesterol and bile pigments.

Deficiencies reported in those receiving biotin-free TPN have resolved with intakes of 200 to 300 µg/d. IV infusion of 30 to 100 µg/d is recommended for adults on TPN and biotin is now in parenteral multivitamin solutions. There are no reports of hypersensitivity.

PANTOTHENIC ACID
Reference Values
- Blood
  > 100 µg/dl
- Urine
  > 2 mg/d

Pantothenic acid is a component of coenzyme A and is important to many enzymatic reactions involved in carbohydrate and lipid metabolism.

Bioavailability of pantathenic acid is about 50% and bacterial synthesis of the vitamin is not considered significant. The liver has the highest concentration. Excess is rapidly excreted in the urine.

There is limited information to help evaluate vitamin status. Urinary excretion is considered a better index of status than blood. Urinary excretions of less than 2 mg/d are considered deficient. Blood levels of less than 100 µg/dl are considered to represent inadequate intake. Elevated blood levels occur in renal dysfunction. Increased urinary excretion is reported in diabetics.

Deficiencies usually do not occur alone but in conjunction with other B vitamin deficiencies. Symptoms of a clinical deficiency are not well described. Volunteers fed vitamin antagonists developed GI distress, fatigue, insomnia, and paresthesias of the hands and feet. Low blood sugar levels and hypersensitivity to insulin have also been reported.

The vitamin is relatively nontoxic but allergic reactions (dermatitis, difficulty breathing) may occur with 250 mg/d or more. Diarrhea may occur with oral doses of 10 grams or more.

The AMA expert panel recommended 15 mg/d in TPN patients over age 11. This level appears to maintain normal blood levels. Those with impaired renal function show high normal levels.

ACID-BASE BALANCE

The arterial blood gas (ABG) profile provides information about acid-base balance. The pH measures the acidity or alkalinity of a solution based on the number of hydrogen ions present. The number of hydrogen ions and pH are inversely related. Blood with a lower pH has a higher number of hydrogen ions present and is acidic. Blood with a higher pH has less hydrogen ions present and is alkalemic. Blood pH must stay within a narrow rate for enzymes to function and normal metabolism to occur. Blood pH also affects oxygen release. Hemoglobin releases oxygen more readily when pH is acidic, and holds on to it when blood pH is alkaline.

Carbon dioxide is a by-product of cell metabolism carried by blood as carbonic acid to the lungs for release. The $PaCO_2$ value represents a direct measure of the partial pressure of CO_2 in the blood. It reflects the respiratory component of the acid-base balance. Depending on the acidity of the blood, the lungs will increase or decrease ventilation to maintain the right amount of carbon dioxide.

The bicarbonate ion (HCO_3^-) reflects the metabolic component of acid-base balance. If blood is alkaline from too much bicarbonate, the kidneys retain hydrogen ions and excrete bicarbonate to restore balance. If blood is too acidic, the kidneys excrete hydrogen ions and retain bicarbonate.

Both diet and metabolism contribute acids and bases. The normal balance of acid and base in the blood is 20 parts base to one part acid. If there is excess base the pH rises (alkalosis), and if there is excess acid pH falls (acidosis). The body has several mechanisms to balance these acids and bases and maintain pH. Their relationship is expressed by the following equation:

$$CO_2 + H_2O = H_2CO_3 = H^+ + HCO_3^-$$

The lungs control the carbon dioxide content of the blood. Carbonic acid (H_2CO_3) can either be created or broken down by the lungs. For example, a patient with COPD can't adequately remove excess carbon dioxide. When the excess CO_2 combines with water it forms carbonic acid making the blood acidic. Over time the kidneys compensate by increasing the excretion of hydrogen ions and retaining bicarbonate ions to raise the pH. In another example, a patient may breathe too rapidly and remove too much CO_2 and the blood becomes alkalemic. The kidneys compensate by retaining hydrogen ions and excreting bicarbonate. This is called compensation. It can be partial as with a partial normalization of pH or complete as with complete normalization of the pH. The lungs can respond quickly (in one to three minutes) to acid-base imbalance. The kidneys may take days to weeks to correct an imbalance. Another system for helping to maintain pH is the bicarbonate buffer system which is capable of accepting or donating hydrogen ions. While the body can compensate the kidneys for an imbalance, it is not the same as correcting the problem.

Metabolic disorders are acid-base disturbances that occur outside the lungs. For example, a patient with severe diarrhea will lose bicarbonate which is present in large quantities in the lower GI tract. In response the lungs will begin to remove more CO_2 to compensate for the increased acidity from loss of bicarbonate. In someone on diuretic therapy who's losing excess hydrogen ions, the lungs will decrease ventilation in order to retain more CO_2 to form carbonic acid and decrease pH.

To assess acid-base balance three values are needed: pH, $PaCO_2$, and HCO_3^-. Using the following chart, determine whether each is acid, base, or normal.

Test	Normal*	Acid	Base
pH	7.35 - 7.45	< 7.35	> 7.45
$PaCO_2$	35 - 45 mm Hg	> 45 mm Hg	< 35 mmHg
HCO_3	22 - 26 mEq/L	< 22 mEq/L	> 26 mEq/L

Normal values will vary somewhat with each institution.

The pH and either the $PaCO_2$ or HCO_3^- will have the same abnormality (i.e., acid or base). If there has been compensation the third value will be opposite (i.e., acid or base) from the other two. If there has not been compensation, the third value will be normal.

Example:

• pH = 7.25 (acid)

• $PaCO_2$ = 64 (acid) (respiratory)

• HCO_3^- = 26 (normal)

Hypoventilation has caused the increased acid and because the bicarbonate value is normal, the patient has uncompensated respiratory acidosis. The kidneys have not yet begun to compensate by retaining HCO_3, thus this is an acute problem.

Example:

• pH = 7.3 (acid)

• $PaCO_2$ = 64 (acid) (respiratory)

• HCO_3^- = 32 (base)

This is chronic respiratory acidosis with renal compensation. Over time the kidneys have been able to excrete excess hydrogen ion and retain bicarbonate to partially compensate for the excess CO_2.

Example:

• pH = 7.6 (base)

• $PaCO_2$ = 25 (base)

• HCO_3^- = 24 (normal)

This is acute or uncompensated respiratory alkalosis. There hasn't been enough time for the kidneys to conserve hydrogen ions and excrete HCO_3-.

Example:

• pH = 7.49 (base)

• $PaCO_2$ = 25 (base) (respiratory)

• HCO_3^- = 19 (acid)

This is compensated (partially) respiratory alkalosis. The kidneys are retaining hydrogen ions and increasing their excretion of bicarbonate. Respiratory alkalosis is caused by hyperventilation and excretion of too much CO_2.

Respiratory problems involve only the lungs Acid-base problems that occur outside the lungs are called metabolic disorders. The imbalance may be due to either an increase or decrease in hydrogen ions (acid) or an increase or decrease in bicarbonate (base).

Example:

- pH = 7.2 (acid)

- $PaCO_2$ = 40 (normal)

- HCO_3^- = 15 (acid) (metabolic)

This is acute metabolic acidosis without respiratory compensation. The lungs will respond quickly to increase respiration and eliminate CO_2 to begin correcting this type of imbalance.

Example:

- pH = 7.3 (acid)

- $PaCO_2$ = 30 (base)

- HCO_3^- = 15 (acid) (metabolic)

These labs reflect metabolic acidosis with partial compensation by the lungs to lower $PaCO_2$ and decrease acid. Two common causes of metabolic acidosis are the inability of the kidneys to remove excess hydrogen ion from metabolism or a significant loss of bicarbonate through the GI tract.

Example:

- pH = 7.51 (base)

- $PaCO_2$ = 40 (normal)

- HCO_3^- = 32 (base) (metabolic)

Disturbances that increase bicarbonate or decrease body acids cause metabolic alkalosis. This is an acute metabolic alkalosis without compensation. The lungs have not yet started to alter CO_2.

Example:

- pH = 7.46 (base)

- $PaCO_2$ = 46 (acid)

- HCO_3^- = 32 (base) (metabolic)

This is metabolic alkalosis with partial compensation. In this example pH is close to normal because of an increase in CO_2 retention by the lungs.

All compensatory responses to acid-base imbalance have limits, and patients with kidney or lung problems have limited capacity to compensation. Furthermore, compensation doesn't mean correction of the problem. And acid-base imbalances frequently don't occur singly, which further complicates interpretation. Potential causes of acid-base imbalances are listed below.

RESPIRATORY ACIDOSIS

Depression of respiratory center

• Drug overdose

• Barbiturate toxicity

• Anesthetics/sedation

Thoracic cage dysfunction

• Deformity

• Kyphoscoliosis

Airway obstruction

• Extrathoracic tumors

• Asthma

• Bronchitis

• Emphysema

Circulatory disorders

• Shock

• Congestive heart failure

METABOLIC ACIDOSIS

Acid Gain

• Renal failures, renal tubular acidosis

• Diabetic ketoacidosis

• Lactic acidosis

• Anerobic metabolism

Hypoxia

• Base loss

• Diarrhea

RESPIRATORY ALKALOSIS

Hypoventilation

Hysteria

Lack of oxygen

Respiratory center stimulation

• High fever

• Cerebral hemorrhage

• Excess artificial respiration

• Salicylates

METABOLIC ALKALOSIS

Acid Loss

• Loss of gastric juice

• Vomiting

Potassium or chloride depletion

• Base gain

• Administration of excess bicarbonate or lactate

References

• Labbé R (ed): Clinics In Laboratory Medicine: Nutrition Support: 13:2, 1993.

• Bernstein, LH: Dietetic Currents 19:2, 1992

• Pagana, K and Pagana, T: Mosby's Diagnostic and Laboratory Test Reference, 2nd ed. Mosby: St Louid, 1995.

• Fischbach, F: A Manual of Laboratory and Diagnostic Tests. 5th ed. Lippincott, 1996.

• Meguid, M and Gray, G: The myth of serum albumin as a measure of nutritional status. Gastroenterology 99:1845, 1990.

• Donahue, S and Phillilps, L: Response of IGF-1 to nutritional support in malnourished hospital patients: a possible indicator of short-term changes in nutritional status. Am. J. Clin. Nutr. 50:962, 1989.

• Hart, W: C-reactive protein: the best laboratory indicator available for monitoring disease activity. Cleveland Clinic Journal of Medicine: 56:2, 1989.

• Courtney, S et al: Rapidly declining serum albumin values in newly hospitalized patients: prevalence, severity, and contributory factors. J. Parent. Enter. Nutr. 6:2, 1982.

• Heymsfield, S et al: Measurement of muscle mass in humans: validity of the 24-hour urinary creatinine method. Am. J. Clin. Nutr 37:478, 1983.

• Bistrian, B et al: Therapeutic index of nutritional depletion in hospitalized patients. Surg., Gyn. and Obstet. 141:512, 1975.

• Konstantinides, F: Nitrogen balance studies in clinical nutrition. Nut. in Clin. Prac. 7:231, 1992.

• Sawicky, D et al: Adequate energy intake and improved prealbumin concentration as indicators of the response to total parenteral nutrition. J. Am. Diet. Assoc. 10:1266, 1992.

• Mears, E: Prealbumin and nutrition assessment. Dietetic Currents 21:1, 1994.

• Hawker, F et al: Relationship of somatomedin-C/insulin-like growth factor I levels to conventional nutritional indices in critically ill patients. Crit. Care. Med. 15:732, 1987.

• Baumgartner, T: Clinical Guide to Parenteral Micronutrition, 2nd ed. Fujisawa, USA, Inc., 1991.

• Vanlandingham, S et al: Prealbumin: a parameter of visceral protein levels during albumin infusion. J.P.E.N. 6:230, 1982.

• Tasota, F and Wesmiller S: Assessing A.B. G.s: maintaining the delicate balance. Nursing 94. May, 1994.

• National Research Council: Recommended Daily Allowances, 10th ed. National Academy Press, Washington, DC, 1989.

• McLaren, D: A Colour Atlas and Text of Diet-Related Disorders, 2nd ed. Mosby-Year Book Europe Limited, 1992.

• Agarwal, N: Predictive ability of various nutritional variables for mortality in elderly people. Am. J Clin Nutr 48:1173, 1988.

• Ross Products Division: Laboratory Utilization for Nutrition Support: Current Practice, Requirements, Expectations. Abbott Laboratories, Columbus, 1994.

• Hull, S: Body Fluid and Electrolyte Balance. Ross Dietetic Currents: Vol. 12. No. 1, 1985.

• Weinberg, A, Pals, J and Campbell, M: Preventing Dehydration in the Elderly. Ross Dietetic Currents. Vol. 21, No. 2, 1994.

- Campbell, S: Maintaining hydration status in elderly persons: problems and solutions. Dietitians in Nutrition Support. Vol. 14, No. 3, 1992.

- Zaloga, G: (ed). Nutrition in Critical Care. Mosby Year Book, Inc.: St Louis, 1994.

- McClatchey, K: Clinical Laboratory Medicine. Williams and Wilkins: Baltimore, 1994.

- Sanders, H et al: Nutritional implications of recombinant human erythropoietin therapy in renal disease. J. Am. Diet. Assoc.: 94: 1023, 1994.

DRUG-NUTRIENT INTERACTIONS

How Drugs Affect Nutritional Status

Drugs and nutrients interact in numerous ways to affect both nutritional status and the effectiveness of drug therapy. Drugs can alter food intake by affecting changes in appetite leading to weight gain or loss. Other side effects such as nausea, vomiting, altered taste, sedation, and depression can reduce food intake. Drug absorption may be altered by the presence of food in the stomach. Food enhances the absorption of some drugs, while others are best absorbed in the fasted state. The relative composition of the diet also influences drug absorption. Fat promotes the absorption of some drugs, while others are adsorbed by fiber. Drugs can produce malabsorption by altering intestinal mucosa, motility, or pH. They also create mechanical barriers to absorption, compete with nutrients for absorption sites, and bind substances such as bile salts and acids that are necessary to proper digestion and absorption.

Some drugs are highly protein-bound. Conditions which reduce serum proteins, (protein malnutrition, stressed states) increase the amount of free drug available and the potential for side effects and interactions. Other drugs can block the normal metabolism and function of certain nutrients and increase the excretion of others. Whether or not an interaction is significant may depend on multiple factors: diet, drug dose, combination drug therapy, chronic disease, age and size of the individual, and length of drug therapy.

Most drugs are best taken on an empty stomach one hour before or two hours after a meal to minimize drug nutrient interactions and to maximize drug absorption. Antacids are the source of the most frequenet nutrient interactions. They should not be taken within two hours of other drugs or food with high nutrient density. Drugs which cause significant GI distress can be taken with a small, low nutrient dense snack (e.g., rice cakes, crackers).

Drug-induced nutrient deficiencies generally develop slowly and are more likely in those using drugs chronically, especially the elderly. Other risk factors include high drug dosages, multiple drug regimes, poor diets, and marginal nutrient stores. A drug history should be part of the nutrition screen. Information should include drug names, dosages, frequencies, reasons for the drugs, how they're taken, and how long they've been taken. This history should include both prescription drugs and over the counter medications.

Drug-Nutrient Interactions in the Elderly

Several additional factors increase the risk of drug-nutrient interactions in the elderly. Four out of five have a chronic disease which increases their exposure to drugs. Two surveys of hospital patients showed an average of four drugs per patient. They take about one-fourth of all prescription medicines. Surveys show that 40 to 90% of them use over-the-counter (OTC) medicines (laxatives, antacids, multivitamins). It is not uncommon for them to have prescriptions written by more than one physician or visit more than one pharmacy, thus increasing their risk of undiscovered interactions. Some may not understand how to take their medicines. "As needed" or "prn" medications have a potential for overuse in institutionalized elderly. The elderly are also more likely to have marginal nutrient intakes than younger persons. Lower socioeconomic groups (often women, blacks, and the elderly) are especially at high risk. Others are on restricted diets (physician or self-prescribed). Decreased organ function may alter drug dissolution, distribution, metabolism, and excretion thus increasing the risk of side effects and interactions. Intervention is best done with a multidisciplinary approach.

The Nutrition Screening Initiative emphasizes the importance of drug nutrient interactions in older Americans. A medication use check list is part of the screening process. Subjects taking three or more prescription or over-the-counter medications or vitamins daily should be evaluated for drug-nutrient interactions.

Drug Therapy in Enteral Feeding

Administering medications to patients receiving enteral feeding can be problematic, especially through small-bore feeding tubes. If not infused properly drugs may clog feeding tubes or else precipitate feeding in the tube causing clogging. Replacement of the tube adds cost and interrupts feeding. Absorption of some drugs is better when the stomach is empty requiring the feeding to be stopped. This may interrupt feeding enough so that the patient doesn't get adequate amounts. Parenteral forms of drugs are usually more costly and have high osmolality causing cramping or diarrhea. Some liquid drugs contain sorbitol which has the potential of producing an osmotic diarrhea. Adding drugs to the formula, especially the acidic forms, may cause coagulation or precipitation of the tube feeding and clogging. It also increases the risk of formula contamination. Recommendations for giving medications to patients on enteral feeding are as follows. Please also see section on enteral nutrition.

- Liquid forms of medications should be used when available.

- Enteric coated drugs should not be crushed. This may increase the rate of absorption and the risk of side effects.

- Medications should not be mixed with the formula if possible. If it must be done, the drug should be added slowly with vigorous mixing.

- Highly concentrated forms should be diluted with 60cc of water to reduce osmolality and risk of cramps or diarrhea.

- The tube should be flushed with at least 30 cc of warm water or saline before and after giving a drug.

- Medications should be given separately one at a time flushing the tube with at least 5 cc of water before and after each. Mixing increases the potential for drug-drug interactions.

- Tablets should be ground finely and mixed in solution with water as should the contents of gelatin capsules.

Drugs which may precipitate tube feeding are listed in the drug-nutrient interaction charts which follow.

ALPHABETICAL LISTING OF DRUGS

5-FLUOROUROCIL – Neoplastic Drug

5-FU – Neoplastic Drug

A-Spas – Gastrointestinal Drug

Accubron – Respiratory Drug

Accupril – Cardiovascular Drug

Accutant – Dermatological Drug

ACETOHEXAMIDE – Endocrine Drug

Acetylsalicylic acid – Musculoskeletal Drug

Achromycin – Respiratory Drug

Achromycin-V – Anti-infective Drug,
    Dermatological Drug

Actinomycin-D – Neoplastic Drug

Actron – Musculoskeletal Drug

Adalat – Cardiovascular Drug

Adriamycin – Neoplastic Drug

Adrucil – Neoplastic Drug

Advil – Musculoskeletal Drug

Aerolate – Respiratory Drug

Airet – Respiratory Drug

ALBUTEROL – Respiratory Drug

Aldactazide – Cardiovascular Drug

Aldactone – Cardiovascular Drug

Aldomet – Cardiovascular Drug

Aleve – Musculoskeletal Drug

ALLOPURINOL – Musculoskeletal Drug

Alophen Pills – Gastrointestinal Drug

Alternagel – Gastrointestinal Drug

Alu-Cap – Gastrointestinal Drug

Alu-Tab – Gastrointestinal Drug

ALUMINUM HYDROXIDE – Gastrointestinal Drug

Ambien – Neuropsychiatric Drug

Amethopterin – Neoplastic Drug

AMILORIDE – Cardiovascular Drug

Amino-Opti-E – Supplement

AMINOPHYLLINE – Respiratory Drug

Aminopterin – Musculoskeletal Drug

AMIODARONE – Cardiovascular Drug

AMITRIPTYLINE – Neuropsychiatric Drug

Amoral – Gastrointestinal Drug

Amphojel – Gastrointestinal Drug

AMPHOTERICIN B – Anti-infective Drug

Anaprox – Musculoskeletal Drug

Antabuse – Neuropsychiatric Drug

Anti-Tuss – Respiratory Drug

Antispas – Gastrointestinal Drug

Anturane – Musculoskeletal Drug

Apo-Ranitidine – Gastrointestinal Drug

Apresoline – Cardiovascular Drug

AquaMEPHYTON Supplement

Aquaphyllin – Respiratory Drug

Aquasol A – Supplement

Aquasol E – Supplement

Aralen – Anti-infective Drug

Artane – Neuropsychiatric Drug

ASCORBIC ACID – Supplement

Ascorbicap – Supplement

ASPIRIN – Musculoskeletal Drug

Astramorph – Neoplastic Drug

ATENOLOL – Cardiovascular Drug

Ativan – Neuropsychiatric Drug

ATTAPULGITE – Gastrointestinal Drug

Aventyl – Neuropsychiatric Drug

Axid – Gastrointestinal Drug

Azidothymidine – Anti-infective Drug

AZITHROMYCIN – Respiratory Drug

AZT – Anti-infective Drug

Azulfidine – Gastrointestinal Drug

Bactrim – Respiratory Drug

Baking Soda – Gastrointestinal Drug

Barbita – Neuropsychiatric Drug

Basajel – Gastrointestinal Drug

BCNU – Neoplastic Drug

Beesix – Supplement

BENAZEPRIL – Cardiovascular Drug

Benemid – Musculoskeletal Drug

Bentyl – Gastrointestinal Drug

BENZTROPINE – Musculoskeletal Drug,
    Neuropsychiatric Drug

ALPHABETICAL LISTING OF DRUGS – CONTINUED

Betapace – Cardiovascular Drug

BiCNU – Neoplastic Drug

BISACODYL – Gastrointestinal Drug

Bismatrol – Gastrointestinal Drug

BISMUTH SUBSALICYLATE – Gastrointestinal Drug

Blenoxane – Neoplastic Drug

BLEOMYCIN – Neoplastic Drug

Blocadren – Cardiovascular Drug

Brethaire – Respiratory Drug

Bronkodyl – Respiratory Drug

BUMETANIDE – Cardiovascular Drug

Bumex – Cardiovascular Drug

BUPRION – Neuropsychiatric Drug

Buspar – Neuropsychiatric Drug

BUSPIRONE – Neuropsychiatric Drug

Calan – Cardiovascular Drug

Calciferol – Supplement

Calcijex – Supplement

CALCIUM ACETATE – Gastrointestinal Drug

CALCIUM CARBONATE – Gastrointestinal Drug

Caltrate – Gastrointestinal Drug

Capoten – Cardiovascular Drug

CAPTOPRIL – Cardiovascular Drug

Carafate – Gastrointestinal Drug

CARBAMAZEPINE – Neuropsychiatric Drug

CARBIDOPA + LEVODOPA – Neuropsychiatric Drug

Cardene – Cardiovascular Drug

Cardioquin – Cardiovascular Drug

Cardizem – Cardiovascular Drug

CARMUSTINE – Neoplastic Drug

Carter's Little Liver Pills – Gastrointestinal Drug

Catapres – Cardiovascular Drug

CCNU – Neoplastic Drug

Ce-Vi-Sol – Supplement

Cebid – Supplement

Cecon – Supplement

CeeNu – Neoplastic Drug

CEFADROXIL – Anti-infective Drug

CEFAZOLIN – Anti-infective Drug

Cemill – Supplement

Cenolate – Supplement

CEPHALEXIN – Anti-infective Drug

CEPHALOTHIN – Anti-infective Drug

CEPHAPIRIN – Anti-infective Drug

CEPHRADINE – Anti-infective Drug

Cephulac – Neuropsychiatric Drug

Cetane – Supplement

Cevalin – Supplement

Cevi-Bid – Supplement

CHLORDIAZEPOXIDE – Neuropsychiatric Drug

CHLOROQUINE – Anti-infective Drug

Chlorpazine – Neuropsychiatric Drug

CHLORPROMAZINE – Neuropsychiatric Drug

CHLORPROPAMIDE – Endocrine Drug

CHLORTHIAZIDE – Cardiovascular Drug

Cholac – Neuropsychiatric Drug

CHOLESTYRAMINE – Cardiovascular Drug

Chooz – Gastrointestinal Drug

Chronulac – Neuropsychiatric Drug

Cibalith-S – Neuropsychiatric Drug

CIMETIDINE – Gastrointestinal Drug

CISAPRIDE – Gastrointestinal Drug

CISPLATIN – Neoplastic Drug

Clinoril – Musculoskeletal Drug

CLONIDINE – Cardiovascular Drug

Clopra – Gastrointestinal Drug

CLOZAPINE – Neuropsychiatric Drug

Clozaril – Neuropsychiatric Drug

Cogentin – Musculoskeletal Drug, Neuropsychiatric Drug

Colace – Gastrointestinal Drug

ColBenemid – Musculoskeletal Drug

COLCHICINE – Musculoskeletal Drug

Colestid – Cardiovascular Drug

COLESTIPOL – Cardiovascular Drug

Compazine – Neuropsychiatric Drug

ALPHABETICAL LISTING OF DRUGS – CONTINUED

Constilac – Neuropsychiatric Drug
Cordarone – Cardiovascular Drug
Corgard – Cardiovascular Drug
Correctol – Gastrointestinal Drug
Cortenema – Musculoskeletal Drug
Cortifoam – Musculoskeletal Drug
CORTISONE – Musculoskeletal Drug
Cosmegen – Neoplastic Drug
Cotazyme – Gastrointestinal Drug
Cotranzine – Neuropsychiatric Drug
Coumadin – Cardiovascular Drug
Crystamine Supplement
Crysti-1000 Supplement
Cuprimine – Musculoskeletal Drug
Cyanoject Supplement
CYCLOPHOSPHAMIDE – Neoplastic Drug
CYCLOSPORINE – Dermatological Drug
Cylert – Neuropsychiatric Drug
Cyomin Supplement
Cytosec – Gastrointestinal Drug
Cytoxan – Neoplastic Drug
Dacodyl – Gastrointestinal Drug
DACTINOMYCIN – Neoplastic Drug
Daraprim – Anti-infective Drug
Deficol – Gastrointestinal Drug
Deltalin Supplement
Deltasone – Respiratory Drug, Gastrointestinal Drug, Musculoskeletal Drug
Depakene – Neuropsychiatric Drug
Depen – Musculoskeletal Drug
DESIPRAMINE – Neuropsychiatric Drug
Desyrel – Neuropsychiatric Drug
Dexedrine – Neuropsychiatric Drug
DEXTROAMPHETAMINE – Neuropsychiatric Drug
DextroStat – Neuropsychiatric Drug
DHT Supplement
DiaBeta – Endocrine Drug
Diabinese – Endocrine Drug

Dialume – Gastrointestinal Drug
Diar-Aid – Gastrointestinal Drug
Diasorb – Gastrointestinal Drug
DIAZEPAM – Neuropsychiatric Drug
Dibent – Gastrointestinal Drug
DICYCLOMINE – Gastrointestinal Drug
DIFLUNISAL – Musculoskeletal Drug
DIGOXIN – Cardiovascular Drug
Dilantin – Neuropsychiatric Drug
DILTIAZEM – Cardiovascular Drug
DIMENHYDRINATE – Gastrointestinal Drug
DIPHENOXYLATE W/ ATROPINE – Gastrointestinal Drug
Diphenylan – Neuropsychiatric Drug
DISULFRAM – Neuropsychiatric Drug
Diuregin – Cardiovascular Drug
Diuril – Cardiovascular Drug
DOCUSATE – Gastrointestinal Drug
Dolgesic – Musculoskeletal Drug
Dolobid – Musculoskeletal Drug
Dopar – Neuropsychiatric Drug
DOSS – Gastrointestinal Drug
DOXEPIN – Neuropsychiatric Drug
DOXORUBICIN – Neoplastic Drug
DPH – Neuropsychiatric Drug
Dramamine – Gastrointestinal Drug
Drisdol Supplement
DRONABINOL – Gastrointestinal Drug
Dulcagen – Gastrointestinal Drug
Dulcolax – Gastrointestinal Drug
Duphalac – Neuropsychiatric Drug
Duramorph – Neoplastic Drug
Duraquin – Cardiovascular Drug
Durlith – Neuropsychiatric Drug
Dyazide – Cardiovascular Drug
Dymelor – Endocrine Drug
Dyrenium – Cardiovascular Drug
E-200, E-400, E-600 Supplement
Easprin – Musculoskeletal Drug

ALPHABETICAL LISTING OF DRUGS – CONTINUED

Ecotrin – Musculoskeletal Drug

Edecrin – Cardiovascular Drug

Edur-Acin – Supplement

Effer-syllium – Gastrointestinal Drug

Effexor – Neuropsychiatric Drug

Efudex – Neoplastic Drug

Elavil – Neuropsychiatric Drug

Eldepryl – Neuropsychiatric Drug

Elixomin – Respiratory Drug

Elixophyllin – Respiratory Drug

Emitrip – Neuropsychiatric Drug

Empirin – Musculoskeletal Drug

ENALAPRIL – Cardiovascular Drug

Endep – Neuropsychiatric Drug

Enkaid – Cardiovascular Drug

Enovil – Neuropsychiatric Drug

Enulose – Neuropsychiatric Drug

Enzymase – Gastrointestinal Drug

Epitol – Neuropsychiatric Drug

Epsom Salt – Gastrointestinal Drug

Equilactin – Gastrointestinal Drug

Esidrix – Cardiovascular Drug

Eskalith – Neuropsychiatric Drug

Espotabs – Gastrointestinal Drug

ESTROGEN – Genitourinary or Contraceptive Drug

ETHACRYNIC ACID – Cardiovascular Drug

ETHINYL ESTRADIOL w/ NORGESTREL –
   Genitourinary or Contraceptive Drug

ETRETINATE – Dermatological Drug

Evac-U-Gen – Gastrointestinal Drug

Evac-U-Lax – Gastrointestinal Drug

Ex-Lax – Gastrointestinal Drug

Ezide – Cardiovascular Drug

FAMOTIDINE – Gastrointestinal Drug

Fansidor – Anti-infective Drug

Feen-a-Mint – Gastrointestinal Drug

Feldene – Musculoskeletal Drug

FELODIPINE – Cardiovascular Drug

Femiron – Supplement

Fenesin – Respiratory Drug

FENOPROFEN – Musculoskeletal Drug

Feosol – Supplement

Feostat – Supplement

Fer-In-Sol Supplement

Fer-Iron Supplement

Fergon Supplement

Ferralet Supplement

Ferrous Fumarate Supplement

Ferrous Gluconate – Supplement

Ferrous Sulfate – Supplement

Fiber-Lax – Gastrointestinal Drug

Fiberall – Gastrointestinal Drug

FiberCon – Gastrointestinal Drug

Flagyl – Anti-infective Drug

Flavorcee – Supplement

FLECANIDE – Cardiovascular Drug

Fleet Laxative – Gastrointestinal Drug

Fleet Mineral Oil – Gastrointestinal Drug

Fletcher's Castoria – Gastrointestinal Drug

Fluoroplex – Neoplastic Drug

FLUOXETINE – Neuropsychiatric Drug

FLUPHENAZINE – Neuropsychiatric Drug

FLUVASTIN – Cardiovascular Drug

Folex – Musculoskeletal Drug, Neoplastic Drug

FOLIC ACID – Supplement

Folvite – Supplement

FOSINOPRIL – Cardiovascular Drug

Fulvicin – Anti-infective Drug

Fumerin – Supplement

Fungizone – Anti-infective Drug

Furadantin – Genitourinary or Contraceptive Drug

Furalan – Genitourinary or Contraceptive Drug

FUROSEMIDE – Cardiovascular Drug

Garamycin – Anti-infective Drug

GEMFIBROZIL – Cardiovascular Drug

Generlax – Neuropsychiatric Drug

Genoptic – Anti-infective Drug

Gentacidin – Anti-infective Drug

ALPHABETICAL LISTING OF DRUGS – CONTINUED

Gentak – Anti-infective Drug

Gentamar – Anti-infective Drug

GENTAMICIN – Anti-infective Drug

Gentrasul – Anti-infective Drug

GLIPIZIDE – Endocrine Drug

Glucophage – Endocrine Drug

Glucotrol – Endocrine Drug

Glucotrol XL – Endocrine Drug

GLYBURIDE – Endocrine Drug

Glynase Pres Tab – Endocrine Drug

GOLD SODIUM THIOMALATE – Musculoskeletal Drug

Grifulvin – Anti-infective Drug

GRISEOFULVIN – Anti-infective Drug

GUAIFENESIN – Respiratory Drug

GUANABENZ – Cardiovascular Drug

GUANETHIDINE – Cardiovascular Drug

Haldol – Neuropsychiatric Drug

Halfprin – Musculoskeletal Drug

HALOPERIDOL – Neuropsychiatric Drug

HCTZ – Cardiovascular Drug

Heart-Trex – Musculoskeletal Drug

Hemocyte – Supplement

Humalin R – Endocrine Drug

HYDRALAZINE – Cardiovascular Drug

Hydrin – Cardiovascular Drug

Hydro-D – Cardiovascular Drug

Hydrochlor – Cardiovascular Drug

HYDROCHLOROTHIAZIDE – Cardiovascular Drug

HYDROCORTISONE – Musculoskeletal Drug

Hydrocortone – Musculoskeletal Drug

Hydrodiuril – Cardiovascular Drug

Hytakerol – Supplement

Ibren – Musculoskeletal Drug

IBUPROFEN – Musculoskeletal Drug

Icortef – Musculoskeletal Drug

Ilozyme – Gastrointestinal Drug

IMIPRAMINE – Neuropsychiatric Drug

Imodium, Immodium A-D – Gastrointestinal Drug

Inderal – Cardiovascular Drug

Indocin – Musculoskeletal Drug

INDOMETHACIN – Musculoskeletal Drug

INH – Respiratory Drug

INSULIN – Endocrine Drug

Ircon – Supplement

IRON – Supplement

Ismelin – Cardiovascular Drug

ISONIAZID – Respiratory Drug

Isoptin – Cardiovascular Drug

ISOTRETINOIN – Dermatological Drug

Jenamicin – Anti-infective Drug

K-Dur – Supplement

K-Lyte – Supplement

K-P – Gastrointestinal Drug

K-Pek – Gastrointestinal Drug

Kao-Spen – Gastrointestinal Drug

KAOLIN/PECTATE – Gastrointestinal Drug

Kaopectate – Gastrointestinal Drug

Kapectolin – Gastrointestinal Drug

KETOCONAZOLE – Anti-infective Drug

KETOPROFEN – Musculoskeletal Drug

KETORALAC – Musculoskeletal Drug

Klorvess – Supplement

Klotrix – Supplement

Kolyum – Supplement

Konakion – Supplement

Kondremul Plain – Gastrointestinal Drug

Konsyl – Gastrointestinal Drug

L-dopa – Neuropsychiatric Drug

LABETALOL – Cardiovascular Drug

LACTULOSE – Neuropsychiatric Drug

Laniazid – Respiratory Drug

Lanophyllin – Respiratory Drug

Lanoxicaps – Cardiovascular Drug

Lanoxin – Cardiovascular Drug

Larodopa – Neuropsychiatric Drug

Lasix – Cardiovascular Drug

ALPHABETICAL LISTING OF DRUGS – CONTINUED

Lescol – Cardiovascular Drug

Levo-T – Endocrine Drug

LEVODOPA – Neuropsychiatric Drug

Levothroid – Endocrine Drug

LEVOTHYROXINE – Endocrine Drug

Levoxyl – Endocrine Drug

Libritabs – Neuropsychiatric Drug

Librius – Neuropsychiatric Drug

Liqui-doss – Gastrointestinal Drug

Liqui-E – Supplement

LISINOPRIL – Cardiovascular Drug

Lithane – Neuropsychiatric Drug

LITHIUM – Neuropsychiatric Drug

Lithonate – Neuropsychiatric Drug

Lithotabs – Neuropsychiatric Drug

Lo-Ovral – Genitourinary or Contraceptive Drug

Lofene – Gastrointestinal Drug

Logen – Gastrointestinal Drug

Lomocot – Gastrointestinal Drug

Lomotil – Gastrointestinal Drug

LOMUSTINE – Neoplastic Drug

Loniten – Cardiovascular Drug

Lonox – Gastrointestinal Drug

LOPERAMIDE – Gastrointestinal Drug

Lopid – Cardiovascular Drug

Lopressor – Cardiovascular Drug

Lopurin – Musculoskeletal Drug

LORAZEPAM – Neuropsychiatric Drug

Lorelco – Cardiovascular Drug

Losec – Gastrointestinal Drug

Lotensin – Cardiovascular Drug

LOVASTATIN – Cardiovascular Drug

Luminal – Neuropsychiatric Drug

Maalox Anticiarrheal Caplets – Gastrointestinal Drug

Macrobid – Genitourinary or Contraceptive Drug

Macrodantin – Genitourinary or Contraceptive Drug

Magnalox – Gastrointestinal Drug

MAGNESIUM HYDROXIDE – Gastrointestinal Drug

MAGNESIUM HYDROXIDE w/ ALUMINUM HYDROXIDE – Gastrointestinal Drug

MAGNESIUM SULFATE – Gastrointestinal Drug

Magnox – Gastrointestinal Drug

Mandelamine – Genitourinary or Contraceptive Drug

Marinol – Gastrointestinal Drug

Maxide – Cardiovascular Drug

Measurin – Musculoskeletal Drug

Meclofen – Musculoskeletal Drug

MECLOFENAMATE – Musculoskeletal Drug

Meclomen – Musculoskeletal Drug

Medipren – Musculoskeletal Drug

Mellaril – Neuropsychiatric Drug

Mephyton – Supplement

MESORIDAZINE – Neuropsychiatric Drug

Metamucil – Gastrointestinal Drug

METFORMIN – Endocrine Drug

METHENAMINE – Genitourinary or Contraceptive Drug

METHOTREXATE – Neoplastic Drug, Musculoskeletal Drug

METHYLDOPA – Cardiovascular Drug

METHYLPHENIDATE – Neuropsychiatric Drug

Meticorten – Gastrointestinal Drug

Meticorten – Musculoskeletal Drug, Respiratory Drug

METOCLOPRAMIDE – Gastrointestinal Drug

METOPROLOL – Cardiovascular Drug

Metric-21 – Anti-infective Drug

MetroGel – Anti-infective Drug

METRONIDAZOLE – Anti-infective Drug

Metryl – Anti-infective Drug

Mevacor – Cardiovascular Drug

Micro-K – Supplement

Micronase – Endocrine Drug

Midamor – Cardiovascular Drug

Milkinol – Gastrointestinal Drug

MINERAL OIL – Gastrointestinal Drug

Minipress – Cardiovascular Drug

ALPHABETICAL LISTING OF DRUGS – CONTINUED

MINOXIDIL – Cardiovascular Drug

Mintox – Gastrointestinal Drug

MISOPROSTOL – Gastrointestinal Drug

Mitrolan – Gastrointestinal Drug

Modane – Gastrointestinal Drug

MOM – Gastrointestinal Drug

Monopril – Cardiovascular Drug

MORPHINE – Neoplastic Drug

Motrin – Musculoskeletal Drug

MS – Neoplastic Drug

MSO$_4$ – Neoplastic Drug

Mutalane – Neoplastic Drug

Myidone – Neuropsychiatric Drug

Myochrisine – Musculoskeletal Drug

Myproic Acid – Neuropsychiatric Drug

Mysoline – Neuropsychiatric Drug

NADOLOL – Cardiovascular Drug

Nalfon – Musculoskeletal Drug

NAPROXEN – Musculoskeletal Drug

Naproxyn – Musculoskeletal Drug

Nardil – Neuropsychiatric Drug

Navine – Neuropsychiatric Drug

NebuPent – Anti-infective Drug

Neoral – Dermatological Drug

Neosar – Neoplastic Drug

Nephrox – Gastrointestinal Drug

Nestrex – Supplement

Neut – Gastrointestinal Drug

Nia-Bid – Supplement

Niac – Supplement

Niacela – Supplement

NIACIN – Cardiovascular Drug, Supplement

NICARDIPINE – Cardiovascular Drug

Nico-400 – Supplement

Nicobid – Cardiovascular Drug, Supplement

Nicolar – Supplement

Nicotinex – Supplement

Nicotinic Acid – Cardiovascular Drug, Supplement

NIFEDIPINE – Cardiovascular Drug

Nitro Bid – Cardiovascular Drug

Nitrofuracot – Genitourinary or Contraceptive Drug

NITROFURANTOIN – Genitourinary or Contraceptive Drug

NITROGLYCERIN – Cardiovascular Drug

Nitroglyn – Cardiovascular Drug

Nitrolin – Cardiovascular Drug

NIZATIDINE – Gastrointestinal Drug

Nizoral – Anti-infective Drug

Nolvadex – Neoplastic Drug

Normodyne – Cardiovascular Drug

Norpanth – Gastrointestinal Drug

Norpramin – Neuropsychiatric Drug

NORTRIPTYLINE – Neuropsychiatric Drug

Novalin – Endocrine Drug

Novo-Diflunisal – Musculoskeletal Drug

Nu-Pirox – Musculoskeletal Drug

Nujol – Gastrointestinal Drug

NuLoras – Neuropsychiatric Drug

Nuprin – Musculoskeletal Drug

Nydrazid – Respiratory Drug

Octamide – Gastrointestinal Drug

OMEPRAZOLE – Gastrointestinal Drug

Oncovin – Neoplastic Drug

Oramorph – Neoplastic Drug

Orasone – Gastrointestinal Drug, Musculoskeletal Drug, Respiratory Drug

Orazinc – Supplement

Oretic – Cardiovascular Drug

Orinase – Endocrine Drug

Orudis – Musculoskeletal Drug

Oruvail – Musculoskeletal Drug

Os-Cal – Gastrointestinal Drug

Ovral – Genitourinary or Contraceptive Drug

OXYTETRCYCLINE – Respiratory Drug

Palmiron – Supplement

Pamelor – Neuropsychiatric Drug

Pancoate – Gastrointestinal Drug

PANCREALIPASE – Gastrointestinal Drug

ALPHABETICAL LISTING OF DRUGS – CONTINUED

Pancrease – Gastrointestinal Drug

Panmycin – Anti-infective Drug, Dermatological Drug, Respiratory Drug

Panwarfarin – Cardiovascular Drug

Parepesctolin – Gastrointestinal Drug

Parnate – Neuropsychiatric Drug

PAROXETINE – Neuropsychiatric Drug

Paxil – Neuropsychiatric Drug

PEMOLINE – Neuropsychiatric Drug

PENICILLAMINE – Musculoskeletal Drug

Pentam – Anti-infective Drug

PENTAMIDINE ISOETHIONATE – Anti-infective Drug

PENTOXIFYLLINE – Cardiovascular Drug, Neuropsychiatric Drug

Pepsid – Gastrointestinal Drug

Pepto-Bismol – Gastrointestinal Drug

Perdiem – Gastrointestinal Drug

Permitil – Neuropsychiatric Drug

PERPHENAZINE – Neuropsychiatric Drug

Petrogalar Plain – Gastrointestinal Drug

PHENELZINE – Neuropsychiatric Drug

PHENOBARBITAL – Neuropsychiatric Drug

Phenolax – Gastrointestinal Drug

PHENOLPHTHALEIN – Gastrointestinal Drug

PHENYTOIN – Neuropsychiatric Drug

Pheryl-E Supplement

Phillips Milk of Magnesia – Gastrointestinal Drug

Phos-Ex – Gastrointestinal Drug

Phoslo – Gastrointestinal Drug

Phyllocontin – Respiratory Drug

PINDOLOL – Cardiovascular Drug

Pink Bismuth – Gastrointestinal Drug

PIROXICAM – Musculoskeletal Drug

Platinol – Neoplastic Drug

Platinol-AQ – Neoplastic Drug

Plendil – Cardiovascular Drug

PMS-Phenidate – Neuropsychiatric Drug

POLYCARBOPHIL – Gastrointestinal Drug

Portalac – Neuropsychiatric Drug

Pravacol – Cardiovascular Drug

PRAVASTATIN – Cardiovascular Drug

PRAZOSIN – Cardiovascular Drug

Predinicen-M – Gastrointestinal Drug, Musculoskeletal Drug, Respiratory Drug

PREDNISONE – Gastrointestinal Drug, Musculoskeletal Drug, Respiratory Drug

Premarin – Genitourinary or Contraceptive Drug

Prilosec – Gastrointestinal Drug

PRIMIDONE – Neuropsychiatric Drug

Prinivil – Cardiovascular Drug

Probalan – Musculoskeletal Drug

ProBanthine – Gastrointestinal Drug

PROBENECID – Musculoskeletal Drug

PROBUCOL – Cardiovascular Drug

PROCAINAMIDE – Cardiovascular Drug

PROCARBAZINE – Neoplastic Drug

Procardia – Cardiovascular Drug

PROCHLORPERAZINE – Neuropsychiatric Drug

Prolixin – Neuropsychiatric Drug

Pronestyl – Cardiovascular Drug

PROPANTHELINE BROMIDE – Gastrointestinal Drug

PROPRANOLOL – Cardiovascular Drug

Propulsid – Gastrointestinal Drug

PROPYLTHIOURIL – Endocrine Drug

Protilase – Gastrointestinal Drug

Protostat – Anti-infective Drug

Proventil – Respiratory Drug

Prozac – Neuropsychiatric Drug

PSYLLIUM GUM – Gastrointestinal Drug

PTU – Endocrine Drug

PYRAZINAMIDE – Respiratory Drug

PYRIDOXINE – Supplement

PYRIMETHAMINE – Anti-infective Drug

Quibron-T – Respiratory Drug

QUINAPRIL – Cardiovascular Drug

QUINIDINE – Cardiovascular Drug

ALPHABETICAL LISTING OF DRUGS – CONTINUED

Quiniglute – Cardiovascular Drug

Quiridex – Cardiovascular Drug

RANITIDINE – Gastrointestinal Drug

RAUWOLFIA – Cardiovascular Drug

Reclomide – Gastrointestinal Drug

Reglan – Gastrointestinal Drug

Regutol – Gastrointestinal Drug

Reserpine – Cardiovascular Drug

Respbid – Respiratory Drug

Retrovir – Anti-infective Drug

Rheaban – Gastrointestinal Drug

Rheumatrex – Musculoskeletal Drug, Neoplastic
Drug

RIBOFLAVIN – Supplement

Rifadin – Respiratory Drug

RIFAMPIN – Respiratory Drug

Rimactane – Respiratory Drug

Risperdal – Neuropsychiatric Drug

RISPERIDONE – Neuropsychiatric Drug

Ritalin – Neuropsychiatric Drug

Robitet – Anti-infective Drug, Dermatological Drug,
Respiratory Drug

Robitussin – Respiratory Drug

Rocaltrol – Supplement

Rodex – Supplement

Rolaids – Gastrointestinal Drug

Roxanol – Neoplastic Drug

Rubesol-1000 – Supplement

Rubex – Neoplastic Drug

Rulox – Gastrointestinal Drug

Sandimmune – Dermatological Drug

SD-Deprenyl – Neuropsychiatric Drug

SELEGILINE – Neuropsychiatric Drug

Senexon – Gastrointestinal Drug

SENNA – Gastrointestinal Drug

Senokot – Gastrointestinal Drug

Senolax – Gastrointestinal Drug

Septra – Respiratory Drug

Serentil – Neuropsychiatric Drug

Serpasil – Cardiovascular Drug

SERTRALINE – Neuropsychiatric Drug

Serutan – Gastrointestinal Drug

Sibilin – Gastrointestinal Drug

Simron – Supplement

SIMVASTIN – Cardiovascular Drug

Sinemet – Neuropsychiatric Drug

Sinequan – Neuropsychiatric Drug

Slo-Phyllin – Respiratory Drug

Slow Fe – Supplement

Slow-Kaylixir – Supplement

Soda Mint – Gastrointestinal Drug

SODIUM BICARBONATE – Gastrointestinal Drug

Solfoton – Neuropsychiatric Drug

Solu-Cortef – Musculoskeletal Drug

SOTALOL – Cardiovascular Drug

Spasmoject – Gastrointestinal Drug

SPRINOLACTONE – Cardiovascular Drug

Stelazine – Neuropsychiatric Drug

Sterapred – Gastrointestinal Drug, Musculoskeletal
Drug, Respiratory Drug

SULCRAFATE – Gastrointestinal Drug

SULFASALAZINE – Gastrointestinal Drug

SULFINPYRAZONE – Musculoskeletal Drug

SULINDAC – Musculoskeletal Drug

Sumycin – Anti-infective Drug, Dermatological
Drug, Respiratory Drug

Surfak – Gastrointestinal Drug

Sustaire – Respiratory Drug

Syllact – Gastrointestinal Drug

Synthroid – Endocrine Drug

T-Phyl – Respiratory Drug

Tagamet – Gastrointestinal Drug

Tagamet HB – Gastrointestinal Drug

Tambocor – Cardiovascular Drug

TAMOXIFEN – Neoplastic Drug

Tegison – Dermatological Drug

Tegretol – Neuropsychiatric Drug

Tenormin – Cardiovascular Drug

ALPHABETICAL LISTING OF DRUGS – CONTINUED

TERAZOSIN – Cardiovascular Drug

TERBUTALINE – Respiratory Drug

Terramycin – Respiratory Drug

TETRACYCLINE – Anti-infective Drug, Dermatological Drug

TETRACYCLINE – Genitourinary or Contraceptive Drug, Respiratory Drug

Tetracyn – Anti-infective Drug, Dermatological Drug, Respiratory Drug

THC – Gastrointestinal Drug

Theo-24 – Respiratory Drug

Theo-Dur – Respiratory Drug

Theo-Sav – Respiratory Drug

Theoclear – Respiratory Drug

Theolair – Respiratory Drug

THEOPHYLLINE – Respiratory Drug

Theospan – Respiratory Drug

Theovent – Respiratory Drug

THIAMIN – Supplement

THIORIDAZINE – Neuropsychiatric Drug

THIOTHIXENE – Neuropsychiatric Drug

Thor-Prom – Neuropsychiatric Drug

Thorazine – Neuropsychiatric Drug

Throchron – Respiratory Drug

TIMOLOL – Cardiovascular Drug

Tipramine – Neuropsychiatric Drug

Titralac – Gastrointestinal Drug

Tofranil – Neuropsychiatric Drug

Tol-Tab – Endocrine Drug

Tolamide – Endocrine Drug

TOLAZAMIDE – Endocrine Drug

TOLBUTAMIDE – Endocrine Drug

Tolectin – Musculoskeletal Drug

Tolinase – Endocrine Drug

TOLMETIN – Musculoskeletal Drug

Topicycline – Anti-infective Drug, Dermatological Drug, Respiratory Drug

Toprol-X – Cardiovascular Drug

Toradol – Musculoskeletal Drug

TRANCYLPROMINE – Neuropsychiatric Drug

TRAZODONE – Neuropsychiatric Drug

Trazon – Neuropsychiatric Drug

Trental – Cardiovascular Drug, Neuropsychiatric Drug

Tri-hexy – Neuropsychiatric Drug

Trialodine – Neuropsychiatric Drug

TRIAMTERENE – Cardiovascular Drug

TRIFLUOPERAZINE – Neuropsychiatric Drug

Trihexane – Neuropsychiatric Drug

TRIHEXYPHENIDYL – Neuropsychiatric Drug

Trilafon – Neuropsychiatric Drug

TRIMETHOPRIM W/SULFAMETHOXAZOLE – Respiratory Drug

TRIMETREXATE – Neoplastic Drug

Truphylline – Respiratory Drug

Tums – Gastrointestinal Drug

Ultrase – Gastrointestinal Drug

Ultrazine – Neuropsychiatric Drug

Uniphyl – Respiratory Drug

Unitussin – Respiratory Drug

Valium – Neuropsychiatric Drug

VALPROIC ACID – Neuropsychiatric Drug

Valrelease – Neuropsychiatric Drug

Vasotec – Cardiovascular Drug

Vazepam – Neuropsychiatric Drug

VENLAFAXINE – Neuropsychiatric Drug

Ventolin – Respiratory Drug

VERAPAMIL – Cardiovascular Drug

Verazinc – Supplement

Verelan – Cardiovascular Drug

Versabran – Gastrointestinal Drug

Vincasar – Neoplastic Drug

Vincrex – Neoplastic Drug

VINCRISTINE – Neoplastic Drug

Viocase – Gastrointestinal Drug

Visken – Cardiovascular Drug

Vita Plus E – Supplement

Vitabee 6 – Supplement

ALPHABETICAL LISTING OF DRUGS

VITAMIN A – Supplement
VITAMIN B$_{12}$ – Supplement
VITAMIN D – Supplement
Vitamin D$_2$ – Supplement
VITAMIN E – Supplement
VITAMIN K – Supplement
Vollmax – Respiratory Drug
WARFARIN – Cardiovascular Drug
Wellbutrin – Neuropsychiatric Drug
Wytensin – Cardiovascular Drug
Zantac – Gastrointestinal Drug
Zestril – Cardiovascular Drug
ZIDOVUDINE – Anti-infective Drug

Zinc 220 – Supplement
ZINC SULFATE – Supplement
Zincate – Supplement
Zinkaps – Supplement
Zithromax – Respiratory Drug
Zolcar – Cardiovascular Drug
Zoloft – Neuropsychiatric Drug
ZOLPIDEM – Neuropsychiatric Drug
Zonalon – Neuropsychiatric Drug
Zyloprim – Musculoskeletal Drug
Zymase – Gastrointestinal Drug
Zymenol – Gastrointestinal Drug

ANTI-INFECTIVE DRUGS

Drug	Interaction
AMPHOTERICIN B Used to treat fungal infections. *Fungizone*	Common side effects: heartburn, nausea, vomiting, hypokalemia, weight loss. Good hydration (2 - 3 L/d) important to reduce nephrotoxicity. Increased potassium and magnesium intake recommended. Potential for causing anemia.
CEFALOSPORIN Used to treat a variety of infections. *Cefadroxil* *Cefazolin* *Cephalexin* *Cephalothin* *Cephapirin* *Cephradine*	Common side effects: nausea, vomiting, diarrhea. Taking with food reduces GI symptoms but food slows absorption. May cause hypokalemia and vitamin K deficiency.
CHLOROQUINE Used to prevent and treat malaria, and to treat amebic liver abscess. *Aralen*	Foods that acidify urine may increase drug excretion. Increased risk of hemolytic anemia in those with glucose-6-phosphate dehydrogenase deficiency.
GENTAMICIN Used to treat or prevent infections. *Garamycin* *Genoptic* *Gentacidi* *Gentak* *Gentamar* *Gentrasul* *Jenamicin*	Potential for magnesium and potassium depletion due to increased excretion. May need increased intake of potassium and magnesium-rich foods or supplement.
GRISEOFULVIN Used to treat fungal infections. *Fulvicin* *Grifulvin*	Take drug with high fat meal to increase absorption. Alcohol intake may cause disulfram reaction (see endocrine drugs).
KETOCONAZOLE Used to treat fungal infections. *Nizoral*	Absorption of drug reduced by food. Best absorption with acidic beverages (pH < 5.0). Avoid taking calcium and magnesium supplements and antacids within 2 hours.

Drug	Interaction
METRONIDAZOLE Used to treat anaerobic infections. *Flagyl* *Metric-21* *MetroGel* *Metryl* *Protostat*	Common side effects: altered taste, anorexia, nausea, vomiting, diarrhea. Alcohol intake may cause disulfram reaction (see endocrine drugs).
PENTAMIDINE ISOETHIONATE Used to treat Pneumocystis carinii pneumonia. *NebuPent* *Pentam*	Common side effects: altered taste, anorexia, nausea, vomiting, diarrhea. Potential for folate deficiency, especially with low intake or malabsorption. Supplement is recommended. May cause hypocalcemia and hyperkalemia. Potential for causing hypoglycemia and hyperglycemia.
PYRIMETHAMINE Used to treat malaria and toxoplasmosis. *Daraprim* *Fansidor*	Risk of megaloblastic anemia from antifolate activity, especially with low intake, malabsorption, and other folate antagonists. Increase intake of folate-rich foods or consider supplement. Adequate intake of vitamin B_{12} also important.
TETRACYCLINE Used to treat a variety of infections and bronchitis. *Achromycin-V* *Panmycin* *Robitet* *Sumycin* *Tetracyn* *Topicycline*	Best taken on an empty stomach. May take with non-dairy food to reduce GI distress. Forms insoluble complexes with calcium, magnesium, iron, and zinc. Separate intake of drug and dairy products, antacids, magnesium-containing laxatives, and calcium, iron, and zinc supplements by 2 - 3 hours. Reduces vitamin K synthesis and increases urinary loss of riboflavin and folate. Potential deficiency with long term use. Increase vitamin intake or consider supplement. Stop tube feeding 1 hour before and 2 hours after drug.
ZIDOVUDINE Used to treat HIV and AIDS infection. *Azidothymidine* *AZT* *Retrovir*	Common side effects: anorexia, nausea, vomiting. Potential for megaloblastic anemia and folate depletion. Moniter folate level. Increase intake of folate-rich foods or consider supplement. Adequate intake of vitamin B_{12} also important.

CARDIVASCULAR DRUGS

Drug	Interaction
AMILORIDE Counteracts potassium loss associated with diuretics used to treat edema. *Midamor*	Take with food to reduce GI distress. Risk of excess potassium retention or sodium loss, and anorexia. Reduce intake of potassium-rich foods. Use potassium supplements, salt sub, and low sodium milk cautiously. Avoid licorice with natural flavoring due to potential for sodium and fluid retention. Use calcium supplements cautiously.
AMIODARONE Management of cardiac arrhythmias. *Cordarone*	Common side effects: altered taste, anorexia, nausea. Potential for hypothyroidism and weight gain due to high iodine content. Hypokalemia and hypomagnesemia reduce drug effectiveness.
ATENOLOL Beta-adrenergic blocking agent (beta-blocker) used to treat hypertension. Tenormin	Common side effects: nausea, vomiting, diarrhea, dry mouth. Sugarless candy and gum or saliva substitute may help dry mouth. Drug absorption increased by food. Potential for hypoglycemia in diabetics. May increase serum triglycerides. Potential for increased CNS effects with low albumin. Take calcium-containing supplements and antacids separately. Avoid licorice with natural flavoring due to sodium and fluid retention.
BENAZEPRIL Angiotensin converting enzyme inhibitor (ACE-I) used to treat hypertension. *Lotensin*	Best taken before meals. Maintain good hydration. Limit alcohol. Avoid licorice with natural flavoring due to potential for sodium and fluid retention. May cause hyperkalemia. Reduce intake of potassium-rich foods. Use potassium supplements, salt sub, and low sodium milk cautiously. Maintain good hydration.
BUMETANIDE Loop diuretic used to treat edema. *Bumex*	Common side effects: nausea, vomiting. May deplete sodium, potassium, magnesium, calcium, and thiamin. Hypokalemia increases digitalis toxicity. Increase intake of potassium, and magnesium-rich foods or consider supplements. Encourage increased milk intake for calcium and vitamin D. Avoid sodium-containing antacids.
CAPTOPRIL Angiotensin converting enzyme inhibitor (ACE-I) to treat hypertension. *Capoten*	Common side effects: altered taste, anorexia, dry mouth. Take one hour before meals as food significantly reduces absorption. Sugarless candy and gum or saliva substitute may help dry mouth. Increased risk of weight loss and hypoalbuminemia. Risk greatest in the elderly, those on high doses, and those also taking digoxin or theophylline. May elevate potassium levels. Reduce intake of potassium-rich foods. Use potassium supplements, salt sub, and low sodium milk cautiously. Avoid concurrent intake of magnesium supplements. Avoid licorice with natural flavoring due to potential for sodium and fluid retention.

Drug	Interaction
CHLORTHIAZIDE Thiazide diuretic used to treat hypertension and edema. *Diuril* *Diuregin*	Take with food to reduce GI distress. Increased sodium, potassium, and magnesium loss. Greatest risk with restricted or poor dietary intake. Increase intake of potassium and magnesium-rich foods. Promotes hyperglycemia and hyperlipidemia, especially in diabetics, and the latter in those with lipid disorders, or who take Acutane for acne. Reduces urinary excretion of calcium. Risk of hypercalcemia with renal disease, calcium supplements, and excess vitamin D. Avoid licorice with natural flavoring due to potential for sodium and fluid retention. Increases uric acid levels and potential for gout attacks.
CHOLESTYRAMINE Lipid-lowering drug used to treat hypercholesterolemia; also used to control itching associated with elevated bile acids. Questran	Common side effects: nausea, vomiting, constipation, heartburn. Best taken on an empty stomach. Increased fluid, fiber, and exercise may help constipation. Risk of malabsorption of multiple nutrients (fat, calcium, magnesium, iron, zinc, folate, vitamins A, D, E, K, and B$_{12}$), especially with prolonged, high doses. Multiple vitamin with minerals may be needed but should be taken separately. Follow good quality, low fat diet.
CLONIDINE Antiadrenergic used to treat hypertension. *Catapres*	Common side effects: dry mouth, nausea, vomiting, constipation. Increased fluid, fiber, and exercise may help constipation. Sugarless candy and gum or saliva substitute may help dry mouth. Niacin supplements may increase vasodilation. Avoid licorice with natural flavoring due to potential for sodium and fluid retention. Maintain good hydration. Avoid alcohol to avoid CNS depression.
COLESTIPOL Lipid-lowering drug used to treat hypercholesteremia; also used to control itching associated with elevated bile acids *Colestid*	Common side effects: nausea, vomiting, constipation, heartburn. Increased fluid, fiber, and exercise may help constipation, Risk of malabsorption of multiple nutrients (fat, calcium, magnesium, iron, zinc, folate, vitamins A, D, E, K, and B$_{12}$), especially with prolonged, high doses. Multiple vitamin with minerals may be needed but should be taken separately. Follow good quality, low fat diet.
DIGOXIN Cardiac stimulant used to treat congestive heart failure. *Lanoxicaps* *Lanoxin*	Common side effects: nausea, vomiting, diarrhea. Take at the same time everyday, one hour before breakfast or else keep breakfast consistent. Bran cereals, high fiber foods, and stool-bulking agents should not be taken with drug due to reduced absorption. May produce anorexia and nausea leading to reduced oral intake and weight loss, especially when heart failure is severe or renal function reduced. High potassium intake may help anorexia. Toxicity increased by hypercalcemia, hypokalemia, and hypomagnesemia. Increase intake of potassium and magnesium-rich foods. Magnesium supplements may reduce absorption, take them separately. Avoid excess calcium and vitamin D intake. Hypercalcemia may cause cardiac arrhythmias. Use laxatives cautiously to avoid excess potassium loss. Avoid herbal preparations which have drug activity (foxglove, dogbane, lily-of-the-valley, and oleander). Avoid licorice with natural flavoring due to potential for sodium and fluid retention.

Drug	Interaction
DILTIAZEM Calcium channel blocker used to treat angina and hypertension. *Cardizem*	If flushing, give with a low fat meal and avoid taking with grapefruit juice. Concurrent nicotinic acid may cause excess vasodilation. Hypercalcemia reduces drug effect. Use caution with calcium and vitamin D supplements. Limit alcohol as drug prolongs the effects. Avoid licorice with natural flavoring due to potential for sodium and fluid retention.
ENALAPRIL Angiotensin converting enzyme inhibitor (ACE-I) used to treat hypertension. *Vasotec*	Take one hour before meals as food significantly reduces absorption. Common side effects: altered taste, anorexia, dry mouth. Sugarless candy and gum or saliva substitute may help dry mouth. Increased risk of weight loss and hypoalbuminemia. Risk greatest in the elderly, those on high doses, and those also taking digoxin or theophylline. May elevate potassium levels. Reduce intake of potassium-rich foods. Use potassium supplements, salt sub, and low sodium milk cautiously. Avoid concurrent intake of magnesium supplements. Avoid licorice with natural flavoring due to potential for sodium and fluid retention.
ETHACRYNIC ACID Loop diuretic used to treat edema. *Edecrin*	May deplete sodium, potassium, calcium, magnesium and thiamin. Hypokalemia increases digitalis toxicity. Increase intake of potassium and magnesium-rich foods. Encourage milk for calcium and vitamin D. May elevate blood sugar or require change in antidiabetic agents. Avoid sodium-containing antacids. Avoid licorice with natural flavoring due to potential for sodium and fluid retention.
FELODIPINE Calcium channel blocker used to treat angina. *Plendil*	Common side effects: diarrhea, constipation, heartburn, weight gain. Increased fluid, fiber, and exercise may help constipation. More rapid absorption when taken with grapefruit juice. To reduce flushing take with a low fat meal. Avoid licorice with natural flavoring due to potential for sodium and fluid retention.
FLECANIDE Used to treat arrhythmias and tachycardia. *Tambocor*	Common side effects: altered taste, heartburn, nausea, vomiting, diarrhea, constipation. Increased fluid, fiber, and exercise may help constipation. Foods that alkalinize urine (strict vegetarian diets) increase blood levels. Foods that acidify urine (acidic juices) increase drug excretion. Hypokalemia and hyperkalemia alter drug effect. Maintain consistent intake.
FLUVASTATIN Lipid-lowering drug used to treat hypercholesterolemia. *Lescol*	Common side effects: nausea, vomiting, heartburn, diarrhea, constipation Increased fluid, fiber, and exercise may help constipation.

Drug	Interaction
FOSINOPRIL Angiotensin converting enzyme inhibitor (ACE-I) to treat hypertension. *Monopril*	Take one hour before meals. Absorption significantly reduced by food. May elevate potassium levels. Use potassium supplements, salt sub, and low sodium milk cautiously. Maintain good hydration. Avoid taking calcium and magnesium supplements within 2 hours of drug. Avoid licorice with natural flavoring due to potential for sodium and fluid retention. Limit alcohol to help control hypertension.
FUROSEMIDE Loop diuretic used to treat edema. *Lasix*	Increases urinary excretion of sodium, potassium, calcium, magnesium, zinc and thiamin. Hypokalemia increases digitalis toxicity. Increase intake of potassium and magnesium-rich foods. Encourage milk for calcium and vitamin D. Avoid sodium-containing antacids. May elevate blood sugar or require change in antidiabetic agents. Avoid licorice with natural flavoring due to sodium and fluid retention.
GEMFIBROZIL Lipid-lowering drug used to treat type II-b hyperlipidemia. *Lopid*	Common side effects: dry mouth, anorexia, and bloating after eating. Sugarless candy and gum or saliva substitute may help dry mouth. May cause hyperglycemia.
GUANABENZ Antiadrenergic used to treat hypertension. *Wytensin*	Common side effects: dry mouth, altered taste. Sugarless candy and gum or saliva substitute may help dry mouth. Maintain good hydration.
GUANETHIDINE Antiadrenergic used to treat hypertension. *Ismelin*	Common side effects: weight gain from edema. Risk of fluid retention especially with high sodium intake.
HYDRALAZINE Vasodilator used to treat hypertension. *Apresoline*	Common side effects: nausea, vomiting, and diarrhea. Best taken after a meal. Potential for peripheral neuropathy due to vitamin B_6 deficiency, especially with low dietary intake or other antagonistic drugs (isoniazid, penicillamine). May need supplement. Avoid licorice with natural flavoring due to potential for sodium and fluid retention.
HYDROCHLOROTHIAZIDE Thiazide used to treat hypertension and edema. *Esidrix* *Hydrodiuril* *Oretic* *Hydrochlor* *HCTZ* *Ezide* *Hydro-D*	Take with food to reduce GI distress. Increases sodium, potassium, and magnesium loss. Greatest risk with restricted or poor dietary intake. Increase intake of potassium and magnesium-rich foods. Promotes hyperglycemia (especially in diabetics), and hyperlipidemia (especially in diabetics, those with lipid disorders, or who take Acutane for acne). Risk of hypercalcemia with renal disease. Use vitamin D and calcium supplements cautiously. Increases zinc and riboflavin excretion. May need increased intake. Avoid licorice with natural flavoring due to potential for sodium and fluid retention. Increased uric acid levels and potential for gout attacks.

Drug	Interaction
LABETALOL Beta-adrenergic blocking agent (beta blocker) used to treat hypertension. *Normodyne*	Drug absorption increased by food. Potential for hypoglycemia in diabetics. May increase serum triglycerides. Potential for CNS effects with low albumin. Take calcium-containing supplements and antacids separately. Avoid licorice with natural flavoring due to potential for sodium and fluid retention.
LISINOPRIL Angiotensin converting enzyme inhibitor (ACE-I) to treat hypertension. *Zestril* *Prinivil*	Common side effects: heartburn, nausea vomiting, diarrhea, edema. May elevate potassium levels. Use potassium supplements, salt substitutes, and low sodium milk cautiously. Avoid licorice with natural flavoring due to potential for sodium and fluid retention.
LOVASTATIN Lipid-lowering drug used in the management of hypercholesterolemia. *Lopid* *Mevacor*	Common side effects: heartburn, nausea, vomiting, diarrhea, and constipation. Most effective when taken with evening meal. Increased fluid, fiber, and exercise may help constipation. Drug absorption may be reduced when taken concurrently with oat bran, and fiber supplements.
METHYLDOPA Antiadrenergic used in the management of hypertension. *Aldomet*	Common side effects: nausea, vomiting, sore tongue, dry mouth. Sugarless candy and gum or saliva substitute may help dry mouth. Drug absorption may be reduced by high protein meals or supplements and iron supplements. Take with a low protein snack or three hours before or after a high protein meal. Do not take iron supplements within 2 hours of drug. Folate and or vitamin B_{12} supplements may be needed with high intakes. Avoid licorice with natural flavoring due to for sodium and fluid retention. Hold tube feeding before and after giving liquid form of drug. Alcohol may increase the potential for hypotension. Limit alcohol.
METOPROLOL Beta-adrenergic blocking agent (beta blocker) used to treat hypertension and angina. *Lopressor* *Toprol-X*	Common side effects: altered taste, dry mouth, nausea, vomiting, heartburn, constipation. Drug absorption increased by food. Increased fluid, fiber, and exercise may help constipation. Potential for hypoglycemia in diabetics. May increase serum triglycerides. Potential for CNS effects with low albumin. Take calcium-containing supplements and antacids separately. Avoid licorice with natural flavoring due to for sodium and fluid retention.
MINOXIDIL Vasodilator used to treat hypertension. *Loniten*	Common side effects: nausea, vomiting, edema. Avoid licorice with natural flavoring due to potential for sodium and fluid retention. Maintain good hydration.

Drug	Interaction
NADOLOL Beta-adrenergic blocking agent (beta blocker) used to treat hypertension. *Corgard*	Drug absorption increased by food. May increase serum triglycerides. Potential for CNS effects with low albumin. Take calcium-containing supplements and antacids separately. Avoid licorice with natural flavoring due to potential for sodium and fluid retention.
NIACIN Vitamin used to treat hyperlipidemia and vitamin deficiency. *Nicotinic acid*	Reduce flushing by giving with aspirin. Reduce GI distress by taking with food. Potential for hyperglycemia in diabetics.
NICARDIPINE Calcium channel blocker used to treat hypertension and angina. *Cardene*	Common side effects: thirst, edema. Do not take with grapefruit juice as this can increase drug effects. Hypercalcemia reduces drug effects. Avoid calcium supplements. Use caution with vitamin D supplements. Avoid licorice with natural flavoring due to potential for sodium and fluid retention. Limit caffeine and alcohol.
NIFEDIPINE Calcium channel used to treat angina and hypertension. *Procardia* *Adalat*	Common side effects: nausea, vomiting, diarrhea, constipation, heartburn, edema. Avoid taking with grapefruit juice due to more rapid absorption and increased drug effect. Reduce flushing by taking with a low fat meal. Avoid licorice with natural flavoring due to potential for sodium and fluid retention. Reduced drug effect with hypercalcemia. Use calcium and vitamin D supplements cautiously. Don't take calcium supplements or antacids within 3 hours of drug.
NITROGLYCERIN (NTG) Antianginal and vasodilator used to treat angina. *Nitro Bid* *Nitroglyn* *Nitrolin*	Alcohol may potentiate problems with faintness and probably should be avoided. May falsely lower serum cholesterol levels. Potential headache and flushing with nitrate-containing foods (ham, hot dogs, etc.)
PENTOXIFYLLINE Blood thinner to increase blood flow in treat peripheral vascular disease. *Trental*	Common side effects: anorexia, nausea, dry mouth, dyspepsia. Take with food to reduce GI distress. Sugarless candy and gum or saliva substitute may help dry mouth. Monitor food intake and weight. Limit beverages with caffeine and xanthines (coffee, tea, caffeinated sodas).
PINDOLOL Beta-adrenergic blocking agent used to treat. hyper-tension. *Visken*	Drug absorption increased by food. Potential for hypoglycemia in diabetics. Potential for CNS effects with low albumin. Take calcium-containing supplements and antacids separately. Avoid licorice with natural flavoring due to potential for sodium and fluid retention.

Drug	Interaction
PRAVASTATIN Lipid-lowering drug used to treat hypercholesterolemia. *Paovacol*	Common side effects: nausea, vomiting, heartburn, diarrhea, constipation. Increased fluid, fiber, and exercise may help constipation. Concurrent high doses of niacin may cause muscle weakness.
PRAZOSIN Alpha-adrenergic used to treat hypertension. *Minipress*	Common side effects: nausea, vomiting, diarrhea, constipation, edema. Risk of fluid retention especially with high sodium intake. Avoid licorice with natural flavoring due to potential for sodium and fluid retention.
PROBUCOL Lipid-lowering drug used to treat hypercholesterolemia. *Lorelco*	Take with meals for better absorption. May cause anorexia. Monitor weight and food intake.
PROCAINAMIDE Used to treat arrhythmias. *Enkaid* *Pronestyl*	Common side effects: altered taste, nausea, vomiting, diarrhea, heartburn. Maintain good hydration.
PROPRANOLOL Beta-adrenergic blocking agent (beta blocker) used to treat hypertension. *Inderal*	Drug absorption increased by food. Best taken after a meal. Potential for hypoglycemia in diabetics. May increase serum triglycerides. Potential for CNS effects with low albumin. Take calcium-containing supplements and antacids at least 2 hours apart. Avoid licorice with natural flavoring due to potential for sodium and fluid retention.
QUINAPRIL Angiotensin converting enzyme inhibitor (ACE-I) to treat hypertension. *Accupril*	Common side effects: altered taste, anorexia, dry mouth. Take one hour before meals as food significantly reduces absorption. Sugarless candy and gum or saliva substitute may help dry mouth. May elevate potassium levels. Reduce intake of potassium-rich foods. Use potassium supplements, salt sub, and low sodium milk cautiously. Avoid alcohol to help control hypertension. Calcium and magnesium supplements may reduce absorption. Take 3 hours apart. Avoid licorice with natural flavoring due to potential for sodium and fluid retention.
QUINIDINE Antiarrythmic used to treat atrial and ventricular arrhythmias. *Duraquin* *Cardioquin* *Quiniglute* *Quiridex*	Common side effects: altered taste, heartburn, nausea, vomiting, diarrhea. Take with food to reduce GI distress. Promotes vitamin K deficiency when given with anticoagulants. May need increased intake. Large intake of citrus juice may promote toxicity (vomiting, diarrhea, tachycardia) by alkalinizing urine. May elevate potassium levels. Reduce intake of potassium-rich foods. Use potassium supplements, salt sub, and low sodium milk cautiously. Maintain good hydration.

Drug	Interaction
RAUWOLFIA Used to treat hypertension. *Serpasil* *Reserpine*	Risk of sodium and potassium depletion, especially with restricted diets. May cause anorexia. Avoid natural licorice due to increased sodium and fluid retention.
SIMVASTIN Lipid-lowering drug used to treat hypercholesterolemia. *Zocar*	Common side effects: nausea, vomiting, heartburn, diarrhea, constipation. Increased fluid, fiber, and exercise may help constipation. Concurrent intake of high doses of niacin may produce muscle weakness.
SOTALOL Beta-adrenergic blocking agent (beta blocker) used to treat arrhythmias. *Betapace*	Common side effects: altered taste, dry mouth, heartburn, nausea, vomiting, diarrhea, edema. Food significantly alters absorption. Be consistent when taking drug. May mask hypoglycemia in diabetics. May elevate serum lipids.
SPIRONOLACTONE Counteracts potassium loss associated with diuretics used to treat edema. *Aldactone*	Common side effects: thirst, dry mouth, heartburn, nausea, vomiting, diarrhea. Take with food to reduce GI symptoms. May produce hyperkalemia or sodium depletion. Reduce intake of potassium-rich foods. Use potassium supplements, salt sub, and low sodium milk cautiously. Avoid licorice with natural flavoring due to potential for sodium and fluid retention.
TERAZOSIN Antiadrenergic used to treat hypertension; also used to treat prostatic hyperplasia. *Hytrin*	Avoid licorice with natural flavoring due to potential for sodium and fluid retention. Maintain good hydration.
TIMOLOL Beta-adrenergic blocking agent (beta blocker) used to treat hypertension. *Blocadren*	Drug absorption increased by food. Potential for hypoglycemia in diabetics. May increase serum triglycerides. Potential for CNS effects with low albumin. Take calcium-containing supplements and antacids separately. Avoid licorice with natural flavoring due to potential for sodium and fluid retention.
TRIAMTERENE Counteracts potassium loss associated with use of diuretics to manage edema. *Dyrenium*	Take with food to reduce GI distress. May lead to hyperkalemia. Reduce intake of potassium-rich foods. Use potassium supplements, salt sub, and low sodium milk cautiously. May also cause folate depletion. Increase intake of folate-rich foods or consider supplement. Adequate intake of vitamin B_{12} important. Potential for causing hyperglycemia in diabetics.
VERAPAMIL Calcium channel blocker used to treat hypertension and angina.	Common side effects: nausea, vomiting, constipation, edema. To reduce flushing take with a low fat meal. Do not take with grapefruit juice as drug effect is increased. Hypercalcemia reduces drug effectiveness. Use vitamin

Drug	Interaction
Calan *Isoptin* *Verelan*	D and calcium supplements cautiously and do not take within 3 hours of drug. Avoid licorice with natural flavoring due to potential for sodium and fluid retention. Drug prolongs effects of alcohol. Limit caffeine intake.
WARFARIN Anticoagulant used to treat and prevent formation of thrombus and embolus. *Coumadin* *Panwarfarin*	Excess intake of vitamin K may reduce drug effect. Consistent intake is important. Check vitamin supplements and tube feedings for vitamin content. Drug anticoagulant effect may be increased by vitamin A and E supplements. Avoid high doses of vitamin A, 400 mg/d vitamin E, and > 500 mg/d ascorbic acid. Antibiotics (which destroy vitamin K-producing bacteria) may also increase drug effect. Avoid herbal products with coumarin activity (horse chestnut, buckeye/aesculus, tonka beans, meililot, and woodruff.) Avoid GI irritants (pepper, alcohol, caffeine, potassium supplements).
COMBINATION DRUGS *Aldactazide* *(spironolactone and thiazide)*	Common side effects: thirst, dry mouth, heartburn, constipation. Sugarless candy and gum or saliva substitute may help dry mouth. Increased fluid, fiber, and exercise may help constipation. Avoid licorice with natural flavoring due to potential for sodium and fluid retention. Reduce intake of potassium-rich foods. Use potassium supplements, salt sub, and low sodium milk cautiously. Hypercalcemia may alter drug effect. Use caution with calcium and vitamin D supplements. (see individual drugs)
Dyazide *Maxide* *(triamterene and hydrochlorothiazide)*	Avoid licorice with natural flavoring due to potential for sodium and fluid retention. Avoid potassium-containing supplements and salt substitutes, and low sodium milk. Increased excretion of magnesium. May need supplement. Anemia may result from folate depletion. (See individual drugs).

DERMATOLOGICAL DRUGS

Drug	Interaction
CYCLOSPORINE Immunosupressant used to treat psoriasis, prevent or treat rejection of transplanted organs. *Neoral* *Sandimmune*	Common side effects: anorexia, nausea, vomiting, diarrhea. Take with milk, chocolate milk or orange juice. Do not take with grapefruit juice. May cause hyperkalemia and hypomagnesemia. May elevate uric acid levels precipitating gout. May elevate cholesterol levels. Absorption increased by high fat meals.
ETRETINATE Used to treat psoriasis. *Tegison*	Common side effects: anorexia, altered taste, oral ulcers, diarrhea. Concurrent intake of milk increases absorption.
ISOTRETINOIN Used to treat acne. *Accutane*	Structurally similar to vitamin A, it may cause same symptoms as vitamin excess. Take with food as it increases absorption. May elevate blood sugar levels. Potential for skeletal changes (bone spurs) with duration greater than 3 months or intakes greater than 1 mg/kg. May elevate plasma lipids (triglycerides, cholesterol). Risks greater with high intake of alcohol, vitamin A supplements, and cholesterol. Try low fat and cholesterol diet before stopping drug. Avoid multivitamin, vitamin A, and beta-carotene supplements. Limit alcohol.
TETRACYCLINE Used to treat a variety of infections and bronchitis. *Achromycin-V* *Panmycin* *Robitet* *Sumycin* *Tetracyn* *Topicycline*	Common side effects: nausea, vomiting and heartburn. Best taken on an empty stomach. May take with non-dairy food to reduce GI distress. Forms insoluble complexes with calcium, magnesium, iron, zinc. Separate drug and dairy products, antacids, magnesium and aluminum-containing laxatives, calcium and iron supplements by 2 - 3 hours. Reduces vitamin K synthesis and increases urinary loss of riboflavin and folate. Potential deficiency with long term use. Increase vitamin intake or consider supplement. Stop tube feeding 1 hour before and 2 hours after drug.

ENDOCRINE DRUGS

Drug	Interaction
ACETOHEXAMIDE Used to control blood sugar in adults with non-insulin-dependent diabetes mellitus when diet therapy is inadequate. *Dymelor*	Appropriate diet is essential. Has mild diuretic effect. Maintain adequate fluid intake. Hypoglycemic effects are greater with hypoalbuminemia due to more free drug. Risk of hyperglycemia with dietary noncompliance, infection, corticosteroids, thiazide diuretics, and high dose nicotinic acid.
CHLORPROPAMIDE Used to control blood sugar in adults with non-insulin-dependent diabetes mellitus when diet therapy is inadequate. *Diabinese*	Common side effects: nausea, vomiting, diarrhea. Appropriate diet is essential. Potential for weight gain from fluid retention or excess food intake. Greater risk of hypoglycemia than with other oral agents due to long-acting effect. Hypoglycemic effects are greater with hypoalbuminemia due to more free drug. Alcohol intake may cause disulfram reaction (see endocrine drugs). Magnesium supplements may increase rate of absorption. Do not take together. Monitor blood sugars and glycosylated hemoglobin. Risk of hyperglycemia with dietary noncompliance, infection, corticosteroids, thiazide diuretics, and high dose nicotinic acid.
GLIPIZIDE Used to control blood sugar in adults with non-insulin-dependent diabetes mellitus when diet therapy is inadequate. *Glucotrol* *Glucotrol XL*	Common side effects: nausea, vomiting, heartburn, diarrhea, constipation. Take 1/2 to 1 hour before breakfast as food delays absorption. Increased fluid, fiber, and exercise may help constipation. Appropriate diet is essential. Risk of hyperglycemia with dietary noncompliance, infection, corticosteroids, thiazide diuretics, and high dose nicotinic acid. High doses of naicin may elevate blood sugar. Hypoalbuminemia increases drug effect due to more free drug.
GLYBURIDE Used to control blood sugar in adults with non-insulin-dependent diabetes mellitus when diet therapy is inadequate. *DiaBeta* *Micronase* *Glynase PresTab*	Common side effects: nausea, vomiting, heartburn. Take an evening snack due to long-acting drug effects. Appropriate diet is essential. Greater risk of hypoglycemia than with other oral agents due to long-acting effects. Hypoglycemia effects are greater with hypoalbuminemia due to more free drug. Risk of hyperglycemia with dietary noncompliance, infection, corticosteroids, thiazide diuretics, and high dose nicotinic acid.
INSULIN Used to control blood sugar in insulin-dependent diabetes mellitus and in non-insulin-dependent diabetes when diet therapy and oral hypoglycemia agents are inadequate. *Humalin R* *Novalin*	Appropriate diet is essential. May increase appetite. May cause hypoglycemia. Insulin needs increase with illness and pregnancy. Monitor blood glucose and glycosylated hemoglobin for adequacy of control. Risk of hyperglycemia with dietary noncompliance, infection, corticosteroids, cold medicines, thiazide diuretics, and high doses of nicotinic acid. Limit alcohol due to hypoglycemic effect.

Drug	Interaction
LEVOTHYROXINE Thyroid hormones used to treat hypothyroidism. *Synthroid* *Levothroid* *Levoxyl* *Levo-T*	Absorption reduced by food. May elevate blood sugar in diabetics. May need to increase insulin or oral hypoglycemic drug. May increase anticoagulant effects of warfarin, promoting bleeding, especially with low vitamin K intake. Iron supplements may reduce absorption. Take 4 hours apart.
METFORMIN Oral hypoglycemia agent used to treat NIDDM. *Glucophage*	Common side effects: nausea, vomiting, diarrhea, bloating. Appropriate diet is essential. Reduces vitamin B_{12} absorption. May need supplement.
PROPYLTHIOURIL Used to control hyperthyroidism. *PTU*	May alter taste acuity. May promote weight gain. May increase effects of anticoagulants, increasing bleeding potential. Greater risk with low vitamin K intake.
TOLAZAMIDE Used to control blood sugar in adults with non-insulin-dependent diabetes mellitus when diet therapy is inadequate. *Tolinase* *Tolamide*	Common side effects: nausea, vomiting, diarrhea, constipation. Appropriate diet is essential. Hypoglycemia effects are greater with hypoalbuminemia due to more free drug. Risk of hyperglycemia with dietary noncompliance, infection, corticosteroids, thiazide diuretics, and high doses nicotinic acid.
TOLBUTAMIDE Used to control blood sugar in adults with non-insulin-dependent diabetes mellitus when diet therapy is inadequate. *Orinase* *Tol-Tab*	Common side effects: nausea, vomiting, diarrhea, constipation. Appropriate diet is essential. Hypoglycemia effects are greater with hypoalbuminemia due to more free drug. Risk of hyperglycemia with dietary noncompliance, infection, corticosteroids, thiazide diuretics, and high doses of nicotinic acid.

GASTROINTESTINAL DRUGS

Drug	Interaction

ALUMINUM HYDROXIDE
Used to lower phosphate levels in renal failure, and treat ulcers, hyperacidity, indigestion, reflux esophagitis.
Alternagel
Alu-Cap
Alu-Tab
Amphojel
Basajel
Dialume
Nephrox

Common side effect: constipation. Increased fluid, fiber, and exercise may help. Excess intake may cause hypophosphatemia and osteomalacia. Low phosphate diet is appropriate if taken as a phosphate binder. May increase viscosity if added to tube feedings and cause clogging. Reduces absorption of several vitamins (vitamin A, folate, riboflavin) and minerals (iron, copper). Inactivates thiamin due to elevated pH. Take vitamin and mineral supplements separately due to formation of complexes with drug. May need folate supplementation with chronic use.

ATTAPULGITE (hydrated magnesium aluminum silicate)
Used to treat diarrhea.
Diar-Aid
Diasorb
Kaopectate
K-Pek
Parepectolin
Rheaban

Potential to cause precipitation of tube feeding if not well blended. Best to give separately. Maintain good hydration.

BISACODYL
Used to treat constipation, empty the bowel before procedures, provide bowel program in spinal cord injured patients.
Carter's Little Liver Pills
Dacodyl
Deficol
Dulcagen
Dulcolax
Fleet Laxative
Theralax

Excess use can cause malabsorption of major nutrients (protein, glucose, fat), producing weight loss. Also malabsorption of fat soluble vitamins D and K, calcium, and potassium. Take dairy products and vitamin and mineral supplements separately. Increased fiber, fluid, and exercise intake may reduce need for drug. Taking with milk or antacids may cause GI irritation by dissolving tablet early. Take separately.

BISMUTH SUBSALICYLATE
Used to treat diarrhea.
Bismatrol
Pepto-Bismol
Pink Bismuth

Risk of GI bleeding from salicylate portion. Avoid other GI irritants (pepper, alcohol, caffeine, potassium supplements). May need folate, iron, and vitamin C supplements with chronic use. Avoid high doses of vitamin C with long term use. See aspirin.

Drug	Interaction
CALCIUM ACETATE Used to bind phosphate preventing absorption and hyperphosphatemia. *Phos-Ex* *PhosLo*	Low phosphate diet is appropriate if taken as a binder. Potential for hypophosphatemia and hypercalcemia. Reduces iron absorption. Take iron supplements separately. Use calcium supplements with caution. Maintain good hydration.
CALCIUM CARBONATE Antacid used to treat hypocalcemia, and osteoporosis. *Caltrate* *Chooz* *Os-Cal* *Rolaids* *Titralac* *Tums*	Take with meals if used as phosphate binder or calcium supplement, between meals if used as antacid. Potential for milk-alkali syndrome (hypercalcemia from excess milk and antacid intake), especially with high intake, chronic use, vitamin D supplements, and renal insufficiency. Take iron supplements separately due to reduced absorption. Do not take with high fiber, oxalate, or phytate foods. Inactivates thiamin by increasing gastric pH. Take 3 hours after meals.
CIMETIDINE Used to treat ulcers, manage gastroesophageal reflux disease. *Tagamet* *Tagamet HB*	May deplete vitamin B_{12} due to decreased acidity and release from binding proteins. Risk increased in vegans and chronic use (> 1 year). Increases vitamin D need. Increases risk of bleeding from vitamin K deficiency when taken with warfarin. Avoid GI irritants (pepper, caffeine, potassium supplements). May potentiate intoxicating effects of alcohol. Liquid form precipitates tube feeding. Reduction of gastric acid along with reduced chewing or high fiber intake may produce food balls in the stomach. Increased risk in the elderly, use with caution. May reduce iron absorption. Take mineral supplements separately.
CISAPRIDE Prokinetic agent used to manage gastroesophageal reflux disease. *Propulsid*	Common side effects: heartburn, nausea, vomiting, diarrhea. Take 15 to 30 minutes before meals. Increases gastric emptying rate. May enhance sedative effects of alcohol.
DICYCLOMINE Used to treat irritable bowel syndrome. *Antispas* *A-Spas* *Bentyl* *Dibent* *Spasmoject*	Common side effects: dry mouth, nausea, vomiting, heartburn, constipation. Sugarless candy and gum or saliva substitute may help dry mouth. Increased fluid, fiber, and exercise may help constipation. Syrup will precipitate tube feeding. Give separately.
DIMENHYDRINATE Used to prevent nausea, vomiting, and symptoms of motion sickness. *Dramamine*	May cause dry mouth. Sugarless candy and gum or saliva substitute may help. May increase effects of alcohol.

Drug	Interaction
DIPHENOXYLATE w/ ATROPINE Used to treat diarrhea. *Lomotil* *Lofene* *Logen* *Lonox* *Lomocot*	Common side effects: heartburn, dry mouth, and sore, swollen gums. Sugarless candy and gum or saliva substitute may help dry mouth. Monitor electrolytes and hydration.
DOCUSATE Used to prevent constipation. *Colace* *Correctol* *DOSS* *Modane* *Regutol* *Surfak*	Common side effects: heartburn. Take with 8 ounces of liquid. Dissolve in flavored liquid to mask taste if needed. Encourage increased fluid, fiber, and exercise to help prevent constipation. Decreases absorption of water and electrolytes. Moniter potassium and hydration.
DRONABINOL Marijuana derivative used to prevent nausea and vomiting with chemotherapy, and treat anorexia. *THC* *Marinol*	Common side effects: nausea, vomiting, heartburn. Monitor food intake and hydration. Potential for CNS depression with alcohol intake.
FAMOTIDINE Used to treat ulcers, manage gastroesophageal reflux disease. *Pepsid*	Common side effect: constipation. Potential for vitamin B_{12} depletion due to reduced gastric acidity. Avoid other GI irritants (pepper, caffeine, potassium supplements). Reduction of gastric acid along with reduced chewing or high fiber intake may result in food balls in the stomach. Use with caution in the elderly.
KAOLIN/PECTATE Used to treat diarrhea. *K-P* *Kao-Spen* *Kapectolin*	Will cause separation of some tube feedings, especially those with intact protein. May need to give separately. Monitor electrolytes and hydration.
LOPERAMIDE Used to treat diarrhea, reduce volume of ileostomy output. *Imodium* *Kaopectate II* *Maalox Antidiarrheal*	Common side effects: heartburn, constipation. May cause dry mouth, and sore, swollen gums. Sugarless candy and gum or saliva substitute may help dry mouth. Monitor electrolytes and hydration.

Drug	Interaction
MAGNESIUM HYDROXIDE Used as antacids, laxatives, and to treat magnesium deficiency. *Phillips Milk of Magnesia* *MOM*	Common side effects: nausea, vomiting, heartburn, diarrhea. Risk of hypermagnesemia in renal patients. May need increased fiber and fluid intake to reduce need. Best taken 3 hours after meals. Do not take concurrently with iron supplement.
MAGNESIUM HYDROXIDE w/ALUMINUM HYDROXIDE Antacid used to treat ulcers. *Alamag* *Gelusil* *Maalox* *Magnalox* *Magnox* *Mintox* *Rulox*	Combined to reduce potential diarrhea from magnesium hydroxide and potential constipation from aluminum hydroxide. Reduces absorption of several vitamins (vitamin A, folate, riboflavin) and minerals (iron, phosphorus, copper). Inactivates thiamin due to high pH. Increased thiamin intake recommended. Best taken 3 hours after meals. Vitamin supplements should be taken separately. Use with caution in renal failure as significant magnesium is absorbed. Phosphorus levels should be monitored. May thicken tube feeding causing clogging. See individual drugs.
MAGNESIUM SULFATE Used as an antacid, laxative, and magnesium supplement. *Epsom Salt*	Risk of dehydration and hypermagnesemia, especially with renal failure. Encourage increased fluid, fiber, and exercise to reduce need.
METOCLOPRAMIDE GI stimulant used to treat nausea, vomiting, esophageal reflux, and diabetic gastric stasis. *Clopra* *Octamide* *Reclomide* *Reglan*	Common side effects: nausea, vomiting, diarrhea. Potential for decreased intake. May increase insulin need. May need to give separately with tube feedings, drug is not compatible with some. May increase sedative effects of alcohol. Monitor electrolytes and hydration.
MINERAL OIL Used to treat constipation. *Amoral* *Fleet Mineral Oil* *Kondremul Plain* *Liqui-doss* *Milkinol* *Nujol* *Petrogalar Plain* *Zymenol*	Chronic use reduces absorption of fat soluble vitamins. Risk greatest with marginal nutrient intake. Best not taken with food or vitamin supplements. Avoid daily use. Increased fiber, fluid, and exercise may reduce need. Do not take at night due to potential aspiration.
MISOPROSTOL Used to treat duodenal ulcers, prevent mucosal injury from NSAIDS. *Cytosec*	Potential for nausea, dyspepsia, and diarrhea. Avoid other GI irritants (pepper, caffeine, potassium supplements).

Drug	Interaction
NIZATIDINE H₂ blocker used for short term treatment of ulcers. *Axid*	Potential to reduce vitamin B_{12} absorption due to reduced acid production. May need increased intake or supplements given separately. Inadequate chewing of food or high fiber intake may cause food balls in the stomach. Use cautiously in the elderly. Avoid other GI irritants (pepper, caffeine, potassium supplements).
OMEPRAZOLE Used to treat gastroesophageal reflex disease, duodenal ulcers, gastric hypersecretion. *Losesc* *Prilosec*	Potential for causing anorexia and dry mouth. Sugarless candy and gum or saliva substitute may help dry mouth. May reduce iron and vitamin B_{12} absorption due to reduced gastric acid.
PANCREALIPASE Used to treat pancreatic insufficiency. *Cotazyme* *Enzymase* *Ilozyme* *Pancoate* *Pancrease* *Protilase* *Ultrase* *Viokase* *Zymase*	Concurrent intake of H₂ blockers (Cimetidine, etc. to reduce enzyme digestion) may reduce folate absorption. May need supplement. Chronic use increases risk of malabsorption of major nutrients, plus vitamins D and K and calcium.
PHENOLPHTHALEIN Used to treat constipation. *Alophen Pills* *Espotabs* *Evac-U-Gen* *Evac-U-Lax* *Ex-Lax* *Feen-a-Mint* *Modane* *Phenolax*	Excess use can cause malabsorption of major nutrients (protein, glucose, fat), producing weight loss. Also malabsorption of fat soluble vitamins D and K, calcium, and potassium. Take vitamin and mineral supplements separately. Increased fiber and fluid intake may reduce need for drug. Taking with milk or antacids may cause GI irritation by dissolving tablet early. Take separately. Maintain good hydration.
POLYCARBOPHIL Bulkformer used to treat irritable bowel syndrome. *Equilactin* *Fiberall* *FiberCon* *Fiber-Lax* *Mitrolan*	Reduces riboflavin absorption. Increased intake recommended. Dilute with at least 8 ounces of fluid to prevent swelling and possible choking. Increased intake of fiber and fluid and exercise may also help constipation. Maintain good hydration with diarrhea.

Drug	Interaction
PREDNISONE Used to treat inflammatory bowel disease. *Deltasone* *Meticorten* *Orasone* *Prednicen-M* *Sterapred*	Common side effect: slowed wound healing. Stimulation of appetite may induce weight gain. Potential for hypokalemia from increased excretion. Increase intake of potassium-rich foods. Potential for hyperglycemia in diabetics and nondiabetics. Increases protein catabolism. May need increased intake. Increases calcium excretion. Chronic use increases risk of osteoporosis, especially when drug dose is high and calcium intake is low (< 500 mg/d). Increased calcium and vitamin D intake recommended. Increases urinary excretion of zinc, and vitamin C. Increases folate and pyridoxine need. May need multivitamin and mineral supplement.
PROPANTHELINE BROMIDE Used to treat peptic ulcers. *Norpanth* *ProBanthine*	Common side effect: dry mouth. Enhances riboflavin absorption due to slowed gastric emptying. Sugarless candy and gum or saliva substitute may help dry mouth. Avoid other GI irritants (pepper, caffeine, potassium supplements).
PSYLLIUM GUM Used to treat constipation and chronic watery diarrhea. *Effer-syllium* *Fiberall* *Konsyl* *Metamucil* *Modane Bulk* *Perdiem* *Serutan* *Sibilin* *Syllact* *Versabran*	Take with 8 ounces of liquid to reduce risk of esophageal or gastric obstruction. Reduces absorption of riboflavin. May need increased intake. May also reduce appetite. Do not use with dysphagia. Increased fiber, fluid, and exercise may reduce need.
RANITIDINE H$_2$ blocker used to treat ulcers, manage gastroesophageal reflux disease. *Apo-Ranitidine* *Zantac*	Reduces vitamin B$_{12}$ absorption. May deplete vitamin, especially in vegans when taken for an extended time (> 1 year). May need increased intake or supplement. Take supplement separately. Use cautiously in the elderly as reduced chewing or increased fiber may induce food balls in the stomach. Avoid other GI irritants (pepper, caffeine, potassium supplements). Potential for bleeding if taken with warfarin. Increased vitamin K intake may be needed.
SENNA Used to treat constipation. *Fletcher's Castoria* *Senexon* *Senokot* *Senolax*	Common side effects: nausea, vomiting, heartburn. Excess use can cause hypokalemia, malabsorption, and weight loss. Risk of electrolyte imbalance with increased use. Increased fluid and fiber may reduce need. Monitor electrolytes and hydration.

Drug	Interaction
SODIUM BICARBONATE Used to treat metabolic acidosis, and to alkalinize urine, and neutralize gastric acidity. *Baking Soda* *Neut* *Soda Mint*	Inappropriate when sodium restriction needed. High sodium content may increase fluid retention. Risk of CHF in cardiac patients. Potential for milk alkali syndrome (hypercalcemia) when taken in large doses with milk. Use calcium supplements cautiously with long term use. High doses reduce folate absorption. May need increased intake. Take iron supplements separately. Inactivates thiamin by reducing gastric pH. Take 1 hour before or 3 hours after meals.
SULCRAFATE Used to manage/prevent duodenal ulcers, and protect gastric mucosa from aspirin and NSAIDS. *Carafate*	Common side effect: constipation. Increased fluid, fiber, and exercise may help constipation. Risk of significant hypophosphatemia, especially when taken with aluminum hydroxide. Do not take concurrently with calcium and magnesium supplements. Avoid other GI irritants (pepper, caffeine, alcohol, potassium supplements). May cause bezoars with enteral feedings. May reduce absorption of fat soluble vitamins. May need supplement.
SULFASALAZINE Used to treat inflammatory bowel disease. *Azulfidine*	Potential risk of folate deficiency, especially with low intake, malabsorption, and concurrent intake of other folate antagonists. Increased intake recommended.

GENITOURINARY AND CONTRACEPTIVE DRUGS

Drug	Interaction
CONJUGATED ESTROGENS Used as a hormone replacement. *Premarin*	Common side effects: nausea, vomiting. Take with food to reduce nausea. Maintain adequate intake of vitamin C but do not exceed 1 gram/day due to possible toxicity. Potential to elevate blood sugar. Increase intake of folate, pyridoxine, and vitamin B_{12}.
ETHINYL ESTRADIOL w/ NORGESTREL Used to prevent pregnancy. *Lo-Ovral* *Ovral*	This and other oral contraceptives may increase vitamin B_6 and folate needs, especially with malabsorption syndromes (gluten enteropathy, inflammatory bowel disease). Increase intake of folate, pyridoxine, and vitamin B_{12}. Potential for riboflavin depletion, especially in malnourished women.
METHENAMINE Used to treat urinary tract infections. *Mandelamine*	Take with cranberry juice to acidify urine and increase drug effect.
NITROFURANTOIN Used to treat urinary tract infections. *Furadantin* *Furalan* *Macrobid* *Macrodantin* *Nitrofuracot*	Common side effects: nausea, headache. Better absorption and less GI distress when taken with food. Magnesium supplements reduce absorption. Take 2 hours apart. Decreases serum folate. May need increased intake.
TETRACYCLINE Used to treat a variety of infections and bronchitis. *Achromycin-V* *Panmycin* *Robitet* *Sumycin* *Tetracyn* *Topicycline*	Best taken on an empty stomach. May take with non-dairy food to reduce GI distress. Forms insoluble complexes with calcium, magnesium, iron, and zinc. Separate intake of drug and dairy products, antacids, magnesium-containing laxatives, and calcium, iron, and zinc supplements by 2 - 3 hours. Reduces vitamin K synthesis and increases urinary loss of riboflavin and folate. Potential deficiency with long term use. Increase vitamin intake or consider supplement. Stop tube feeding 1 hour before and 2 hours after drug.

MUSCULOSKELETAL DRUGS

Drug	Interaction

ALLOPURINOL
Used to prevent attacks of gouty arthritis, treat hyperuricemia during chemotherapy.
Lopurin
Zyloprim

Common side effects: nausea, vomiting, diarrhea. Taking with food reduces GI symptoms. Low protein diet slows drug clearance. Action of vitamin K antagonists (warfarin) are prolonged with concurrent intake. High fluid intake recommended to prevent renal stones. Limit alcohol due to diuretic effect. Limit citrus fruits/juices and high dose ascorbic acid to keep urine alkaline. Decreases iron absorption. May need increased intake.

ASPIRIN
Nonsteroidal anti-inflammatory drug used to treat inflammatory disorders, prevent myocardial infarct and transient ischemic attacks.
Acetylsalicylic acid
Easprin
Ecotrin
Empirin
Halfprin
Heart-Trex
Measurin

Common side effect: heartburn. Take with food or 8 ounces of beverage to reduce GI symptoms. Potential for anemia due to GI blood loss, especially with low iron intake. Increased risk of bleeding with vitamin K deficiency. Reduces ascorbic acid absorption. Increase ascorbic acid intake but avoid high doses. May reduce serum folate with chronic use. May need iron and folate supplements. Adequate hydration important to prevent urine crystals. Limit other GI irritants (pepper, alcohol, caffeine, potassium supplements).

BENZTROPINE
Used to treat Parkinson's disease.
Cogentin

Common side effects: dry mouth, constipation. Sugarless gum or candy or saliva substitute may help dry mouth. Increased fluid, fiber, and exercise may help constipation. Maintain good hydration.

COLCHICINE
Used to treat or prevent attacks of gouty arthritis.
Colchicine
ColBenemid

May cause malabsorption of sodium, potassium, fat, carotene, and vitamin B_{12} with extended use, especially with other causes of malabsorption (gluten-insensitivity, excess alcohol intake). Supplements may be needed. Avoid high doses of ascorbic acid. Limit alcohol.

CORTISONE
Used to treat inflammatory conditions.

Potential for GI bleeding and iron deficiency anemia. Potential for causing hyperglycemia, muscle wasting, and osteoporosis. Increases urinary loss of potassium, nitrogen, zinc, ascorbic acid, and calcium. May need increased protein, potassium, intake plus multivitamin. Take supplements separately.

DIFLUNISAL
Nonsteroidal anti-inflammatory drug used to treat pain, inflammatory disorders.
Dolobid
Novo-Diflunisal

Common side effects: nausea, vomiting, heartburn, diarrhea, constipation. Take with food to reduce GI distress. Increased fluid, fiber, and exercise may help constipation. Potential for anemia due to GI bleeding, especially with low iron intake. Increase iron intake. Potential for hyperkalemia, especially with renal disease, high potassium intake (supplements, salt substitutes) or potassium-sparing diuretics. Use caution with other GI irritants (pepper, alcohol, caffeine, potassium supplements).

Drug	Interaction
FENOPROFEN Nonsteroidal anti-inflammatory drug used to treat pain, inflammatory disorders. *Nalfon*	Potential for anemia due to GI bleeding, especially with low iron intake. Potential for hyperkalemia, especially with renal disease, high potassium intake (supplements, salt substitutes) or potassium-sparing diuretics. Use caution with other GI irritants (pepper, alcohol, caffeine). May cause edema.
GOLD SODIUM THIOMALATE Used to treat rheumatoid arthritis. *Myochrisine*	May cause nephrosis and protein deficiency.
HYDROCORTISONE Short-acting glucocorticoid used as an anti-inflammatory or immunosupressive agent. *Icortef* *Cortenema* *Cortifoam* *Hydrocortone* *Solu-Cortef*	Potential for ulcers, bleeding, and iron deficiency anemia. Take with meals to minimize GI irritation. May cause hyperglycemia and impaired wound healing. Increases urinary loss of potassium, nitrogen, glucose, zinc, vitamin C, and calcium. Encourage a high protein, calcium, and potassium diet. Vitamin and mineral supplement may be needed. May cause growth retardation in children. Moniter height and weight.
IBUPROFEN Nonsteroidal anti-inflammatory agent used to treat pain and inflammatory disorders. *Advil* *Dolgesic* *Ibuprofen* *Ibren* *Medipren* *Motrin* *Nuprin*	Common side effects: nausea, vomiting, heartburn, diarrhea, constipation. Increased fluid, fiber, and exercise may help constipation. Potential for ulcers, GI bleeding, and iron deficiency anemia with chronic use. Increase iron intake. Avoid other GI irritants (caffeine, alcohol, pepper, potassium supplements).
INDOMETHACIN Used to treat inflammatory disorders. *Indocin*	Common side effects: heartburn. Take with food to reduce GI distress. May increase blood sugar in diabetics. Potential for anemia due to GI bleeding, especially with low iron intake. Reduces absorption of vitamin C. Increase intake of iron and vitamin C. Potential for hyperkalemia, especially with renal disease, high potassium intake (supplements, salt substitutes) or potassium-sparing diuretics). Avoid other GI irritants (pepper, caffeine, potassium supplements).

Drug	Interaction
KETOPROFEN Nonsteroidal anti-inflammatory drug used to treat pain, inflammatory disorders. *Actron* *Orudis* *Oruvail*	Potential for anemia due to GI bleeding, especially with low iron intake. Potential for hyperkalemia, especially with renal disease, high potassium intake (supplements, salt substitutes) or potassium-sparing diuretics. Use caution with other GI irritants (pepper, alcohol, caffeine, potassium supplements). May cause edema.
KETORALAC Nonsteroidal anti-inflammatory drug used to treat pain. *Toradol*	Common side effects: nausea, vomiting, heartburn, diarrhea, constipation. Take with food to reduce GI distress. Increased fluid, fiber, and exercise may help constipation. Potential for anemia due to GI bleeding, especially with low iron intake. Use caution with other GI irritants (pepper, alcohol, caffeine, potassium supplements).
MECLOFENAMATE Nonsteroidal anti-inflammatory drug used to treat pain, inflammatory disorders, and dysmenorrhea. *Meclofen* *Meclomen*	Potential for anemia due to GI bleeding, especially with low iron intake. Potential for hyperkalemia, especially with renal disease, high potassium intake (supplements, salt substitutes) or potassium-sparing diuretics. Use caution with other GI irritants (pepper, alcohol, caffeine, potassium supplements). May induce edema.
METHOTREXATE Used to treat tumors, leukemia, psoriasis, rheumatoid arthritis. *Aminopterin* *Folex* *Rheumatrex*	Common side effects: anorexia, vomiting, diarrhea, stomatitis. Antifolate activity leads to acute effects (stomatitis, enteritis, leukopenia) and chronic effects (megaloblastic anemia, malabsorption, liver toxicity). Potential for malabsorption of fat, calcium, vitamin B_{12}, and folate. Folate supplement (1 mg/d) can reverse GI effects with low drug dose. Maintain good hydration.
NAPROXEN Nonsteroidal anti-inflammatory drug used to treat pain, inflammatory disorders, dysmenorrhea. *Naproxyn* *Aleve* *Anaprox*	Common side effects: nausea, vomiting, heartburn, diarrhea, constipation. Take with food to reduce GI distress. Increased fluid, fiber, and exercise may help constipation. Avoid other GI irritants (pepper, caffeine, potassium supplements). Potential for anemia due to GI bleeding, especially with low iron intake. Potential for hyperkalemia, especially with renal disease, high potassium intake (supplements, salt substitutes) or potassium-sparing diuretics).
PENICILLAMINE Used to treat rheumatoid arthritis and recurrent cystine calculi and to chelate copper in Wilson's disease. *Cuprimine* *Depen*	Food significantly reduces drug absorption. Increases urinary excretion of zinc and may cause zinc deficiency, especially with high alcohol intake and previous use of nephrotoxic drugs. May need supplement, but take separately. Complexes with vitamin B_6 and increases excretion. A 25 mg/d supplement is recommended. Maintain good hydration if used for renal calculi. Limit copper intake if taken for Wilson's disease.

Drug	Interaction
PIROXICAM Nonsteroidal anti-inflammatory drug used to treat inflammatory disorders, dysmenorrhea. *Feldene* *Nu-Pirox*	Common side effect: nausea, vomiting, heartburn, diarrhea, constipation. Take with food to reduce GI distress. Increased fluid, fiber, and exercise may help constipation. Potential for anemia due to GI bleeding, especially with low iron intake. Increase intake of iron-rich foods. Include a good source of ascorbic acid to increase absorption. Potential for hyperkalemia, especially with renal disease, high potassium intake (supplements, salt substitutes) or potassium-sparing diuretics. Use caution with other GI irritants (pepper, alcohol, caffeine, potassium supplements).
PREDNISONE Used to treat inflammatory bowel disease. *Deltasone* *Meticorten* *Orasone* *Prednicen-M* *Sterapred*	Common side effects: slowed wound healing. Stimulation of appetite may induce weight gain. Potential for hypokalemia from increased excretion. Increase intake of potassium-rich foods. Potential for hyperglycemia in diabetics and nondiabetics. Increases protein catabolism. May need increased intake. Increases calcium excretion. Chronic use increases risk of osteoporosis, especially when drug dose is high and calcium intake is low (< 500 mg/d). Increased calcium and vitamin D intake recommended. Increases urinary excretion of zinc, and vitamin C. Increases folate and pyridoxine need. May need multivitamin and mineral supplement. Increases vitamin A transport from the liver depleting stores.
PROBENECID Used to treat gouty arthritis, hyperuricemia. *Benemid* *Probalan*	Increased risk of renal stones with high protein or purine intake. Reduces riboflavin absorption. Maintain adequate intake. Increase fluid intake to produce dilute urine (2 - 3 L/d). Limit citrus fruits/juices, and large doses vitamin C to help keep urine alkaline.
SULFASALAZINE Anti-inflammatory used to treat GI disease. *Azulfidine*	Common side effects: anorexia, nausea, vomiting, diarrhea. Take with food or 8 ounces of water to reduce GI symptoms. Reduces folate absorption. Increase intake of folate-rich foods but avoid high doses as supplements. Maintain adequate hydration with 1.5 L/d.
SULFINPYRAZONE Used to treat gout. *Anturane*	Avoid high intakes of citrus juices or ascorbic acid to keep urine alkaline. Maintain good hydration. May potentiate effects of oral hypoglycemic drugs and insulin.
SULINDAC Used to treat gouty arthritis, inflammatory disorders. *Clinoril*	Take with food to reduce GI distress. Avoid other GI irritants (pepper, caffeine, potassium supplements, alcohol). Potential for anemia due to GI bleeding. Increase intake of iron-rich foods. Include a good source of ascorbic acid to increase absorption. Potential for hyperkalemia, especially with renal disease, high potassium intake (supplements, salt substitutes) or potassium-sparing diuretics.

Drug	Interaction
TOLMETIN Nonsteroidal anti-inflammatory drug used to treat inflammatory disorders. *Tolectin*	Potential for anemia due to GI bleeding, especially with low iron intake. Increase intake of iron-rich foods. Include a good source of ascorbic to increase absorption. Potential for hyperkalemia, especially with renal disease, high potassium intake (supplements, salt substitutes) or potassium-sparing diuretics. Use caution with other GI irritants (pepper, alcohol, caffeine, potassium supplements). May cause edema.

NEOPLASTIC DRUGS

Drug	Interaction
BLEOMYCIN Used to treat a variety of malignancies. *Blenoxane*	Oral ulcers, vomiting, and pneumonitis/shortness of breath may limit food intake. Greatest risk of nausea and vomiting with large food intake within a few hours of taking the drug. Maintain good hydration.
CARMUSTINE Used to treat a variety of malignancies. *BCNU* *BiCNU*	Greatest risk of nausea and vomiting with large food intake within a few hours of taking the drug. May cause renal toxicity with hypophosphatemia and glucosuria. Maintain good hydration.
CISPLATIN Used to treat a variety of malignancies. *Platinol* *Platinol-AQ*	Common side effects: altered taste, nausea, vomiting, diarrhea. Greatest risk of nausea and vomiting with large food intake within a few hours of taking the drug. May cause magnesium depletion, especially with renal dysfunction, dehydration, and loop diuretics. Increased urinary loss of potassium, calcium, zinc, copper, and amino acids. May need mineral supplement. Maintain good hydration.
CYCLOPHOSPHAMIDE Used to treat a variety of malignancies. *Cytoxan* *Neosar*	May cause vomiting. Take with food to reduce GI distress. Greatest risk of nausea and vomiting with large food intake within a few hours of taking the drug. Maintain good hydration.
DACTINOMYCIN Used to treat a variety of malignancies. *Actinomycin-D* *Cosmegen*	Common side effects: nausea, vomiting, diarrhea. Greatest risk of nausea and vomiting with large food intake within a few hours of taking the drug. Maintain good hydration. Posssible malabsorption of calcium, iron, and fat. May increase vitamin B_{12} need.
DOXORUBICIN Used to treat solid tumors, leukemia, lymphomas. *Adriamycin* *Rubex*	Common side effect: cardiomyopathy. Greatest risk of nausea and vomiting with large food intake within a few hours of taking the drug. Maintain good hydration.
5-FLUOROUROCIL Used to treat a variety of malignancies. *Adrucil* *Efudex* *Fluoroplex* *5-FU*	Anorexia, vomiting, diarrhea, and stomatitis may limit food intake. Greatest risk of nausea and vomiting with large food intake within a few hours of taking the drug. Mild anti-folate activity. May increase thiamin requirement.

Drug	Interaction
LOMUSTINE Used to treat a variety of malignancies. *CCNU* *CeeNu*	Greatest risk of nausea and vomiting with large food intake within a few hours of taking the drug. Maintain good hydration.
METHOTREXATE Used to treat a variety of malignancies, psoriasis, rheumatoid arthritis. *Amethopterin* *Folex* *Rheumatrex*	Greatest risk of nausea and vomiting with large food intake within a few hours of taking the drug. Weight loss from anorexia, stomatitis, diarrhea, and malabsorption are common. Blocks metabolism of folate. Risk of folate depletion increased without folinic acid (citrovorum factor) rescue. Maintain good hydration. Possible malabsorption of calcium, fat, and vitamin B_{12}. Avoid taking with dairy products.
MORPHINE Used to treat pain, pulmonary edema. *Astramorph* *Duramorph* *MS* *MSO4* *Oramorph* *Roxanol*	Common side effects: anorexia, nausea, vomiting, constipation. Take with food to reduce GI distress.. Increased fluid, fiber, and exercise may help constipation. Greatest risk of nausea and vomiting with large food intake within a few hours of taking the drug. Maintain good hydration. Alcohol increases CNS effects.
PROCARBAZINE Used to treat Hodgkin's disease. *Mutalane*	Greatest risk of nausea and vomiting with large food intake within a few hours of taking the drug. Drug is a vitamin B_6 antagonist. As a monoamine oxidase inhibitor (MAOI) may cause hypertension with similar drugs or tyramine-containing foods. Potential disulfram reaction with alcohol (see endocrine drugs). Avoid alcohol.
TAMOXIFEN Used to treat breast cancer. *Nolvadex*	Potential for hypercalcemia if bone metastases. Take calcium and magnesium supplements separately by 2 hours.
TRIMETREXATE Used to treat a variety of malignancies.	May cause anemia due to folate antagonism. Risk of folate depletion increased without folinic acid rescue.
VINCRISTINE Used to treat a variety of malignancies. *Oncovin* *Vincasar* *Vincrex*	Common side effect: constipation. Increased fluid, fiber, and exercise may help constipation. Maintain good hydration.

NEUROPSYCHIATRIC DRUGS

Drug	Interaction
AMITRIPTYLINE Used to treat depression. *Elavil* *Emitrip* *Endep* *Enovil*	Common side effect: constipation. Increased fiber, fluid, and exercise may reduce constipation. Increased fiber may reduce drug effect so take high fiber foods separately. Reduced coordination and tremors may interfere with eating, especially in the elderly. Increase riboflavin intake. Avoid alcohol as it may increase sedation.
BENZTROPINE Anticholinergic used to treat Parkinson's disease. *Cogentin*	Common side effects: reduced appetite, dry mouth, constipation. Use sugarless gum or candy or saliva substitute for dry mouth. Increased fiber, fluid, and exercise may reduce constipation. Maintain good hydration.
BUPROPION Used to treat depression. *Wellbutrin*	Common side effects: dry mouth, heartburn, nausea, vomiting, constipation Use sugarless gum or candy or saliva substitute for dry mouth. Maintain good hydration. Increased fiber, fluid, and exercise may reduce constipation. Potential for GI bleeding and anemia with chronic use. May need to avoid other GI irritants (pepper, caffeine, alcohol) if taken chronically. Alcohol may increase CNS effects.
CARBAMAZEPINE Anticonvulsant used to treat seizures. *Epitol* *Tegretol*	Common side effects: dry mouth, nausea, vomiting, diarrhea. Take with food to reduce GI distress. Sugarless gum or candy or saliva substitute may help dry mouth. May produce altered taste and decreased food intake. Drug clearance reduced with excess weight. Weight reduction may require reduced dose. Alcohol may increase CNS effects.
CARBIDOPA + LEVODOPA Used to treat Parkinson's disease. *Sinemet*	Common side effects: altered taste, dry mouth, anorexia, heartburn, nausea, vomiting. Take with food to reduce GI distress. Sugarless candy or gum or saliva substitute may help dry mouth. Drug may cause vitamin B_6 deficiency. Inversely, vitamin B_6 may interfere with drug activity. Risk is less than with levodopa alone. Use caution with vitamin supplements. Do not take concurrently with high protein foods which can reduce absorption. Large, high fat, or high fiber meals slow gastric emptying increasing drug breakdown. Potential for hypertensive crises when taken with MAOI drugs or high tyramine-containing foods. Potential for hypokalemia. Risk of iron deficiency anemia due to GI bleeding from ulcers. Take iron supplements separately.
CHLORDIAZEPOXIDE Used to treat anxiety and alcohol withdrawal. *Libritabs* *Librius*	Common side effects: nausea, vomiting. Take with food to minimize GI distress. Avoid concurrent intake with alcohol. Hypoalbuminemia increases drug effect due to more free drug. Take calcium and magnesium supplements separately.

Drug	Interaction
CHLORPROMAZINE Antipsychotic used to treat psychoses, antiemetic used to treat nausea, vomiting. *Thorazine* *Thor-Prom*	Common side effects: dry mouth, appetite stimulation, constipation, weight gain. Sugarless candy and gum or saliva substitute may help dry mouth. Increased fluid, fiber, and exercise may help constipation. Increases excretion of riboflavin. Increased intake recommended. Stimulates appetite and may cause excess weight gain, especially with unlimited access to food. Reduces vitamin B_{12} absorption. Take vitamin and mineral supplements separately. Liquid form may precipitate, clogging feeding tubes.
CLOZAPINE Used to treat schizophrenia. *Clozaril*	Common side effect: dry mouth, nausea, vomiting, constipation. Sugarless candy and gum or saliva substitute may help dry mouth. Increased fluid, fiber, and exercise may help constipation. Hypoalbuminemia increases drug effect due to more free drug.
DEXTROAMPHETAMINE CNS stimulant used to treat narcolepsy, attention deficit hyperactivity disorder. *Dexedrine* *DextroStat*	Common side effects: dry mouth. Sugarless candy and gum or saliva substitute may help dry mouth. Large doses of ascorbic acid may acidify urine increasing drug excretion and reducing drug effect. Potential for increased drug levels with calcium and magnesium supplements. Take separately. Avoid large amounts of caffeine. Potential for growth supression. Monitor weight and height in children.
DIAZEPAM Anticonvulsant used to treat status epilepticus sedative used to provide sedation, muscle relaxant. *PMS-Diazepam* *Valium* *Valrelease* *Vazepam*	Potential for reduced food intake from dry mouth, especially with high doses. Sugarless gum or candy or saliva substitute may help. Large, high fiber, or high fat meals delays gastric emptying increasing drug breakdown. Limit caffeine intake to < 500 mg/d. Hypoalbuminemia increases drug effect due to more free drug.
DESIPRAMINE Tricyclic antidepressant used to treat depression. *Norpramin*	Common side effects: dry mouth, nausea, vomiting, constipation. Sugarless gum or candy or saliva substitute may help dry mouth. Increased fiber, fluid, and exercise may reduce constipation. Increased urinary loss of riboflavin. Increased intake recommended. Increased fiber may reduce drug effect. Do not take with high fiber foods.
DISULFRAM Used for prevention of alcohol abuse. *Antabuse*	Produces disulfram reaction (nausea, vomiting, headache, chest pain) with alcohol intake. Avoid alcohol and alcohol-containing foods, beverages, and medicines (e.g. cold medications). Read labels carefully. Drug increases caffeine effects. Limit caffeine.

Drug	Interaction
DOXEPIN Used to treat depression and anxiety. *Sinequan* *Zonalon*	Common side effects: dry mouth, constipation. Sugarless gum or candy or saliva substitute may help dry mouth. Increased fluid, fiber, and exercise may help constipation. Potential for weight gain. High fiber intake may reduce drug effect. Don't take with high fiber foods. Don't take with carbonated drinks or grape juice. Limit caffeine. Potential riboflavin deficiency from increased urinary loss. Increased intake recommended.
FLUOXETINE Used to treat depression and obsessive compulsive disorder. *Prozac*	Common side effects: dry mouth, heartburn, nausea, vomiting, diarrhea. Sugarless gum or candy or saliva substitute may help dry mouth. Tryptophan supplements taken concurrently will increase drug side effects.
FLUPHENAZINE Used to treat psychoses. *Prolixin* *Permitil*	Common side effects: appetite stimulation, dry mouth, nausea, vomiting, constipation, weight gain. Sugarless gum or candy or saliva substitute may help dry mouth. Increased fiber, fluid, and exercise may reduce constipation. Potential for riboflavin depletion. Increased intake recommended. Concurrent intake of tryptophan supplements will increase drug side effects. If concentrate form mixed with caffeinated beverages or fruit juice, drug may precipitate.
HALOPERIDOL Used to treat psychoses and nausea and vomiting. *Haldol*	Common side effects: dry mouth, constipation. Sugarless gum or candy or saliva substitute may help dry mouth. Increased fluid, fiber, and exercise may help constipation. If concentrate form mixed with caffeinated beverages or fruit juice, drug may precipitate. Maintain good hydration.
IMIPRAMINE Used to treat depression. *Tipramine* *Tofranil*	Common side effects: increased appetite, weight gain, dry mouth, nausea, vomiting, constipation. Sugarless gum or candy or saliva substitute may help dry mouth. Increased fluid, fiber, and exercise may help constipation. High fiber intake may reduce drug effect so take drug separate from high fiber foods. Potential riboflavin deficiency from increased urinary loss. Increased intake recommended.
LACTULOSE Laxative used to treat constipation, hepatic encephalopathy. *Cephulac* *Cholac* *Chronulac* *Constilac* *Duphalac* *Enulose* *Generlax* *Portalac*	Common side effects: heartburn. Contains galaclose and lactose. Should not be used with a lactose or galactose restricted diet. Increase fiber and fluid intake if used as a laxative. Needs dilution before adding to tube feeding. Increased loss of electrolytes and water soluble vitamins. Vitamin supplement recommended.

Drug	Interaction
LEVODOPA Used to treat Parkinson's disease. *Dopar* *L-dopa* *Larodopa*	Common side effects: altered taste, anorexia, dry mouth, nausea, vomiting, heartburn. Sugarless gum or candy or saliva substitute may help dry mouth. Take with food to reduce GI distress. Drug may cause vitamin B_6 deficiency. Inversely, vitamin B_6 reverses drug effect. Use caution with vitamin supplements. Limit intake to < 5 mg/d. Do not take concurrently with high protein foods which can reduce absorption. Take with a low protein breakfast. Large, high fiber, or high fat meals slow gastric emptying, thus increasing drug breakdown in the stomach reducing the amount available for absorption. Potential for hypertensive crises when taken with MAOI drugs or high tyramine-containing foods. Potential for hypokalemia, especially with laxatives or non potassium-sparing diuretics. Take iron supplements separately.
LITHIUM Used to treat a variety of psychiatric disorders, especially bipolar affective disorders. *Cibalith-S* *Duralith* *Eskalith* *Lithane* *Lithonate* *Lithotabs*	Common side effects: dry mouth, nausea, vomiting, heartburn, diarrhea, constipation. Take with food to reduce GI distress. May promote increased appetite and weight gain. Sugarless gum or candy or saliva substitute may help dry mouth. Increased fiber, fluid, and exercise may reduce constipation. Inadequate sodium intake or diuretics can increase drug toxicity. Avoid acute changes in sodium intake. Maintain adequate hydration. Limit caffeine. Potential risk of hypothyroidism with iodine supplement. Syrup form precipitates tube feedings.
LORAZEPAM Used to treat anxiety and insomnia. *Ativan* *NuLoras*	Sleepiness may reduce food intake. Limit caffeine to < 500 mg/d.
MESORIDAZINE Used to treat psychoses. *Serentil*	Common side effects: dry mouth, constipation. Sugarless candy and gum or saliva substitute may help dry mouth. Increased fluid, fiber, and exercise may help constipation. Liquid form precipitates tube feeding. Increase riboflavin intake due to increased excretion.
METHYLPHENIDATE Used to treat attention-deficit hyperactivity disorder and narcolepsy. *PMS-Methylphenidate* *Ritalin*	Common side effects: heartburn. Potential for anorexia, reduced food intake, weight loss or growth retardation in children with chronic use. Monitor height and weight or intake. Reduce anorexia by taking with meals. Limit caffeine intake due to CNS effects.
NORTRIPTYLINE Tricyclic antidepressant used to treat depression. *Aventyl* *Pamelor*	Common side effects: constipation. Increased fiber, fluid, and exercise may reduce constipation. Agitation and tremors may interfere with eating. Limit caffeine intake. Increased riboflavin intake recommended due to increased urinary excretion. Large, high fiber, or high fat meals delay gastric emptying, allowing greater drug breakdown in the stomach.

Drug	Interaction
PAROXETINE Used to treat depression. *Paxil*	Common side effects: dry mouth, nausea, vomiting, constipation. Sugarless candy and gum or saliva substitute may help dry mouth. Increased fluid, fiber, and exercise may help constipation. Avoid tryptophan supplements.
PEMOLINE Used to treat attention deficit hyperactivity disorder in children. *Cylert*	Potential for growth suppression. Monitor height and weight with chronic use. Avoid large amounts of caffeine due to CNS effects.
PENTOXIFYLLINE Blood thinner used to treat peripheral vascular disease, increase cerebral circulation. *Trental*	Potential reduced food intake from anorexia and nausea. Take with food to reduce GI distress. Limit caffeine intake.
PERPHENAZINE Used to treat psychoses, also nausea, vomiting, and hiccoughs. *Trilafon*	Common side effects: dry mouth, nausea, vomiting, constipation. Stimulates appetite and may cause excess weight gain, especially with unlimited access to food. Take with food to reduce GI distress. Sugarless candy and gum or saliva substitute may help dry mouth. Increased fluid, fiber, and exercise may help constipation. Potential for causing riboflavin depletion. Increased intake recommended.
PHENELZINE Monoamine oxidase inhibitor used to treat depression. *Nardil*	Common side effects: dry mouth, heartburn, constipation. Increased fluid, fiber, and exercise may help constipation. Potential for acute hypertensive crises with concurrent intake of foods high in tyramine and other pressor amines. Avoid tryptophan supplements. Potential vitamin B_6 deficiency. May need supplementation. Concentrated form should not be mixed with caffeinated beverages or fruit juice as it may precipitate drug. Limit caffeine due to CNS effects.
PHENOBARBITAL Anticonvulsant used to treat seizures. *Barbita* *Luminal* *Solfoton*	Potential for folate deficiency and megaloblastic anemia, especially with low folate intake, other anticonvulsant drugs, and malabsorption. Increase intake of folate and vitamin B_{12}-rich foods. Use caution with vitamin supplements as excess folate and vitamin B_6 may reduce drug effect. Risk of vitamin D deficiency (increased breakdown) and osteomalacia with chronic intake, especially with little sun exposure, poor dietary intake, and other anticonvulsants. Encourage intake of fortified dairy products. May increase effect of anticoagulants by inducing vitamin K deficiency (due to increased metabolism) and bleeding. Excess vitamin B_6 (80-400 mg/d) may reduce drug effect. Increase intake of vitamin C-rich foods due to lower serum levels.

Drug	**Interaction**
PHENYTOIN Anticonvulsant used to treat seizures. *DPH* *Dilantin* *Diphenylan*	Common side effects: nausea, vomiting, constipation. Take with food to reduce GI distress. Increased fluid, fiber, and exercise may help constipation. Potential folate and megaloblastic anemia, especially with low folate intake, other anticonvulsant drugs, and malabsorption. High intakes of folate (> 5 mg/week) reduces drug availability. Risk of vitamin D deficiency (increased breakdown) with chronic intake, especially with little sun exposure, poor dietary intake, and other anticonvulsants. Supplementation with 1000 to 2000 IU/d is recommended. Reduces calcium absorption. Take calcium and magnesium supplements and antacids separately. May increase effect of anticoagulants by inducing vitamin K deficiency and bleeding. Increase vitamin intake. Vitamin K supplements may be needed in the third trimester of pregnancy. Stop enteral feeding at least one hour before and after giving due to reduced drug absorption.
PRIMIDONE Anticonvulsant used to treat seizures. *Myidone* *Mysoline*	Potential for folate deficiency and megaloblastic anemia. Increase intake of folate-rich foods. Supplements may interfere with drug action. Increased risk of vitamin D deficiency, calcium malabsorption, and decreased bone density. Increase intake of vitamin D and calcium.
PROCHLORPERAZINE Antipsychotic and antiemetic used to treat psychosis and nausea and vomiting. *Chlorpazine* *Compa-Z* *Compazine* *Cotranzine* *Ultrazine*	Common side effects: dry mouth, constipation. Stimulates appetite and may cause excess weight gain, especially with unlimited access to food. Sugarless candy or gum or a saliva substitute may help dry mouth. Increased fluid, fiber, and exercise may help constipation. Potential for causing riboflavin depletion from increased excretion. Increased intake recommended. Limit caffeine intake due to CNS effects.
RISPERIDONE Used to treat psychoses. *Risperdal*	Common side effects: dry mouth, nausea, vomiting, heartburn, diarrhea, constipation. Sugarless candy and gum or saliva substitute may help dry mouth. Increased fluid, fiber, and exercise may help constipation. Maintain good hydration.
SELEGILINE Used in conjunction with levodopa and carbodopa to treat Parkinson's disease. *Eldepryl* *SD-Deprenyl*	Potential for hypertensive reactions with tyramine-containing foods with drug dose of > 10 mg/d. Limit intake of foods high in tyramine and other pressor amines.
SERTRALINE Used to treat depression. *Zoloft*	Common side effects: altered taste, dry mouth, nausea, vomiting, heartburn, diarrhea, constipation. Take regularly with or without food for consistent absorption. Sugarless candy or gum or a saliva substitute may help dry mouth. Increased fiber, fluid, and exercise may help constipation.

Drug	Interaction
THIORIDAZINE Antipsychotic used to treat psychosis and depression. *Mellaril*	Common side effects: appetite stimulation, weight gain, dry mouth, constipation. Sugarless gum or candy or saliva substitute may help dry mouth. Increased fiber, fluid, and exercise may reduce constipation. Stimulates appetite and may cause excess weight gain, especially with unlimited access to food. Potential for causing riboflavin depletion. Increased intake recommended. Do not give liquid form with tube feeding due to precipitation and risk of clogging.
THIOTHIXENE Used to treat psychoses. *Navane*	Common side effects: appetite stimulation, weight gain. Potential for causing riboflavin depletion. Increased intake recommended.
TRANCYLPROMINE Used to treat depression. *Parnate*	Common side effects: dry mouth, heartburn, nausea, vomiting, diarrhea, constipation. Sugarless candy and gum or saliva substitute may help dry mouth. Increased fluid, fiber, and exercise may help constipation. Potential hypertensive crises with high tyramine-containing foods. Avoid foods high in tyramine and other pressor amines. Avoid tryptophan supplements. Limit caffeine intake due to CNS effects. Maintain good hydration.
TRAZODONE Used to treat depression. *Desyrel* *Trazon* *Trialodine*	Common side effects: dry mouth, nausea, vomiting, constipation. Sugarless candy or gum or saliva stimulant may reduce dry mouth. Increased fiber, fluid, and exercise may reduce constipation.
TRIFLUOPERAZINE Used to treat psychoses, anxiety. *Stelazine*	Common side effects: dry mouth, nausea, vomiting, constipation. Take with food to reduce GI distress. Sugarless candy or gum or saliva stimulant may reduce dry mouth. Increased fiber, fluid, and exercise may reduce constipation. Concentrate form should not be mixed with caffeinated beverages or fruit juice. Increased riboflavin intake recommended due to increased excretion. Maintain good hydration. Limit caffeine intake due to CNS effects.
TRIHEXYPHENIDYL Used to treat Parkinson's disease. *Artane* *Trihexane* *Tri-hexy*	Common side effects: dry mouth, nausea, vomiting, constipation. Take with food to reduce GI distress. Sugarless candy or gum or saliva stimulant may reduce dry mouth. Increased fiber, fluid, and exercise may reduce constipation. Avoid concurrent intake of calcium or magnesium supplements.
VALPROIC ACID Anticonvulsant used to treat seizures. *Depakene* *Myproic Acid*	Common side effects: dry mouth, nausea, vomiting, heartburn, constipation. Take with food to reduce GI distress. Sugarless candy and gum or saliva substitute may help dry mouth. Increased fluid, fiber, and exercise may help constipation. May cause carnitine deficiency with elevated ammonia levels. Potential for bleeding and anemia due to

Drug	Interaction
	coagulation defects. Potential for megaloblastic anemia with or without folate deficiency. Avoid taking syrup form with carbonated beverages; drug is released causing oral irritation or bad taste. Do not take with milk. Maintain good hydration. Hypoalbuminemia increases drug effect due to more free drug.
VENLAFAXINE Used to treat depression. *Effexor*	Common side effects: anorexia, dry mouth, nausea, vomiting, constipation. Sugarless candy and gum or saliva substitute may help dry mouth. Increased fluid, fiber, and exercise may help constipation. Potential for ulcers with bleeding and anemia. Monitor weight and food intake.
ZOLPIDEM Hypnotic used to treat insomnia. *Ambien*	Common side effects: reduced appetite, dry mouth, nausea, vomiting, heartburn, diarrhea, constipation. Absorption reduced by food. Increased fluid, fiber, and exercise may help constipation. Sugarless candy and gum or saliva substitute may help dry mouth.

RESPIRATORY DRUGS

Drug	Interaction

ALBUTEROL
Bronchodilator used to treat airway obstruction in COPD, asthma.
Airet
Proventil
Ventolin
Vollmax

May need increased dose of insulin or oral hypoglycemia agent due to hyperglycemic effect. Limit caffeine.

AMINOPHYLLINE
Bronchodilator used to treat airway obstruction from asthma or COPD.
Phyllocontin
Truphylline

Common side effects: nausea, vomiting, constipation. Increased fluid, fiber, and exercise may help constipation. Food slows drug absorption. Taking slow release forms (e.g. Theo-24) with a high fat meal increases risk of dizziness due to rapid absorption. High protein, low carbohydrate diets reduce blood levels of drug. Keep protein and carbohydrate intake consistent. Charbroiled foods reduce duration of drug effect. Avoid regular intake of charbroiled foods. Excess intake of xanthine or caffeine-containing foods (tea, coffee, colas, chocolate) may increase cardiovascular (tachycardia) or CNS side effects (insomnia, nervousness) due to chemical similarity. Drug is metabolized to caffeine in the liver. Liquid forms are not compatible with common commercial tube feedings. Give separately. Maintain good hydration (2 liters/d) to decrease viscosity of airway secretions.

AZITHROMYCIN
Antibiotic used to treat respiratory infections.
Zithromax

Food reduces absorption by about 50%. Take 1 hour before or 2 hours after meals. Take magnesium supplements separately.

GUAIFENESIN
Expectorant used to treat cough and reduce viscosity of secretions.
Amonidrin
Anti-Tuss
Breonesin
Fenesin
Robitussin
Unitussin

Precipitates tube feeding. Give separately.

ISONIAZID
Antitubercule used to treat or prevent tuberculosis.
INH
Laniazid
Nydrazid

Take with food to reduce GI distress. High carbohydrate meals reduce absorption; best taken between meals unless GI symptoms. May produce vitamin B6 deficiency due to increased excretion especially with multidrug therapy, extended use, and low vitamin intake. A 25 - 50mg/d supplement is recommended. Potential for pellagra with low protein and niacin intake. May need vitamin D supplement with extended use due to altered metabolism of the vitamin, especially with multidrug therapy, low intake,

Drug	Interaction
	and minimal sun exposure. Drug has monoamine oxidase inhibitor activity. Avoid high tyramine and histamine containing foods.
OXYTETRACYCLINE Antibiotic used to respiratory infections. *Terramycin*	Forms nonabsorbable complexes with calcium, magnesium, iron, and zinc. Avoid concurrent intake with dairy products and substances (laxatives, antacids, vitamin and mineral supplements) containing these minerals. Take at least one hour apart.
PREDNISONE Used to treat inflammatory bowel disease. *Deltasone* *Meticorten* *Orasone* *Prednicen-M* *Sterapred*	Common side effect: slowed wound healing. Stimulation of appetite may induce weight gain. Potential for hypokalemia from increased excretion. Increase intake of potassium-rich foods. Potential for hyperglycemia in diabetics and nondiabetics. Increases protein catabolism. May need increased intake. Increases calcium excretion. Chronic use increases risk of osteoporosis, especially when drug dose is high and calcium intake is low (< 500 mg/d). Increased calcium and vitamin D intake recommended. Increases urinary excretion of zinc, and vitamin C. Increases folate and pyridoxine need. May need multivitamin and mineral supplement.
PYRAZINAMIDE Antitubercule used to treat tuberculosis.	May produce vitamin B_6 deficiency, especially with multidrug therapy, extended use, and low vitamin intake. A 25 mg/d supplement is recommended.
PYRIMETHAMINE Used to treat malaria, toxoplasmosis, and Pneumocystis Carinii pneumonia. *Daraprim*	Take with food to reduce GI symptoms. Interferes with folate metabolism. Reduces serum vitamin B_{12} levels. Supplement recommended if platelet and WBC counts fall.
RIFAMPIN Antitubercule used to treat tuberculosis. *Rifadin* *Rimactane*	Common side effects: heartburn, diarrhea. Take between meals as food reduces absorption. May elevate blood sugar in diabetics. Interferes with folate and vitamin B_{12} testing. Potential for osteomalacia due to interference with vitamin D metabolism. Encourage increased calcium and vitamin D intake. Maintain good hydration.
TERBUTALINE Bronchodilator used to treat airway obstruction in COPD, asthma. *Brethaire* *Bricanyl*	May need increased dose of insulin or oral hypoglycemia agent due to hyperglycemic effect.

Drug	Interaction

TETRACYCLINE
Used to treat a variety of infections and bronchitis.
Achromycin
Panmycin
Robitet
Sumycin
Tetracyn
Topicycline

Best taken on an empty stomach. May take with non-dairy food to reduce GI distress. Forms insoluble complexes with calcium, magnesium, iron, and zinc. Separate intake of drug and dairy products, antacids, magnesium-containing laxatives, and calcium, iron, and zinc supplements by 2 - 3 hours. Reduces vitamin K synthesis and increases urinary loss of riboflavin and folate. Potential deficiency with long term use. Increase vitamin intake or consider supplement. Stop tube feeding 1 hour before and 2 hours after drug.

THEOPHYLLINE
Bronchodilator used to treat airway obstruction in COPD, asthma.
Aquaphyllin
Bronkodyl
Elixophyllin
Lanophyllin
Quibron-T
Respbid
Slo-Phyllin
Sustaire
Theo-24
Theo-Dur
Theolair
Theovent
T-Phyl
Uniphyl

Common side effects: anorexia, nausea, vomiting, constipation. High protein intake and char-broiled meats increase metabolism and reduce drug levels. Keep diet consistent and avoid daily intake of charbroiled meats. Potential for increased side effects with high fat intake (Theo-24) due to more rapid absorption. Minimize intake of xanthine-containing foods (colas, coffee, chocolate) or be consistent. Because of chemical similarity with the drug (90% of which is metabolized to caffeine) cardiovascular and CNS effects may be increased. Fiber slows absorption but increases the amount of drug absorbed. Liquid version not compatible with tube feedings. Stop tube feeding before and after giving drug. Adequate hydration important to reduce viscosity of airway secretions. May complex with minerals reducing absorption of both. Take mineral supplements separately. May increase blood sugar with high doses.

TRIMETHOPRIM w/ SULFAMETHOXAZOLE
Antibacterial used in combination with sulfamethoxazole to prevent or treat Pneumocystis carinii pneumonia (PCP).
Bactrim
Septra

Potential for folate depletion, especially with inadequate intake, and other folate antagonists (methotrexate, phenobarbital, phenytoin sulfasalazine) or double strength products. Increase intake of folate-rich foods or consider supplement. Adequate intake of vitamin B_{12} important for folate metabolism. Maintain good hydration.

SUPPLEMENTS

Drug	Interaction
VITAMIN A Used to treat deficiency, or prevent deficiency in fat malabsorption. *Aquasol A*	Take with or after meals. Can mix with food or juice. Reduced absorption when taken with mineral oil. Avoid taking concurrently. Encourage intake of vitamin A-rich foods.
VITAMIN D Calcitriol: used to treat hypocalcemia in renal failure, or hypoparathyroidism. *Calcijex* *Rocaltrol* *Vitamin D$_3$* Dihydrotachysterol: used to treat hypophosphatemia, hypocalcemia, vitamin D deficiency. *DHT* *Hytakerol* Ergocalciferol: used to treat vitamin D deficiency, hypophosphatemia, hypocalcemia, osteomalacia, osteodystrophy. *Calciferol* *Deltalin* *Drisdol* *Vitamin D$_2$*	Take with or without food. May cause hypercalcemia with high calcium intake. Mineral oil interferes with absorption. Do not take together. Potential delayed growth with high doses. Monitor height and weight with chronic use. Encourage intake of calcium and vitamin D-rich foods plus sun exposure. Take magnesium-containing antacids and supplements separately.
VITAMIN E Used as to treat or prevent deficiency or as an antioxidant and to treat hemolysis in low-birthweight infants. *Amino-Opti-E* *Aquasol E* *E-200, E-400, E-1000* *E-Complex-600* *E-Vitamin* *Liqui-E* *Pheryl-E* *Vita Plus E*	Take with or after meals. Liquid may be mixed with food or juice. Increased risk of bleeding in vitamin K deficiency or warfarin therapy. Reduced absorption when taken with mineral oil. May reduce response to iron supplements. Use cautiously with iron deficiency. Encourage intake of a good quality diet and intake of vitamin E-rich foods. Increased need in those who smoke or chew tobacco.

Drug	Interaction
VITAMIN K (Phytonadione) Used to treat hypoprothrombinemia, prevent hemorrhagic disease of the newborn. *AquaMEPHYTON Konakion Mephyton*	Large doses will counteract the effects of warfarin. Large doses of salicylates and some antibiotics may increase vitamin K requirements. Mineral oil may reduce absorption. Take separately.
THIAMIN Used to treat deficiency and prevent Wernicke's encephalopathy.	Usually given in combination with other B vitamins as single deficiencies are rare. Encourage intake of a good quality diet. Needs increased by alcohol, and high carbohydrate intake.
RIBOFLAVIN Used to treat or prevent deficiency.	Usually given in combination with other vitamins. Encourage intake of a good quality diet. Alcohol reduces vitamin absorption. Do not take together.
NIACIN Used to treat or prevent vitamin deficiency, or to treat hyperlipidemia. *Edur-Acin Nia-Bid Niac Niacela Niacor Nico-400 Nicobid Nicolar Nicotinex Nicotinic Acid*	Common side effects: GI upset, flushing, pruritis. Only nicotinic acid (not niacinamide) reduces serum lipids. Take with meals to reduce GI symptoms. Flushing may be reduced by taking aspirin 30 minutes before drug. High doses may elevate blood sugar or uric acid levels. Encourage a good quality or low fat, low cholesterol diet.
PYRIDOXINE Used to treat or prevent deficiency or neuropathy when taking with isoniazid, penicillamine, or hydralazine. *Beesix Nestrex Rodex Vitabee 6*	High protein intake increases vitamin requirements. Encourage increased intake of pyridoxine-rich foods. Neuropathy (unsteady gait, numbness in feet, poor hand coordination) reported with chronic intake of more than 2 grams per day.

Drug	Interaction
FOLIC ACID Used to treat or prevent megaloblastic anemia and to promote normal fetal development. *Folvite*	Absorption is reduced by sulfasalazine. Requirements are increased by estrogens, phenytoin and glucocorticoids. Encourage intake of a good quality diet. If given in pernicious anemia, will correct anemia but neurological damage will continue. Take zinc supplements separately.
VITAMIN B$_{12}$ Used to treat vitamin deficiency and pernicious anemia. *Crystamine* *Crysti-1000* *Cyanoject* *Cyomin* *Rubesol-1000*	Take with meals to improve absorption. Only 5 μg/d is absorbed. Absorption may be decreased by excess alcohol and vitamin C. Response to vitamin will be impaired if folate or iron deficiency present. Encourage intake of a good quality diet. Will need to take parenterally or IM and chronically with gastric and/or ileal resection, and malabsorption syndromes.
ASCORBIC ACID Used as a supplement or to treat deficiency. *Ascorbicap* *Cebid* *Cecon* *Cemill* *Cenolate* *Cetane* *Cevalin* *Cevi-Bidd* *Ce-Vi-Sol* *Flavorcee*	Large doses may reduce effectiveness of oral anticoagulants. Needs may be increased by smoking, salicylates, and primidone. Encourage intake of a good quality diet. Taper large doses when starting and discontinuing. Potential for reducing vitamin B$_{12}$ absorption. Take vitamin supplements separately. Take with iron supplements to increase iron absorption.
IRON Used to treat iron deficiency anemia. Ferrous fumarate *Femiron* *Feostat* *Fumerin* *Hemocyte* *Ircon* *Palmiron* Ferrous Gluconate *Fergon* *Ferralet* *Simron* Ferrous Sulfate *Feosol* *Fer-In-Sol* *Fer-Iron* *Slow Fe*	Common side effects: heartburn, nausea, vomiting, constipation. Best taken on an empty stomach 1 to 2 hours before or after meals. Taking with food reduces GI distress but absorption is reduced 1/3 to 1/2. Taking with ascorbic acid improves absorption. Increased fluid, fiber, and exercise may help constipation. Absorption of nonheme iron increased with concurrent intake of meat or vitamin C. Avoid taking with coffee, tea, dairy products, eggs, or high fiber or phytate foods or supplements due to reduced absorption. Should be avoided with hemachromatosis, thalassemia, or hemolytic anemia. Potentially fatal toxicity with a single high dose (> 200 to 250 mg) or chronic intake. Liquid forms of ferrous sulfate precipitate tube feeding. Give separately. Take other mineral supplements separately because of potential competition for absorption. May destroy vitamin E. Take supplement separately.

Drug	Interaction
ZINC SULFATE Used to treat or prevent zinc deficiency. *Orazinc* *Verazinc* *Zinc 220* *Zincate* *Zinkaps*	Normally 20 - 30% absorption. Absorption reduced by taking with caffeine, dairy products, and bran. Competes with copper for absorption. Avoid taking with meals or other mineral supplements. Regular use may produce copper deficiency. Encourage intake of zinc-rich foods.
POTASSIUM SUPPLEMENTS Used to treat or prevent potassium depletion. *Klorvess* *K-Lyte* *K-Dur* *Klotrix* *Micro-K* *Slow-Kaylixir* *Kolyum*	Common side effects: nausea, vomiting, heartburn, diarrhea. High osmolality may produce diarrhea with tube feeding. Some liquid forms precipitate tube feeding. Avoid other GI irritants (pepper, alcohol, caffeine). Reduce GI irritation by taking with meals. Avoid other high potassium sources (low sodium milk, salt substitute) unless allowed.

TYRAMINE

Some drugs produce adverse reactions when taken with foods containing tyramine and other pressor amines (dopamine, norepinephrine, serotonin, histamine). Normally tyramine is rapidly oxidized in the body by the enzyme monoamine oxidase (MAO). Drugs which inhibit MAO metabolism (monoamine oxidase inhibitors) elevate tyramine levels and produce mood elevation. When taken along with foods containing tyramine and other pressor amines these drugs increase the release of catecholamines producing vasoconstriction, elevated blood pressure, and other unpleasant symptoms (headache, chest pain, heart palpitations, photosensitivity, nausea, and vomiting.) The severity of the reaction depends on the drug dose, the amount of amine in the food, the timing of the food in relation to the drug, and the individual. Offending foods are usually high protein foods that have been dried, aged, fermented, pickled, smoked, cured, or bacterially contaminated. Foods high in tyramine should be avoided while on these drugs. Those with low to moderate amounts should be used cautiously. Fresh foods that have been stored more than 2 days after purchase should also be consumed cautiously. Caffeine-containing foods should also be limited due to potential for arrhythmias.

High Tyramine Foods

- Aged cheeses, products made with aged cheese (cheese spreads, salad dressings).
- Aged, dried, fermented, salted, smoked, and pickled meats and fish (bacon, sausage, liverwurst, hot dogs, corned beef, pepperoni, salami, bologna, ham, smoked salmon, pickled herring, sardines).
- Fermented soybean products (miso).
- Fava beans, broad beans, Italian beans, chinese pea pods.
- Sauerkraut, kim-chee.
- Overripe fruits.
- Chianti, burgundy, sherry, vermouth, beer, ale.
- Sourdough bread, homemade yeast breads.
- Brewer's yeast, yeast extracts, meat extracts .

Lower Tyramine Foods

- Cultured dairy products (yogurt, buttermilk, sour cream).
- Caviar, paté.
- Chocolate-containing foods (milk, ice cream, pastries).
- Soy sauce, teriyaki sauce.

VITAMIN AND MINERAL SOURCES

Below are some of the best sources of the major vitamins and minerals.

Nutrient	Good Sources		
VITAMIN A	liver sweet potato milk kale	tomatoes spinach broccoli carrots	pumpkin winter squash cantaloupe apricots
VITAMIN D	liver sardines salmon tuna	fortified milk Mazola margarine fortified yogurt ready-to-eat cereals	oysters mackerel shrimp herring
VITAMIN E	wheat germ almonds almond oil cottonseed oil	sunflower seeds Mazola margarine spinach avocado	sweet potato fortified oatmeal Best Foods mayonnaise eggs
VITAMIN K	beef liver spinach cabbage turnip greens	spinach (frozen) cabbage sweet potato cauliflower	broccoli Product 19 cereal Total cereal green tea
VITAMIN C	broccoli Brussels sprouts mango cranberry juice	citrus fruits citrus juices kiwi cantaloupe	red/yellow peppers papaya strawberries mango
THIAMIN	lean beef lean pork whole grain products soybeans	sunflower seeds peanuts ready-to-eat cereals beans	split peas Product 19 Total cereal instant oatmeal (fortified)
RIBOFLAVIN	lean beef lean pork liver milk	ricotta cheese cottage cheese eggs enriched white flour	spinach, cooked Product 19 Total cereal chicken
NIACIN	lean beef lean pork liver turkey	peanuts whole grains Pacific oysters salmon	halibut mackerel chicken tuna
PYRIDOXINE	lean meat liver fish eggs	chicken bananas Brussels sprouts oatmeal	whole grains carrots sunflower seeds brown rice
FOLATE	liver lentils dry beans asparagus	cooked spinach peanuts orange juice lima beans	Total cereal Product 19 cereal instant oatmeal (fortified) avocado
VITAMIN B$_{12}$	oysters mackerel tuna crab	Product 19 cereal Total cereal clams clamato juice	cottage cheese liver yogurt salmon

Nutrient	Good Sources		
POTASSIUM	orange juice grapefruit juice prune juice tomato juice	avocado papaya cantaloupe banana	dried fruit dried beans lentils baked potato
MAGNESIUM	All-Bran cereal Bran Buds cereal dried beans dried fruits	halibut mackerel tofu soybean products	cooked spinach sunflower seeds almonds baked beans
PHOSPHORUS	liver milk yogurt cheese	nuts dried beans lentils split peas	meats fish oatmeal All-Bran cereal
IRON	clams oysters soybean products tofu	liver dried beans lentils Product 19 cereal	Total cereal grapenuts cereal instant oatmeal spinach, cooked
CALCIUM	cheddar cheese mozzarella cheese ricotta cheese milk	yogurt tofu spinach, cooked. turnip greens, cooked.	instant oatmeal (fortified) custard salmon with bones orange juice (fortified)

References

• Davis's Drug Guide For Nurses, 5th ed., FA. Davis Company: Philadelphia, 1997.

• Roe, D: Handbook on Drug and Nutrient Interactions, 5th ed. The American Dietetic Association: Chicago, 1994.

• Roche-Dudek, M, Roche-Klemma, K and Nyquist, L: Drug-Nutrient Resource. 1st ed. Roche Dietitians, L.L.C.: Riverside, 1996.

• Cook, MC and Taren, DL: Nutritional implications of medication use and misuse in elderly. J. Florida MA: 77:606, 1990.

• Murray, J and Healy, M: Drug-mineral interactions: A new responsibility for the hospital dietitian.

• Gora, ML et al: Considerations of drug therapy in patients receiving enteral nutrition. Nutrition in Clinical Practice 4:105-110, 1989.

• Nutrition Interventions Manual for Professionals Caring for Older Americans. Washington, D. C., 1992.

• Shils, M et al: Modern Nutrition in Health and Disease. 8th ed. Lea and Febiger: Philadelphia, 1994.

• Manual of Clinical Dietetics. American Dietetic Association. Chicago, 1992.

MEDICAL NUTRITION THERAPY

NUTRITION SUPPORT OF THE CRITICALLY ILL

Trauma is the leading cause of death in the first four decades of life. Complications accompaning trauma often play a significant role in the outcome of the individual. The preservation of nutritional status is a major factor that may improve outcome. Adequate nutrition support is essential to the care of the severely stressed patient; also standard nutrition principles are not always applicable due to the metabolic response to stress. Before nutrition support is instituted, the critically ill patient should be hemodynamically stable with full blood volume, adequately oxygenated and have near normal electrolytes. The benefits of nutrition support (three to five days) for critically ill surgical patients have not been demonstrated. Nutrition support prior to surgery only lends to repletion of liver glycogen and correction of blood volume. Repletion of body cell mass deficits requires a minimum of two to three weeks.

Biochemically evaluating the critically ill patient is difficult, as test results can be altered by stress and injury. Transport proteins (i.e., albumin, prealbumin, transferrin and retinol-binding protein) decrease while creatinine excretion and white blood cell count increase. These changes probably reflect the degree of injury and not nutritional depletion. Laboratory values must be reviewed routinely.

An increase rather than a decrease in weight usually follows injury. This is secondary to resuscitation with large quantities of fluid. A weight history should be obtained from the patient when possible. Recent weight loss prior to injury may indicate a nutritional risk factor. A five percent weight loss in one month or a ten percent loss over six months puts the patient at high risk. A nutrition history taken at this time helps identify reasons for the weight loss.

During stress the first goal of nutrition support is to provide calories and protein to maintain body weight and reduce nitrogen losses. Exogenous calories and protein have a marked sparing effect on the patient's own reserves. At this time hormonal changes favor catabolism. Positive nitrogen balance and anabolism are therefore difficult, if not impossible, to achieve, so large quantities of nutrients may increase metabolic complications.

Calorie and protein requirements can vary throughout the various stages of illness or trauma. A source of protein is necessary to support hepatic protein synthesis even though positive nitrogen balance usually is unattainable during the hypercatabolic phase. Protein requirements can range from 1.5 to 2.5 gms/kg/day. Protein recommendations for the septic or severely traumatized patient can range up to 2.0 gms/kg/day or more, with a nitrogen calorie ratio of 1:100. Between the fifth and tenth days post-injury, a turning point occurs when the body becomes anabolic. Negative nitrogen balance is reduced sharply and lean body mass begins to be synthesized as corticosteroid and other hormone levels return to normal. These changes may take up to three weeks. Albumin usually starts to increase in the second week. Repletion of body fat follows restoration of lean body mass and normal body weight is regained approximately 50 days after the initial trauma provided there are no complications.

Nutrition support augments the metabolic response to injury by providing nutrients for protein synthesis, immune response, energy needs and by reducing protein catabolism. The major goal of nutrition therapy is the maintenance of body cell mass and the provision of adequate nitrogen and fuel to heal tissues, meet metabolic needs and support the immune system. Nutrition therapy must be individualized for each patient and must avoid the complications of overfeeding.

COMPOSITIONAL AND METABOLIC CHANGES IN STARVATION AND SEVERE INJURY

BODY COMPOSITION

In the words of Ancel Keys, "The body is, in the most literal sense, the product of its nutrition." The body itself can be a source of nutrition support as shown by the approximate breakdown of the major body components.

Lean Body Mass	70%
Water	55%
Protein	15%
Fat	25%
Other (bones, collagen, etc.)	5%

Body energy stores are not endless, however. Energy needs can be met from within for a only limited time before excess tissue catabolism occurs. The following table shows the available energy stores of a man weighing 65 kg.

Table 1: Available Energy Stores of a 65 Kg Man

	Total Body Content Grams	Available Stores Calories	Daily Utilization Grams	Exhaustion Days
Carbohydrates	500	600	120/24 hours	1
Fat	9,000	58,500	150	40
Protein	11,000	9,600	60	40 *

Death can occur when one third of body protein has been lost rapidly.

These stores are available to preserve life, assuming the availability of adequate water and oxygen. The usual BMR is 24 kcal/kg/day, providing 23 days of reserves if these calories are used to exhaustion.

STARVATION WITHOUT INJURY

Metabolic response to simple starvation differs from that of starvation with superimposed trauma. This in turn influences how rapidly body stores are depleted.

When inadequate protein and/or calorie intake occurs without injury, the body's metabolic response shows three distinct phases of adaptation.

Phase 1: Lasts 2 - 4 days. Urinary nitrogen loss gradually increases from 5 - 7 gms/day to 8 - 11 gms/day. Increase apparently is due to increased gluconeogenesis from body protein.

Phase 2: Lasts 20 - 40 days. Urinary nitrogen excretion gradually declines. May be due to decreased lean body mass, decreased calorie needs and increased fat oxidation.

Phase 3: Ketoadaptation. Urinary nitrogen loss decreases to 2 - 4 gms/day. Glucose burning tissues have adapted to metabolizing ketones.

When calorie intake is zero, the average daily weight loss is approximately 500 gms or one pound and can be divided among fat and muscle tissue as follows.

Muscle tissue	180 - 300 gms (36 - 60%)
Fat tissue	150 - 200 gms (30 - 40%)

After three to four days of starvation, the body begins to conserve sodium and water. This may lead to water retention and edema if water is unrestricted. This water retention may obscure weight changes reflecting loss of body tissue. Serum proteins may also appear low due to dilution by excess water. Fat mobilization increases slowly and is dependent on the body's energy needs. Energy needs are determined by basal energy requirements (maintenance of body temperature, body function, etc.) and physical activity. Glycogen stores and muscle protein also contribute to the energy pool in late starvation. Death generally occurs from infection. Failure of the respiratory muscles, secondary to severe muscle wasting, leads to the inability to clear the lungs of infectious secretions and pneumonia. When a prior infection exists, the starvation process is accelerated by resulting hypermetabolism. If weight loss has been modest, the patient should be able to take nutrients through the gastrointestinal tract.

STARVATION WITH INJURY

In contrast to simple starvation, significant changes in hemodynamics and metabolism occur during trauma. A post-traumatic state is invoked by a massive injury, severe volume reduction (a bleed of 500 ml or more), infection or a combination of these. Changes include urinary nitrogen loss, immediate conservation of sodium and water and increased fat oxidation, plus, the protein sparing effect of carbohydrate is not evident. Bodily response to injury has been divided into two phases:

Phase 1, The Ebb, or acute phase, is initiated by direct trauma and is referred to as shock. Within the first twenty-four hours, infection, stress and trauma can produce multiple metabolic responses, including hyperglycemia (due to glucocorticoids and other hormones antagonizing the action of insulin in the peripheral tissues) and changes in plasma proteins (due to redistribution of body reserves to meet amino acid requirements for synthesis of protein). Other responses include decreased heat production and decreased oxygen consumption (as a result of low blood volume), decreased cardiac output, vasoconstriction, pooling of blood in the tissues, increased blood viscosity, increased hematocrit and occlusion of vessels by emboli. Urinary excretion of nitrogen, sulfur, phosphorus, potassium and frequently magnesium, zinc and creatinine are also increased.

Phase 2 The flow or adaptive phase usually occurs past the eighth day. During this phase increased heat production and protein oxidation (equivalent to the extra nitrogen and sulfur in the urine) occur. This is "Traumatic Fever" after injury but without infection. Increased oxidation of fat does not occur at this time. In response to injury there is a decrease in appetite which may be complicated by the inability to ingest, digest or absorb nutrients adequately. Accompanied by increased heat production this results in rapid loss of lean body tissue.

Nitrogen losses during trauma can range as high as 15 - 25 grams per day. Nitrogen loss peaks between 5 - 10 days after the onset of stress. The use of a high protein, high calorie diet during peak catabolic response cannot eliminate nitrogen losses but can help replenish lost protein. Therefore, a positive nitrogen balance cannot be attained during peak response to severe stress.

Table 2 compares bodily response to starvation and trauma.

Table 2: Response to Starvation and Trauma

Starvation	Trauma
Gradual lysis of body protein (8 - 11 grams per day)	Rapid lysis of body protein (15 - 25 grams per day)
Slow acceleration of fat oxidation	Fat oxidation quickly achieves maximum rate
Delayed water and sodium conservation at onset	Immediate and prolonged water and sodium conservation
Late decrease in albumin	Early decrease in albumin synthesis
Hypoglycemia	Hyperglycemia
Decreased basal metabolic rate	Increased basal metabolic rate
Remarkable sparing of body protein with a small amount of carbohydrate	Minor sparing of body protein with a small amount of carbohydrate

The stimulus from trauma must be reduced or eliminated for recovery and repair to begin. A phase during trauma is described as the "anabolic opportunity," during which the insulin/glucagon ratio, blood sugar levels and glucose utilization return to normal. Levels of catecholamines decrease and insulin levels rise. If adequate nutrition support is provided at this time, protein synthesis should occur. Oral support can be started when peristalsis and bowel sounds return and the gastrointestinal tract is functional. Premature feeding leads to vomiting and aspiration.

The following guidelines have been suggested for nutrition intervention when oral intake is inadequate:

	Stressed	Unstressed
Malnourished	1 - 3 days	3 - 5 days
Well nourished	3 - 5 days	5 - 7 days

These guidelines are based on a minimum of available data and facts and a maximum of clinical experience. The goal of therapy is to minimize catabolism and restore body cell mass.

Certain body systems show changes during starvation and injury. Some of these are listed below.

GI Tract

Decreased size

Increased gastric emptying time

Increased intestinal transit time

Impaired digestion from reduced pancreatic enzymes

Slower turnover of mucosal cells

Flattened villi and decreased absorptive area

Possible decreased enzyme activity, especially lactase

Possible impaired fat and carbohydrate absorption

Bacterial overgrowth of intestines

Cardiovascular System
- Decreased heart size
- Decreased heart function
- Decreased cardiac output
- Decreased ability to handle fluid overload
- Bradycardia
- Hypotension
- Decreased RBC
- Decreased blood pressure
- Diminished venous return

Liver
- Altered drug metabolism
- Decreased liver size
- Decreased production of clotting factor
- Enlarged liver in PCM
- Decreased albumin synthesis
- Fatty infiltration
- Large glycogen depletion

Kidney
- Reduced concentrating ability with resulting diuresis
- Altered glomerular filtration rates and renal plasma flow
- Polyuria and nocturia
- Impaired ability to excrete acid load

Respiratory/Lungs
- Reduced respiratory muscle function (dependent upon adequate supply of nutrients)
- Diminished vital capacity, respiratory rate, minute ventilation and total volume

Immune System
- Decreased resistance to infection
- Possible post-operative sepsis

Hematologic System
- Progressive anemia
- Leukopenia, thrombocytopenia, acanthocyte formation and hypoplasia of the cellular elements of the marrow

Pancreas
- Pancreatitis, acinar atrophy and fibrosis
- Malabsorption syndrome caused by pancreatic insufficiency and disaccharide intolerance

Musculoskeletal
- Diminution of skeletal muscle mass
- Increased muscle fallibility
- Altered pattern of muscle contraction and relaxation associated with bone loss and an osteopathic effect

Drug Metabolism

Compromised /decreased tissue concentration of drug-metabolizing enzymes

Increased drug toxicity

Altered drug absorption and drug clearance

FLUID AND ELECTROLYTE BALANCE

The total body water ranges from 45 - 80% of the body weight, depending upon sex, age and fat composition. The more fat present the smaller the percentage of water. The total amount of water is divided into the intracellular (ICF) and extracellular (ECF) compartments.

Example: 70 kg man

60% of body weight = total body water (42 liters)

ECF 1/3   ICF 2/3

14 L   28 L

Water moves in and out of both compartments. Osmotic force, along with blood pressure, determines the fluid movement.

Serum sodium reflects water balance. It does not reflect salt (saline) status. Serum sodium is used to detect disturbances of water balance, not sodium needs. The following demonstrates the effect of adding water and adding isotonic saline.

140 mEq Na

ECF		ICF	
14 L		28 L	
3 L water ↓ 130 mEq Na		3 L isotonic saline ↓ 140 mEq Na	
ECF	ICF	ECF	ICF
15 L	30 L	17 L	28 L
Water passes freely.		Sodium stays in ECF. ICF puts it back due to the sodium pump.	
10 mEq below normal is equal to 3 L water excess.		Patients with excess or deficiency of salt and water isotonically may have no alteration in serum Na.	

The following formula can be used to calculate water status.

$$\text{Water} = \frac{\text{Nl serum Na} - \text{abnormal serum Na} \times \text{total body wt} \times 0.6}{\text{abnormal serum sodium}}$$

Example: normal serum sodium = 140 mEq/L

abnormal serum sodium = 130 mEq/L

body weight = 70 kg

$$\text{Water} = \frac{140 - 130 \times 70 \times 0.6}{130} = 3.2 \text{ L water excess}$$

Water excess is a decrease in serum sodium and the therapy is to restrict free water. An increase in serum sodium indicates water depletion and therapy is to add water slowly, one liter per day. **Table 3** below further illustrates laboratory/clinical findings with water and saline deficits.

Table 3: Characteristics of Water and Salt Deficits

Degree	Clinical Signs	Lab Data
Hypertonic (Water Loss Without Salt)		
Mild	Possibly thirst	2 - 4% wt loss *Na 147 - 151 mEq/L
Moderate	Dry mucous membrane Thirst, oliguria, weakness	6 - 8% wt loss Na 156 - 162 mEq/L
Severe	Mental, physical incapacity possibly decreased skin turgor	8 - 14% wt loss Na 162 - 174 mEq/L
Isotonic (Acute Fluid Loss)		
Mild	Skin turgor loss	*Hematocrit 52%
Moderate	Mental slowing	5 - 6% wt loss Hematocrit 56 - 59% 430 - 520 mEq Na loss
Severe	Stupor, recumbent hypotension, soft eyeballs, dry mucous membranes, oliguria	6 - 7% wt loss Hematocrit 56 - 59% 500 - 600 mEq Na loss
Hypotonic (Chronic Salt Loss with Free Water Ingestion)		
Mild	Mild skin turgor	600 mEq Na loss
		Sodium 132 mEq/L
Moderate	Mental slowness, orthostatic hypotension, poor skin turgor, weakness, tachycardia	600 - 800 mEq Na loss Sodium 127 - 132 mEq/L

140 mEq/L used as normal serum sodium
45% used as normal hematocrit

FLUID REQUIREMENTS

Assessment of water balance is critical in evaluating and providing appropriate fluid therapy. The patient's ability to ingest, absorb, secrete, metabolize and excrete water must be evaluated frequently.

Approximately 2500 ml per day is considered the general requirement for a normal adult. An individualized requirement may be calculated as 35 ml per Kg for adults. The RDA is 1 ml/kcal of energy expenditure can be recommended for adults under average conditions. The recommendations is 150 ml/kg in infants or 1500 ml/m^2 body surface area is needed because of large surface area per unit of body weight, a higher percentage of body water, a higher rate of turnover, the kidneys limited capacity for handling solute loads from high protein intake and susceptibility to dehydration secondary to inability to express thirst. For children the recommendation is 50 to 60 ml/kg UBW. The elderly need special attention because their thirst sensation may be blunted. Also, for the markedly overweight or underweight person the following methods can be used to determine fluid requirements.

Calculating Fluid Requirements

1) Incremental Kg method

		mL/kg/24 hour	ml fluid
First 10 Kg		100	1000
Next 10 Kg		50	500
Remaining kg	(Age < 50)	20	1000
	(Age > 50)	15	NA

2) Per Kg – 35 mL/Kg/24 hour

3) BSA – 1500 mL/m²/24 hours

Water requirements are increased when extrarenal fluid losses are high, (e.g., fever, excessive sweating, fistula drainage, profuse vomiting and severe diarrhea). Water deficit can develop when the daily intake is inadequate to meet the body's fluid needs. Daily patient weights may indicate water loss. Other symptoms include dry skin, parched tongue, urine output of less than 500cc per day and a urine specific gravity of 1.020.

FLUID INTAKE

The majority of daily fluid intake, 1200 - 1500 ml, is provided by water and other beverages. Foods provide 700 - 1000 ml of preformed water per day. The body also obtains an amount of water as the oxidation end product of metabolism, but the quantity of metabolic water produced varies with different nutrients.

Water Yield in Metabolism

100 g fat yields 107 g water

100 g CHO yields 55 g water

100 g Pro yields 41 g water

On the average, 200 - 300 ml of water are produced by the body's metabolic activity. Postsurgically, catabolism of tissue alone may be responsible for approximately 900 - 1000 ml of endogenous water, which usually is excreted. However, in stress or wasting illness, the endogenous water is retained by the body.

FLUID EXCRETION

In a normal adult patient, water without salt is lost through insensible loss at the rate of approximately 15 ml per Kg per day. Water is excreted through the kidneys, skin and feces. This represents both obligatory water excretion and facultative losses. The kidney provides a margin of safety for the conservatory and excretory mechanisms of body which utilize water. Obligatory water excretion is the quantity of water the kidney is "obligated" to excrete in order to remove the load of urinary solutes from the body. This is also referred to as the renal solute load.

Water Balance – Adult

Input (Obligatory ml)		Output (Obligatory ml)	
Fluids	750	Urine	750
Foods	750	Sweat	500
Metabolism	300	Lungs	400
		Feces	150

Input (Facultative ml)	Output (Facultative)
1000	1000

Total Input (ml)	Total Output (ml)
2800	2800

Daily insensible water losses have been estimated to be 15 ml per Kg for adults; infants 30 ml per Kg.

HYPONATREMIA

Hyponatremia reflects a below normal serum sodium level or any drop in serum sodium exceeding the rate of 0.5 mmol/L/hour. It is due to a relatively greater concentration of water than sodium. It may be a result of an excessive loss of sodium (serum Na < 135 mEq/L) or an excessive water gain.

Hyponatremia with ECF volume **excess** may occur in:
- Cardiac failure
- Cirrhosis of the liver
- Nephrotic Syndrome

Hyponatremia with ECF volume **deficit** may occur in:
- Loss of GI fluids
- Diuretic abuse
- Salt-losing nephritis
- Osmotic diuresis

Etiological factors
Sodium **loss** may be due to:
- GI fluid loss
- Use of diuretics
- Adrenal insufficiency

Gain of water may be due to:
- Excessive administration of IVs
- SIADH (Syndrome Inappropriate Antidiuretic Hormone Secretion)
- Psychogenic polydipsia

Hyponatremia characteristics are dependent upon the cause, magnitude and rapidity of onset. The following lists the clinical symptoms.

Clinical Symptoms

Weight gain over short period of time:
- 2% mild excess, 2 - 4 lb/55 kg person
- 5% moderate excess, 5 - 6 lb/55 kg person
- 8% or > severe excess, 10 lb or > in a 55 kg person

Chronic (sodium loss/water gain):
- Anorexia
- Muscle cramps
- Feeling of exhaustion, DOE
- Dulling sensorium (Na < 115 mEq/L)
- Lethargy, weakness, confusion
- Muscular twitching
- Focal weakness, hemiparesis, ataxia, Babinski's sign, convulsions, papilledema coma

Acute (water overload):
- Same as above plus
- Neurological manifestations more severe
- Serum Na falls rapidly

Lab Data
- Serum Na < 135 mEq/L
- Urinary Na < 10 mEq/L
- Specific Gravity low (1.002 - 1.004)
- Urinary Na > 20 mEq/L and SG > 1.012 in SIADH

A free water restriction generally is used as the initial management for hyponatremia due to diseases associated with an ECV excess such as cirrhosis, nephrotic syndrome and congestive heart failure. It also occurs in diseases associated with inappropriate ADH release. Free water restriction is best used as sole management for asymptomatic patients whose serum Na is > 118 mEq/L. For patients with more severe hyponatremia, or who are symptomatic, other therapies also should be considered.

"Free water" means water and other hypotonic solutions. Hypertonic solutions should not be restricted except as they provide electrolytes limited by a diet prescription.

A free water restriction limits consumption of water and other hypotonic fluids. Hypotonic fluids include those which are hypotonic relative to plasma. Plasma is 0.9% sodium chloride and is the isotonic standard.

Chronic hyponatremia may be corrected more slowly ($\geq$ 0.5 mmol/L/hr) and acute hyponatremia (Na < 125 mEq/L) requires prompt treatment. Hypertonic saline (3 or 5% NaCl) is given over a six to eight hour period with a maximal rate of administration of 200 ml over four hours.

HYPERNATREMIA

Hypernatremia is defined as a greater than normal serum sodium level at greater than 145 mEq/L. caused by a sodium gain in excess of water or a water loss in excess of sodium. Usually both causes are present. With sodium retention, sodium diuresis, induced by hypernatremia, leads to a secondary loss of water. With primary water loss, the volume depletion leads to secondary renal retention of sodium, which can occur with normal fluid volume or with fluid volume excess or deficit. Hypernatremia may be attributed to one or a combination of: excessive sodium administration, inadequate water intake and excessive water loss, It can be prevented through the administration of adequate water.

Hypernatremic States:

Hypernatremia Associated with a Near Normal ECF Volume
- Loss of water causes elevation of serum sodium level; does not lead to volume contraction unless water losses are massive
- May occur in increased insensible water loss (hyperventilation)

Hypernatremia Associated with ECF Volume Deficit
- Loss of both sodium and water but relatively greater loss of water
- May occur through profuse sweating and diarrhea, particularly in children and aged individuals with poor water intake

Hypernatremia Associated with Fluid Volume Excess
- Gains of both sodium and water, but relatively greater gain of sodium
- May occur in administration of hypertonic sodium solutions

Etiological Factors
- Deprivation of water
- Hypertonic tube feedings without adequate water
- Increased insensible water loss
- Watery diarrhea
- Ingestion of salt in unusual amounts
- Excessive hypertonic saline, $NAHCO_3$ or $NaCl$.
- Diabetes Insipidus (if patient does not respond to thirst)
- Heatstroke and drowning in seawater

Clinical Symptoms
- Thirst
- Elevated body temperature
- Tongue dry and swollen; dry and sticky mucous membranes
- Restlessness and weakness
- Disorientation, delusions and hallucinations in severe hypernatremia
- Lethargy, stupor, or coma. Level of consciousness depends upon the sodium levels and rate of development.
- Muscle irritability and convulsions can occur
- Laboratory data
- Serum sodium greater than 145 mEq/L
- Serum osmolality greater than 295 mOsm/kg
- Urinary SG greater than 1.015

Treatment consists of infusion of a hypotonic electrolyte solution to gradually lower the serum sodium level. Recommendations vary for the rate. Some suggest that the sodium level should not be lowered more than 15 mEq/L in any eight hour period. Others recommend the serum sodium level be dropped no faster than 0.5 mEq/hr in severely hypernatremic children. It is important to allow sufficient time to readjust through diffusion across fluid compartments. **Table 4** summarizes the signs of fluid and electrolyte imbalances.

Table 4: Signs of Fluid and Electrolyte Imbalances

Imbalance	Symptoms
Water Deficiency	Soft eyeballs and loss of skin turgor Dry mucous membranes Increased temperature and pulse Delirium and coma Concentrated urine Thirst
Water Excess	Pulmonary and peripheral edema Abdominal and skeletal muscular twitching and cramps Stupor, coma, or convulsions
Hyponatremia	Lethargy, delirium, coma, seizures Muscle weakness, cramps Edema Postural hypotension Decreased urine output
Hypernatremia	Lethargy, delirium, coma, convulsions Loss of skin turgor Dry mucous membranes Muscular weakness Fever, tachycardia
Hypokalemia	Muscle weakness, cramps and paralysis Hyporeflexia Paralytic ileus Parasthesias, latent tetany Cardiac arrhythmias Hyposthenuria
Hyperkalemia	Muscle weakness Paresthesias Cardiac arrhythmias, heart block and cardiac standstill
Acidosis (metabolic and respiratory)	Hyperventilation Lethargy, stupor, or coma Asterixis Abdominal pain Usually signs of dehydration
Alkalosis (metabolic)	Hypoventilation Stupor, progressing to coma Tetany and convulsions Muscle cramps Usually signs of hypokalemia
Alkalosis (respiratory)	Hyperventilation Stupor progressing to coma Tetany and convulsions Muscle cramps

CLINICAL ASSESSMENT OF FLUID BALANCE

The following parameters should be considered when evaluating fluid balance:

- Comparison of I & O
- Urine volume and concentration
- Skin and tongue turgor
- Dry mucous membrane
- Body weight
- Thirst
- Tearing and salivation
- Appearance and temperature of skin
- Edema
- Temperature, pulse and respiration
- Blood pressure
- Neck vein filling
- Hand vein filling
- Facial appearance

The following blood and urine tests can be used to evaluate fluid and electrolyte status:

Blood and Urine Tests: Fluid and Electrolyte Status

Test	Significance	Comments
Serum (K)	Changes in potassium in relation to pH levels: • Potassium is higher in acidosis (due to shift of K out of cells) • Potassium is lower in alkalosis (due to shifts in the cell) Potassium values may be artificially low if the specimen is anticoagulated	There are a number of causes of factitious hyperkalemia • Tight tourniquet on an exercising extremity (can elevate K as much as 2.7 mEq/L) • Leukocytosis (70,000) • Hemolysis of sample • Platelets > one million
Serum Na	Each 3 mEq/L above usual represents a deficit of one liter water. Each 3mEq/L below usual represents the gain of one liter of pure water.	Evaluate level in relation to water of gain and loss. Sodium levels may be artificially low when serum contains contains abnormal constituents (TGs).
Serum Ca	Each fall or rise of albumin beyond Nl is associated with a fall or rise of Ca concentration of 0.8mg/dl.	Consider albumin level and pH: • Total Ca drops when albumin level is decreased; the ionized fraction does not. • Alkalosis causes a decrease in the ionized fraction of Ca.
Serum Mg	Some of the effects of hypomagnesemia are due to the low levels of Mg; others are due to secondary changes in K and Ca metabolism.	Hemolysis results in falsely high serum levels of cellular ions. Hypomagnesemia can cause hypocalcemia because it interferes with the calcium-elevating effects of parathyroid hormone; it may also cause hypokalemia.

Serum Phosphorus	Hypophosphatemia results from deficiency of either ATP or 2,3 DPG or both. Hyperphosphatemia is usually the result of renal disease.	Intravenous glucose running prior to or at the time of the test causes a lowered PO_4 level (due to CHO metabolism).
Serum Osmolality	Determined mainly by serum Na concentration. Decreased in overhydration. Increased in dehydration. Decreased in hyperglycemia and in presence of elevated BUN	
Blood Urea Nitrogen (BUN)	Elevated BUN due to: • Reduced renal blood flow secondary to fluid volume deficit (causing reduced urea clearance). • Excessive protein intake. • Increased catabolism due to starvation, bleeding into the intestines, or catabolic drugs. Low BUN is often associated with overhydration; may be due to low protein intake.	Evaluate in relation to hydration status.
Creatinine	Elevated in kidney diseases in which 50% or more of the nephrons are destroyed. Slightly elevated in severe volume depletion, which results in a reduction of GFR. May be slightly over Nl in patients with large muscle mass or acromegaly.	Creatinine is a more specific and sensitive indicator of renal disease than is BUN.
BUN Creatinine Ratio (10:1)	When ratio increases in favor of the BUN (> 10:1) the following conditions may be present: hypovolemia, low perfusion pressure to the kidney or increased protein metabolism. When ratio is < 10:1, conditions such as low protein intake, hepatic insufficiency or repeated dialysis may be present.	Useful in evaluating hydration status.
Hematocrit (HCT)	Elevates one point for each 100 ml loss of pure plasma. Elevates one point for each 500 ml loss of isotonic extra-cellular fluid. cellular fluid.	Changes are interpretable in terms of fluid balance when no changes in red blood cell mass. Sometimes used to assess degree of third-space fluid shifts.
Serum Glucose	Markedly elevated glucose causes osmotic diuresis and fluid volume deficit	Results will be elevated above baseline if patient is receiving parenteral glucose.
Serum Proteins	Decreased protein level causes osmotic pull in intravascular space, allowing fluid to shift to the interstitial space (edema).	Levels may be reduced falsely high when dehydration is present.

Serum Osmolality	Determined mainly by serum Na concentration. Increased in dehydration. Decreased in overhydration. Increased in hyperglycemia and in presence of elevated BUN.	Can be measured by lab or calculated.
Urinary Sodium	Less than 10 mEq/L in hypovolemia. Less than 10 mEq/L in hyponatremia. Greater than 20 mEq/L in hypovolemia associated with: • Adrenal insufficiency • Osmotic diuresis • Early diuretic use • Salt-wasting renal disease Greater than 20 mEq/L in SIADH and psychogenic polydipsia.	Need a 24 hour collection. Values of urinary Na need to be evaluated in view of the total clinical picture.
Urinary Potassium	Increased in hyperaldosteronism (the normal Na:K ratio of 2:1 may be reversed). Decreased in adrenal insufficiency (Na:K ratio may be 10:1)	Need a 24 hour collection. Normal Na:K ratio is 2:1.
Urinary Chloride	Helps in differentiating between types of metabolic alkalosis: • Less than 10 mEq/L when alkalosis is due to vomiting, gastric suction or diuretic use. • Usually greater than 20 mEq/L when metabolic alkalosis due to profound potassium depletion.	Need a 24 hour collection.
Urinary Calcium	May be as high as 800 - 900 mg/24 hr in hypercalcemia associated with metastatic tumors. May be low when hypocalcemia is present.	Need a 24 hour collection.
Urinary Specific Gravity	Elevated in fluid volume deficit. Decreased in fluid volume excess. SG persistently below 1.015 is a sign of significant renal disease. The following values are roughly equivalent: **Specific** **Osmolality** **Gravity** **(mOsm/Kg)** 1.000 0 1.010 350 1.020 700 1.030 1050	Heavy molecules such as glucose, albumin, or dyes, will elevate SG out excess. of proportion to the actual concentration. Thus, it is more accurate to measure urine osmolality in patients with glycosuria, proteinuria, or recent use of radiopaque dyes. The aged may have a lower range due to concentrating decreased renal ability.
Urinary Osmolality	Elevated in fluid volume deficit (healthy kidneys conserve needed fluid, causing urine to be more concentrated). Decreased in fluid volume excess (healthy kidneys excrete unneeded fluid causing dilute urine).	More accurate than SG in measuring urine concentration in patients with glycosuria, protein uria or dyes. After a fast of 12 hours, the urine osmolality should be at least three times the serum osmolality.

	Simultaneous measurement of serum and urine osmolality is a more accurate way of measuring renal concentrating ability than is urinary SG.	
Urinary pH	Usually increased (more alkaline) in alkalotic states however urine may be acidic when alkalosis is accompanied by severe hypokalemia.	Alkalinization of urine is recommended for acid stone formers (pH > 6.5) and for cystine stone formers (pH > 7.5).
	Acidification of urine is increased (more alkaline) in urea-splitting infections.	Calcium phosphate and struvite stone formers.
	Increased with use of alkalinizing agents such as: • Sodium bicarbonate • Potassium citrate Decreased with acidifying agents: •Ascorbic acid •Sodium acid phosphate •Methenamine mandelate	Urinary pH fluctuates throughout the day.

Adapted from Matheny

Dehydration in the elderly is a significant problem and is the most common fluid and electrolyte disorder. The signs are confusion, lethargy and poor skin turgor. All of these symptoms may be confused with aging.

OBRA (Omnibus Budget Reconciliation Act)

Minimum Data Set for the elderly dehydration/fluid maintenance triggers include:

- Deterioration in cognitive status, skills, or abilities in the last 90 days
- Failure to eat or take medications
- UTI in the last 30 days
- Current diagnosis of dehydration
- Dizziness/vertigo
- Fever
- Internal bleeding
- Vomiting, diarrhea
- Weight loss (5% in last 30 days; or 10% in last 180 days)
- Insufficient fluid
- Poor consumption of liquids (all/almost all) last 30 days
- 25% of most meals uneaten
- Parenteral/IV fluids

THIRD-SPACING

Third space fluid refers to a distributed shift of fluid into a space from which it not easily exchanged with the extracellular fluid. Fluid can be sequestered into the peritoneal, pericardial and joint cavities, bowel by obstruction or in the interstitial space (as edema).

Third-spacing occurs in the following:

- Acute intestinal obstruction (as much as 5 - 10 L)
- Ascites

- Acute peritonitis (extensive: as much as 4 - 6 L)
- Pancreatitis (as much as 6 - 10 L)
- Acute gastric dilatation
- Pleural effusion
- Burns
- Crushing injuries
- Blockage of lymphatic system
- Hypoalbuminemia
- Fractured hip

Obvious considerations in differentiating fluid volume deficit from third-spacing are observable, measureable fluid losses. Third-spacing cannot be observed and measured and changes in body weight do not occur. Even though the fluid is in the body, it is functionally unavailable for use. Expectations may be:

- Tachycardia and hypotension
- Urine volume < 30 ml/hr
- High urinary SG and osmolality (conservation)
- Elevated hematocrit
- Postural hypotension
- Low central venous pressure
- Poor skin turgor

First, correct the cause of the third-space shift of body fluids. It is important to correct the reduced plasma before renal damage occurs (decreased plasma volume causes reduced renal blood flow). Fluid replacement is accomplished with an isotonic electrolyte solution.

ELECTROLYTE IMBALANCE

Table 6 is a differential diagnosis of single electrolyte changes.

Table 6: Differential Diagnosis of Single Electrolyte Changes

Hypokalemia

Decreased Intake
- Increased secretion

Gastrointestinal losses
- Vomiting
- Pyloric and other forms of intestinal obstruction
- Biliary or gastrointestinal fistulas
- Suction
- Diarrhea or repeated enemas

Increased excretion
- Chronic or regulatory disorders
- Potassium-losing nephritis
- Renal tubular acidosis
- Diuretics

Hormonal or regulatory disorders
- Aldosteronism
- Cushing's syndrome
- Steroid therapy
- Diabetic acidosis

Miscellaneous
- Acidosis of any cause
- Trauma or burns with tissue breakdown
- Intravenous administration of potassium-free liquids

Hyperkalemia

Increased intake or IV administration

Decreased excretion
- Acute renal disease
- Dyrenium diuretic therapy
- Spironolactone therapy
- Adrenal insufficiency

Redistribution from intracellular to extracellular fluid
- Acidosis (H^+ moves into cell. K^+ moves out)
- Anoxia
- Hyponatremia (K^+ moves out of cell to replace Na^+)

Hypochloremia

Disorders of intake
- Decreased intake with normal or increased water intake

Decreased absorption
- Malabsorption syndrome
- Diarrhea

Increased secretion
- Pyloric and other forms of intestinal obstruction
- Biliary and intestinal fistulas
- Excessive sweating with normal water intake
- Vomiting

Increased excretion
- Chronic renal failure
- Diuretics

Disorders of transport
- Congestive heart failure

Disorders of regulation
- Inappropriate ADH secretion
- Respiratory acidosis
- Adrenal insufficiency
- Primary aldosteronism

Miscellaneous
- Diabetic acidosis
- Lactic acidosis

Hyperchloremia

Disorders of intake
- Lack of water intake (dehydration)
- Ingestion of ammonium chloride

Disorders of secretion
- Pathologic diaphoresis without water ingestion

Disorders of excretion
- Renal tubular acidosis
- Diamox diuretics
- Salicylate intoxication
- Acute renal failure

Disorders of regulation
- Diabetes Insipidus

Decreased Bicarbonate

Disorders of intake
- Starvation (leading to ketonemia)
- Dehydration
- Ingestion of acids

Disorders of secretion
- Diarrhea
- Biliary and lower intestinal fistulas

Disorders of excretion
- Acute and chronic renal failure
- Renal tubular acidosis
- Salicylate intoxication
- Diuretics

Disorders of regulation
- Addison's disease

Miscellaneous
  • Diabetic acidosis
  • Lactic acidosis
  • Specific toxin ingestion (e.g., methyl alcohol)

Increased Bicarbonate

Disorders of intake
  • Ingestion of bicarbonate and antacids
  • Intravenous administration of bicarbonate, lactate and citrate

Disorders of secretion
  • Pyloric and upper intestinal obstruction
  • Vomiting

Disorders of excretion
  • Mercurial diuretics
  • Pulmonary emphysema and other causes of respiratory acidosis

Disorders of regulation
  • Primary aldosteronism

Monitoring

It is extremely important to understand all aspects of fluid balance and imbalance when recommending nutrition support. It also is important to recognize increased or decreased electrolytes and ABGs not influenced by nutrition support. Nutrition support modalities should not change when the electrolytes and/or ABGs are abnormal as a result of a non-nutritional cause.

ACID-BASE BALANCE

Normal plasma pH (7.35 - 7.45) is maintained by chemical buffering mechanisms, the kidneys and the lungs. Chemical buffering mechanisms are substances to prevent changes in pH of body fluids by removing or releasing hydrogen ions. Bicarbonate (HCO_3) <−> Carbonic acid (H_2CO_3) is the major buffer system (20 parts of bicarbonate to one part of carbonic acid). Acid-base imbalance results when either bicarbonate or carbonic acid is increased or decreased. The following are examples of pH changes with alterations in the bicarbonate:carbonic acid ratio.

Balance	Change/ratio	pH
Normal	HCO_3 = 24 mEq/L H_2CO_3 = 1.2 mEq/L Ratio = 20:1	7.4
Metabolic Acidosis	HCO_3 = 12 mEq/L H_2CO_3 = 1.2 mEq/L Ratio = 10:1	7.1
Metabolic Alkalosis	HCO_3 = 36 mEq/L H_2CO_3 = 1.2 Ratio = 30:1	7.58
Respiratory Acidosis	HCO_3 = 24 mEq/L H_2CO_3 = 1.84 Ratio = 13:1	7.21

Respiratory Alkalosis	HCO_3 = 21 mEq/L	7.7
	H_2CO_3 = 0.6	
	Ratio = 40:1	

Kidneys regulate the bicarbonate level in ECF and can regenerate bicarbonate ions as well as reabsorb them from the renal tubular cells.

Lungs control the carbon dioxide (and thus carbonic acid) by adjusting ventilation in response to the amount of carbon dioxide in the blood.

Evaluation of acid-base balance is measured by arterial blood gases (ABGs). **Table 5** exhibits normal values and implications.

Table 5: Arterial Blood Gases

Normal Value	Comments
pH: 7.37 - 7.45	Reflects H^+ concentration: acidity increases as H^+ concentration increases pH decreases as acidity increases pH < 7.35 (acidosis) pH > 7.45 (alkalosis)
PaCO₂: 38 - 42 mm Hg	Partial pressure of CO_2 < 38 mm Hg, hypocapnia (respiratory alkalosis) 42 mm Hg, hypercapnia (respiratory acidosis)
PaO₂: 80 - 100 mm Hg	Partial pressure of O_2 in arterial blood (decreases with age) 80 mm Hg (on room air) is acceptable Adults < 60 year (room air) < 80 mm Hg - mild hypoxemia < 60 mm Hg - moderate hypoxemia < 40 mm Hg - severe hypoxemia > than 60 years - slightly lower levels are acceptable as normal secondary to loss of ventilatory function
Stnd HCO₃: 22 - 26 mEq/L	HCO_3 concentration that has been equilibrated at a $PaCO_3$ of 40 mm Hg and with O_2, in order to fully saturate the hemoglobin.
Base Excess: -2 mEq ± 2 mEq	Reflects metabolic (nonrespiratory) body disturbances Always negative in metabolic acidosis Always positive in metabolic alkalosis

Adapted from Metheny, N: Fluid and Electrolyte Balance

The four primary acid-base disturbances are as follows:

Metabolic acidosis is associated with a fall in plasma pH and a decrease in plasma bicarbonate. It may arise from removal of bicarbonate from the body in alkaline fluids or by addition of the hydrogen ion, which reacts with bicarbonate to form carbon dioxide and water. The following are the etiological factors and clinical symptoms.

	Etiological Factors	Clinical Symptoms
Normal Anion Gap	• Intestinal fistulas • Ureterosigmoidostomy • PN • Acidifying drugs • Renal tubular acidosis	• Headache • Diarrhea • Confusion • Drowsiness • Increased respiratory rate

High Anion Gap	• Nausea and vomiting • Diabetic ketoacidosis • Starvation ketoacidosis • Starvation ketoacidosis • Lactic acidosis • Renal failure • Poisons (salicylates, ethylene glycol and methanol) • Arterial blood gases: fall in pH (< 7.35) $HCO_3 < 22$ mEq/L (primary) $PaCO_3 < 38$ mm Hg (compensation by lungs)	• Peripheral vasodilation (warm flushed skin) • Decreased cardiac output when pH falls below 7: bradycardia
	• Base always negative	• Hyperkalemia (except in RTA, diarrhea and use of acetazolamid

The treatment is to correct the pH to 7.2. and correct the metabolic defect. If the problem is excessive chloride, treatment focuses on eliminating the source. When necessary, bicarbonate is administered.

Metabolic alkalosis is associated with a rise in pH and an increase in the plasma bicarbonate and is usually caused by loss of HCL through vomiting or gastric secretion. The following lists the etiological factors and clinical symptoms.

Etiological Factors	Clinical Symptoms
Vomiting or gastric suction	As related to decreased calcium ion such as:
Hypokalemia	• Dizziness • Tingling of fingers and toes
Hyperaldosteronism	• Circumoral paresthesia • Carpopedal spasm
Potassium-losing diuretics	• Hypertonic muscles
Alkali ingestion	Depressed respiration
Parenteral $NaHCO_3$ administration for cardiopulmonary resuscitation	Arterial blood gases: • pH > 7.45 • Bicarbonate > 26 mEq/L(primary)
Abrupt relief of chronic respiratory acidosis	• $PaPCO_2 > 42$ mm Hg (compensatory) • Base excess always positive
	Hypokalemia often present
	Serum Cl relatively lower than Na

Treatment is to reverse the underlying disorder. Sufficient chloride has to be supplied for the kidney to absorb the excess bicarbonate. The bicarbonate excess equals the chloride deficit.

Respiratory acidosis is associated with fall in pH due to a primary increase in PCO_2 as a result of pulmonary insufficiency. It is always due to inadequate excretion of carbon dioxide.

Listed are the etiological factors and clinical symptoms.

Etiological Factors	Clinical Symptoms
Acute Respiratory Acidosis:	**Acute Respiratory Acidosis:**
• Acute pulmonary edema	• Feeling of fullness in head
• Aspiration of a foreign body	• ($PaCO_2$ causes cerebrovascular vasodilation and increased cerebral blood flow)

• Atelectasis
  • Pneumothorax, hemothorax
  • Overdosage of sedatives or anesthetic
  • Position in OR that interferes with respiration
• Cardiac arrest
• Severe pneumonia
• Laryngospasm
• Improper regulation of mechanical ventilation
	• Mental cloudiness
	• Dizziness
	• Palpitations
	• Muscular twitching
	• Convulsions
	• Warm, flushed skin
	• Unconsciousness

Chronic Respiratory Acidosis:
  • Emphysema
  • Cystic Fibrosis
  • Advance multiple sclerosis
  • Bronchiectasis
  • Bronchial asthma
	• Ventricular fibrillation
	• ABGs
	• pH < 7.35
	• $PaCO_2$ > 42 mm Hg (primary)
	• HCO_3 Nl or slightly elevated

Factors favoring hypoventilation
  • Obesity
  • Tight abdominal binders/dressings
  • Postoperative pain
  • Abdominal distention
	Chronic Respiratory Acidosis
	• Weakness
	• Dull headache
	• Symptoms of underlying disease
	• ABGs
	• pH < 7.35
	• $PaCO_3$ > 42 mm Hg (primary)
	• HCO_3 > 26 mEq/L

Treatment is improved ventilation and adequate hydration. The elevated $PaCO_3$ needs to be decreased slowly because rapid excretion of carbon dioxide prevents the kidneys from eliminating excess bicarbonate with sufficient rapidity to prevent alkalosis and convulsions.

Respiratory alkalosis is associated with a rise in pH from a decrease in PCO_2 due to primary hyperventilation, which causes excessive "blowing off carbon dioxide."

Listed below are the etiological factors and clinical symptoms of respiratory alkalosis.

Etiological Factors	Clinical Symptoms
Extreme anxiety	Lightheadedness
Hypoxemia	Inability to concentrate
High fever	Numbness and tingling of extremities caused by rapidly decreased calcium ionization
Early salicylate intoxication	
Gram-negative bacteremia	Hyperventilation syndrome
CNS lesions involving respiratory center	• Tinnitus
Pulmonary emboli	• Palpitations

Thyrotoxicosis	• Sweating
Excessive ventilation by mechanical means	• Dry mouth
Pregnancy	• Tremulousness • Precordial pain • Nausea and vomiting • Epigastric pain • Blurred vision • Convulsions and loss of consciousness ABGs • pH > 7.45 • $PaCO_3$ < 38 mm Hg (primary) • HCO_3 < 22 mEq/L (compensatory)

Treatment: If the patient is anxious, they need to breathe more slowly (to cause the accumulation of carbon dioxide) or to breathe into a closed system. Treatments for other causes are directed at correcting the underlying problem(s).

Each disturbance is accompanied by a compensating change in the other in a similar direction. The compensating change is always smaller than the primary change.

RESPIRATORY MANAGEMENT

Respiratory failure is the severe impairment of gas exchange in the lungs, preventing the absorption of oxygen and the excretion of carbon dioxide. Symptoms include malaise, difficulty sleeping, headaches, weakness, palpitations, cough, tachycardia, arrhythmia's, ascites and edema. Arterial blood gases and pH are measured for diagnosis of respiratory failure.

Malnutrition can cause or worsen respiratory failure by impairing respiratory muscle function and pulmonary defense mechanism and decreasing ventilatory drive. Respiratory muscle function can be impaired by isolated mineral and electrolyte deficiencies as follows:

- Hypophosphatemia reduces diaphragmatic contractile strength in mechanically ventilated patients with acute respiratory failure.
- Hypocalcemia is associated with decreased diaphragmatic function.
- Sodium depletion leads to appetite depression and then slowing of the ventilatory drive.

Diagnosis:

- Auscultation: Listening for sounds of congestion or evidence of collapsed lung
- Chest X-ray: Evidence of pneumonia, heart failure, trauma, fibrosis, emphysema
- Arterial Blood Gases: Blood drawn from an artery instead of a vein
- ABGs measure the status of the body's respiratory environment

Measures include:

- pH: Reflecting acid-base balance
- pCO_2: The partial pressure of oxygen in the blood. A good value is 75 - 100mmHg. Low values mean the patient is not oxygenating well and needs supplemental O_2.
- pCO_2: The pressure of CO_2 in blood. Normal value is 35-45. High values mean the patient is not ventilating or excreting CO_2 adequately. A low CO_2 means the patient is hyperventilating. Hyperventilation occurs because oxygenation is poor (low pO_2) and more breaths are needed to get the needed O_2.

Indications for respirator therapy are:

- Hypoxia: Low oxygen, usually a pO_2 of 55 or less (normal 75 - 100)
- Hypercarbia: Too much CO_2, usually at a pCO_2 of 50 - 55 (normal 35 - 45)
- Tachypnea: The patient is simply wearing out because of respiratory effort
- Acidosis: Blood is acidic due to increased pCO_2

Definitions:

- Vt: Tidal volume, or amount of air delivered on each breath. Usually 10 - 15cc/kg BW

- FiO_2: Percentage of oxygen the patient is breathing. Room air is 21% (or an FiO_2 of 0.21), 70% oxygen would be an FiO_2 of 0.7

- PEEP: Positive End Expiratory Pressure - the respirator keeps up a certain pressure at the end of expiration by not letting all the air out. It improves oxygenation but decreases ventilation (pCO_2 goes up) and decreases cardiac output by impeding venous return to the chest

- IMV: Intermittent Mandatory Ventilation - the number of breaths the machine delivers per minute. The patient can take more on their own

- IRV: Inspiratory Reserve Volume amount of air maximally inhaled from resting inspiration

- VC: Vital capacity

Example: On an FiO_2 of 0.6, an IMV of 12 with a Vt of 700 with patient blood gases of:

pH	7.5
pO_2	60
pCO_2	30

This means the patient is breathing 60% oxygen, the respirator is delivering 12 breaths a minute and the volume of the breath is 700 cc.

From the ABG, the pH is slightly high. The patient is hyperventilating trying to increase pO_2. As a result the CO_2 is low (hyperventilation decreases pCO_2 and decreased pCO_2 increases pH). The FiO_2 needs to be increased.

Seriously ill patients may have a decreased ability to utilize carbohydrates. Excess calories are stored as fat and accompanied by a high RQ (~8.0), which yields a proportionally higher production of CO_2. RQ is the ratio of carbon dioxide production to oxygen consumption during substrate utilization. A higher CO_2 can lead to hypercapnia.

Substrate	Cal	02	RQ
Protein	4 kcal/gm	1L	.8
Carbohydrate	4 kcal/gm	1L	1.0
Fats	9 kcal/gm	1L	.7

There is a question as to whether the total CHO load or total calorie load is producing excessive CO_2. To avoid an increase in CO_2 production, excess total calories should be avoided.

WOUND HEALING

The relationship between general catabolism in muscle and rapid synthesis of new tissue in the wound is part of the general adaptation to severe injury. Nutritional factors have pronounced effects on wound healing. Following injury, changes occur in energy, protein, carbohydrate, fat, vitamins, mineral and water metabolism. Severe injuries (burns, septic shock) have the most changes in metabolism. The changes are modified by many factors (age, gender, previous nutritional status, type and severity of injury and nutrient intake) and effect nutrition, wound healing, the immune response and other defense mechanisms. The malnourished patient often has delayed wound healing. When wound healing is impaired, wound infection is a frequent complication.

The phases in wound healing include inflammation with recruitment of polymorphonuclear leukocytes, macrophages and lymphocytes; fibroblast proliferation and collagen production; and collagen remodeling and epithelization when appropriate. The strength and integrity of repair depend on collagen cross-linking and deposition.

Wound healing occurs in several phases. Early wound healing occurs readily during a period of negative energy balance because the wound has high biological priority. New tissue is synthesized within the fibroblasts using nutrients donated by other body tissues through catabolism. Initial wound healing occurs between the fifth and fifteenth day after surgery or trauma. Failure to heal is commonly result of infection. Malnutrition also may contribute to alterations in normal wound healing. If exogenous nutrients are not provided at this stage, wound healing is delayed. The muscle cells become avid to replete catabolized tissues and wound healing loses its high biological priority. Prolonged starvation or continued catabolism at this point causes the wound to become a protein donor and compete with other tissues for nutrients. Sufficient calories, protein, zinc and vitamin C are necessary for continued wound healing after the initial stage.

PCM or clinically evident nutrient deficiencies interfere with wound healing. Effects of specific nutrients are as follows:

Protein: Deficiency contributes by prolonging the inflammatory response and impairing fibroplasia. Edema also may occur secondary to hypoalbuminemia. This slows oxygen diffusion flow from capillaries to the cell membrane and causes further insult to tissue.

Carbohydrate and Fat: Carbohydrate deficiencies affect phagocytic activity of WBC prior to fibroplasia. Fat deficiencies cause decreased cellular proliferation.

Vitamin C: Plays a key role in the synthesis of collagen and maintenance of immune function. Deficiency causes capillary fragility, decreased collagen synthesis, decreased fibroblast mitosis and delayed healing of pressure sores. More vitamin C is required to maintain wound integrity than to maintain developmental collagen.

Vitamin A: Plays a role in cell differentiation and epithalization. Deficiency causes decreased fibroplasia, decreased collagen accumulation in wounds and decreased tensile strength.

Zinc: Required for protein synthesis, DNA synthesis, mitosis and cell proliferation. Deficiencies decrease rates of epithelialization and collagen synthesis. If body levels are low, wound healing slows.

Iron: Required for hydroylation of proline and lysine in collagen synthesis and is a component of a variety of cellular enzymes. Deficiencies decrease formation of collagen. Severe and acute iron deficiency anemia adversely effects oxygen transport and thus wound healing.

Copper: A constituent of a number of metalloenzymes important in wound healing. Deficiencies interfere with oxygen transport thus decreasing the formation in the cross-linking in collagen and decreased wound strength.

Thiamine and Riboflavin: Essential for adequate collagen production and cross-linking. Deficiencies can cause problems in protein, carbohydrate and fat metabolism.

IMMUNE RESPONSE

Protein-calorie malnutrition (PCM) can have a profound impact on immune function. It is the most common cause of immunodeficiency worldwide. Prolonged protein deficiency impairs immune mechanisms leading to increased wound infections, urinary tract infections and pneumonia. Response to chemotherapy also is impaired. Significantly reduced immune response also may occur with a deficiency of vitamins B and C, magnesium and zinc.

Protein-energy malnutrition hampers the phagocytic process and predisposes the patient to infection. Infection in turn can impact immune response by altering vitamin and iron metabolism, muscle metabolism and electrolyte and water balance. Infection also may precipitate significant negative nitrogen balance. In surgical patients impaired host defense mechanisms can be a major cause of increased morbidity.

Nutritional losses due to the infectious process can be absolute or functional. Absolute losses are measurable, occur shortly after the onset of fever or infection and can be sustained during the entire illness. They include loss of body protein leading to negative nitrogen balance and loss of potassium, magnesium, phosphorus and possible sulfur and zinc. The magnitude of tissue loss is proportional to the severity of the infection and total body weight loss. Provision of increased protein and calorie intake reverses the negative nitrogen balance and the body begins to retain nutrients. This usually occurs after two weeks of improved nutrition. If the illness continues, daily nitrogen balance gradually becomes less negative as the body goes into a new equilibrium but is still wasted and cachectic.

Functional losses result from altered metabolic processes and may be due to overutilization, diversion or sequestration of essential body nutrients. Fever and infection increase the rate at which nutrients are utilized thus leading to depletion. An example is the increased utilization of amino acids in muscle tissue to meet the fever-induced need for increased carbohydrate when glucose stores are depleted. Nutrients also can be diverted into other metabolic pathways. While some amino acids are transported to the liver for glucose synthesis others are transformed into ketones by hepatic enzymes, a less efficient energy source. Still others are sequestered, rendering them useless for normal metabolic activities. Sodium and iron are sequestered during infection.

In the presence of fever, a ten percent increase over normal requirements are recommended along with adequate fluid. There have been recommendations that 20 to 25 percent of calories be given as protein. During fever and infection a greater percentage of protein is diverted for glucose synthesis. For this reason a 1:100 to 1:150 nitrogen to calorie ratio may be necessary.

The supporting amino acids in immune function are arginine, glutamine and the branch chain amino acids. Rapidly growing tissues, such as intestinal epithelium, require purines and pyrimidines for synthesis of DNA and RNA. If liver function becomes impaired during critical illness, exogenous sources of nucleotides may prove essential for maintenance of cell-mediated immunity. The lipid composition of the immune cell reflects the fatty acid composition of lipids in the diet. MCT and some LCT or structured lipids should be used in feeding. MCT can be absorbed into portal circulation and metabolized by the hepatic oxidative processes, even in patients with abnormal liver function and systemic sepsis. This mixture of MCT and structured lipids provides calories that will not clog the macrophages or cause hepatic dysfunction.

Immunosuppression from PCM is reversed with proper nutrition support. The feeding route should be carefully considered and the effect of a number of nutritional substrates on the critically ill and infected should be evaluated.

EXERCISE

Exercise enhances the utilization of nutrients and promotes synthesis of lean body mass. Exercise has been shown to reduce muscle breakdown and promote increased muscle bulk. Studies show that losses of body protein can occur in normal healthy individuals who are suddenly immobilized and in stroke patients who have impaired mobility. The resulting protein losses are equivalent to a loss of 1 1/2 to 2 pounds of muscle per week. Follow up studies showed that these losses could be reduced by exercise and ambulation. Albert, et al observed daily submaximal exercise produced a systematic enhancement of tissue/amino acid uptake therefore improving nitrogen balance. Whenever possible, exercise should become part of the patient's therapy plans.

SKIN TESTING

A review of reports on skin testing has shown lack of supporting data and uniformity in skin testing. Studies do not account for the effects of disease (e.g., cancer, immune diseases), infection or therapy (e.g., radiation, surgery, immunosuppression), which are known to influence skin test reactivity. Evaluation of immune competence in relation to nutritional status requires precise knowledge of a patient's nutritional intake, metabolic state, current illness, previous exposure to infectious agents, duration of the immune deficit as well as genetic factors. We believe the question still remains as to whether skin testing correlates well with nutritional status. We suggest keeping abreast of the current and future developments in the literature with regard to skin testing.

NUTRIENT REQUIREMENTS

ESTIMATING CALORIC NEEDS

Energy requirements are highly individualized and can vary widely. Patients may be hypometabolic, hypermetabolic or normal metabolic. The depleted patient who has adapted to starvation has a decreased basal metabolic rate (BMR) while the hypermetabolic patient has an elevated BMR. Nourished patients undergoing nonstressful procedures have normal metabolic rates. The least changes in BMR are seen in female, elderly or poorly nourished patients, whereas the largest changes occur in well-nourished, young, muscular males.

Total caloric needs depend on the basal energy expenditure (BEE) as well as the presence of trauma, surgery, infection, sepsis and other factors. When estimating caloric needs attention must be given to age, development, prior and present nutritional status and metabolic rate. After injury, the body requires energy to respond to heightened demands and fuel repairs.

Caloric needs can be estimated several ways. The characteristics of the patient population at each institution should guide the method choice. For example, a tertiary care center may need to assess caloric needs more precisely than a community hospital. The average age in a tertiary facility care is usually lower and the degree of injury is higher for a greater share of the population. The characteristics of the patient population must be evaluated constantly in this era of patients "coming sicker and leaving quicker."

The following are useful parameters in assessing a patient's nutritional status based on weight:

- Height
- Weight: current, normal on admission
- Weight for height
- Percent weight change over amount of time (weight patterns)
- Percent above/below ideal body weight

Various methods exist for calculating energy needs, both in the hospital and outpatient setting:

Harris-Benedict Formula

The Harris-Benedict formula is useful and accurate for calculating basal energy requirements. This formula accounts for difference in age, sex, height and current weight (AB wt). The BEE is appropriate for adolescents as well as adults.

HB Formula:

Males:

66.5 + 13.8 (AB wt) + 5.0 (ht) - 6.8 (age)

Females:

655.1 + 9.6 (AB wt) + 1.8 (ht) - 4.7 (age)

Additional calories are added to the basal energy needs depending the presence of the following factors. The additions are based on percentage of basal calories.

Factor	Percent of Basal Calorie Adjustment

Activity
    Bedrest
    Ambulatory
	
	5 - 10
	5 - 20

Elevated temperature	C° - 13% per degree above normal
Surgery	10 - 15
Infection, stress, trauma	20
Sepsis	40
Growth	500 extra calories/day

Monitoring weight helps determine if the caloric estimates are adequate. Body surface area (BSA) is another method. BSA is proportional to the BMR.

$$BMR = BSA \times Kcal/m^2 \text{ per hour} \times 24 \text{ hours.}$$

Another method suggested based on the Harris-Benedict (B.E.E.) formula is:

Harris-Benedict formula:

B.E.E. x (A.F.) x (I.F.)

A.F. (Activity Factor) I.F. (Injury Factor)

Bedrest	1.2	Minor surgery	1.2
Ambulatory	1.3	Skeletal trauma	1.35
		Major sepsis	1.60
		Severe burns	2.10

> *Example:*
> B.E.E. (1200) x 1.2 x 1.6 = 2300 kcal

The Mayo Clinic Nomogram also can be used. It relates basal metabolic rate to surface area, age and sex. To calculate energy needs, determine surface area from the individual's height and weight, then multiple by the estimated calories per square meter per hour (Cal/m²/hr). For individuals requiring tube feeding and who have severe developmental delay and are inactive, this method may be more appropriate, especially if the individual is a child.

> *Example:*
> Cal/m²/24° 40 x 1.75 x 24 = 1680

Yet another method of estimating calories is as follows:

Status	Kcal/kg/IBW
Basal energy needs	25 - 30
Ambulatory with weight maintenance	30 - 35
Malnutrition with mild stress	35 - 40
Severe injuries and sepsis	40 - 50
Extensive burns	50+

Calorimetry

Calorimetry can be defined as the measurement of energy. **Direct calorimetry** measures the amount of heat produced by a patient in a sealed, insulated chamber. The energy produced by the body can be accounted for by the heat lost and/or stored in the body. This is a slow and arduous process and is rarely used. The preferred method, **Indirect calorimetry,** determines the heat produced by measuring the amount of oxygen consumed and the quantity of nitrogen and carbon dioxide eliminated. Individualized medical nutrition therapy for the critically ill patient is enhanced by monitoring nitrogen balance and resting energy expenditure (REE) which provides a more accurate way to determine protein and energy needs for anabolism. Through indirect calorimetry, calories needed for maintenance, repletion or depletion of a patient's energy stores can be determined. The are two types: circulatory indirect, which measures oxygen utilization from arterial and mixed venous blood and respiratory indirect, which measures oxygen from inhaled and exhaled gases. Indirect is a more accurate, cost-effective means of determining calories. It's use helps avoid overfeeding and the accompanying costs of excess nutrient solutions, toxicities and extensive monitoring. Clinical situations that may require indirect calorimetry are as follows:

- Hypermetabolic patients (trauma, sepsis, burns)
- Malnourished or starvation adapted
- Greatly obese (> 200% IBW)
- Peripheral edema
- Hypoalbuminemia
- Limb amputation
- Inappropriate response to standard nutrition support
- Difficulty in weaning
- Non healing wounds
- Postoperative organ transplant

Many equations can be applied:

The *FICK equation* is used in patients who have a Pulmonary artery/Swan catheter to measure cardiac output. Arterial and venous blood gas should be drawn at the same time the cardiac output is measured.

$$\textbf{VO}_2 = CO \times (CaO_2 - CvO_2) \times 10$$

$$\textbf{REE} = (CO) \times (\% \text{ sat artery } O_2 - \% \text{ sat venous } O_2) \times (Hgb) \times (95.18)$$

World Health Organization - kJ/24 hour

Men   18 - 30 year: EE = 64.4 x wt (kg) - 113.0 x ht (m) + 3000
30 - 60 year: EE = 19.2 x wt (kg) + 66.9 x ht (m) + 3769

Women   18 - 30 year: EE = 55.6 x wt (kg) + 1397.4 x ht (m) + 146
30 - 60 year: EE = 36.4 x wt (kg) - 1104.6 x ht (m) + 3619

Weir Formula

REE (kcal/day) = [(3.9 x O_2 + 1.1 x VCO_2) x 1.44] - (2.17 x TUN)

Modified Weir: REE = 3.9 VO_2 + 1.1 VCO_2

Calories for **outpatients** can be determined as follows (by activity level):

1. Convert the ideal body weight to kilograms.
2. Multiple the number of kg by the figure obtained from below at the intersection of columns representing the patient's weight status and level of activity.

	Sedentary	Light	Moderate	Marked
Overweight	20	25	30	35
Normal Weight	25	30	35	40
Under Weight	30	35	40	45 - 50

Activity levels are determined according to the type of activity composing the major portion of the waking hours.

Activity	Description
Sedentary	Confined to chair or bedrest, convalescence from debilitating illness
Light	Mostly seated or standing, with arm movements
Moderate	Frequent movements involving arms and legs, walking briskly
Marked	Walking uphill, activities involving intermittent but frequent spurts of energy

Whatever method used, the most important factor is the outcome. Monitoring the patient's weight and labs will helps verify the effectiveness of the method chosen.

Calorie Requirements of the Critically Ill Obese

The relation between mortality and nutrient intake occurs above and below the maintenance range of energy intake. In critically ill patients, hyperglycemia becomes more common and blood glucose control becomes more difficult with high glucose loads.

Energy expenditure from indirect calorimetry indicates that daily energy expense in adults ranges from 1700 - 2500 (30 - 35 kcal/kg) or less than that of healthy subjects. The basal hypermetabolism of disease often is offset by decreased physical activity.

Hypocaloric feeding may be prudent in the early stage of injury to minimize the risk of metabolic instability and its consequences. This limits the loss of lean or fat tissue. Repletion can be emphasized in the recovery phase of injury.

It is estimated that 15 to 23 percent of critically ill patients are obese. The relative proportions of metabolically active lean body mass decreases as the percentage of body weight fat increases. The lean body mass may be significantly depleted or adequate. Therefore, in the obese patient, normal parameters of nutritional assessment may be difficult to interpret.

Volume status may be more difficult to evaluate in severely obese patients because they may be fluid overloaded. Evaluation includes measurement of orthostatic blood pressure, estimation of jugular venous pressure and presence of edema.

The chronically ill obese may develop protein depletion and weight loss, thus creating the diagnosis of malnutrition and/or undernutrition. It is difficult to predict energy requirements in this patient population. Overfeeding must be avoided since the predisposition of stressed obese patients is to develop carbohydrate intolerance, weak diaphragmatic musculature, blunted carbon dioxide sensitivity and cardiac insufficiency. The severely obese patient may be insulin resistant and glucose intolerant. Also, fatty liver infiltration may be common. A careful nutrition assessment can be made following these parameters: nutrition history (intake, weight, functional status); physical exam (muscle mass, volume status, signs of micronutrient deficiencies); laboratory data (serum albumin, prealbumin, TLC); and observation (weight changes, energy intake and protein intake).

Studies of moderate and morbidly obese patients have shown that equations using current body weight significantly over or underestimates energy expenditure in 60 percent of patients. The morbidly obese are usually underestimated.

Several methods can be used to estimate energy requirements for these patients. Each critically ill obese patient must be assessed as an individual.

    1. Adjustment formula for obesity (> 125% of IBW)

The obese person has a greater percentage of body fat, which is much less metabolically active. Using actual body weight skews the caloric needs to the high side. The following formula may be used:

    { (ABW - IBW) x 0.25} + IBW = wt in Kg for BEE

    where:

    ABW = actual body weight

    IBW = ideal body weight

    0.25 = 25% of body fat tissue is metabolically active

    2. BEE - using the IBW and adjusting upwards as indicated by patient's clinical condition and level of activity. Normally this method is not recommended.

    3. 16 to 19 kcal/kg of current body weight

    4. 21 kcal/kg ABW $\pm$ 400 (obese, ventilated)

    5. 25 to 30 kcal/kg/IBW

    6. Indirect calorimetry

    EEE (V) = 1925 - 10 (A) + 5 (W) + 281 (S) + 292 (T) + 851 (B)

    EEE (S) = 629 - 11 (A) + 25 (W) - 609 (O)

whereas V = ventilator dependent; S = spontaneously breathing, A = age, W = weight (kg), S= sex (m = 1, f =0), T= trauma, B = burn and O = obesity (present 1, absent 0).

Hypocaloric Feeding of the Obese

Data supports hypocaloric feeding of the moderately stressed obese patient. The observation is that endogenous energy can supply the body cell mass with sufficient energy to support mechanical and chemical work. Therefore, protein and micronutrients need to be added to support protein synthesis. Approximately 2 gm protein/kg/IBW and 52 percent of measured resting energy expenditure (approximately 880 kcal per day) are recommended.

Severly obese patients with related hypoventilation and respiratory failure may respond by the hypocaloric feeding regimen with the 2 gm pro/kg/IBW. This would promote short-term weight loss with minimal loss of lean body mass.

It must be remembered that few critically ill obese patients require immediate weight loss. Therefore, proceed with caution. Standard nutrition support modalities may result in greater rates of complications. For further information, refer to the obese patient under the enteral and parenteral sections.

Evaluating Weight Change

Monitoring weight helps determine if the patient's calorie needs were estimated accurately. Weight gain appears to follow a pattern. Early weight gain is rapid, approximately 250 to 500 grams per day and is mainly due to water retention. For this reason the preadmit or usual dry weight should be used for nutrition assessment of the critically ill patient. During the second, stage patients experience a period of minimal weight gain despite adequate protein and calorie intake. This is secondary to some diuresis or loss of retained fluid. Once the diuretic phase has passed weight gain occurs as lean tissue and fat is repleted. A period of rapid protein synthesis occurs initially as 18 - 30 grams of protein (90 - 150 grams of muscle per 70 kilograms of body weight) are synthesized per day. Increases in muscle mass are limited to 250 grams per day or less. Weight gains of more than 250 grams are due to either adipose tissue or fluid retention. Fat is not usually deposited until after cell mass is restored.

Weight Loss

Weight loss usually is due to increased basal energy expenditure, decreased oral intake or both. With uncomplicated mild trauma (such as elective surgery), patients lose less than 250 grams per day. The severely traumatized patient loses up to 500 grams per day. The extent of loss is influenced by sex, body build, preoperative nutritional status, degree of injury and complicating factors such as infection. Weight loss is more rapid and prolonged following serious infection or injury. Losses greater than 500 grams per day are associated with loss of lean body mass in addition to water loss. Morbidity and/or mortality may be predicted from weight loss as shown below.

% Weight Loss	% Usual Body Weight	Morbidity/mortality
0%	100%	None
10%	90%	Limited
20%	80%	Significant
30%	70%	Serious
40%	60%	Life threatening
< 40%	< 60%	Lethal

Because rapid weight loss is more detrimental than gradual loss, the rate and percent of weight loss are important factors in nutrition assessment.

The following can be used as guidelines for determining percentage weight loss (severe weight loss would be anything greater):

Significant weight losses are as follows:

Time	Percent Loss
1 week	1 - 2 %
1 month	5.0 %
3 months	7.5 %
6 months	10 %

Estimating Protein Needs

Metabolic rate, body protein reserves, caloric intake (i.e. nitrogen: calorie ratio), nutritional status and age must be considered when estimating protein needs. Normal, depleted and hypermetabolic individuals all vary in protein requirements. Hypermetabolic patients have a marked inefficiency in utilizing dietary protein whereas normal and depleted patients conserve protein. Positive nitrogen balance can be achieved in the normal and depleted patient when 7 to 10 percent of total adequate calories are protein. The hypermetabolic patient requires 16 to 20 percent to achieve positive nitrogen balance. Excessive protein intake may be associated with an elevated BUN and increased urinary urea nitrogen excretion. Death may occur from loss of lean body mass as muscle protein is catabolized to meet energy demands in the stressed, critically ill patient.

Provision of amino acids, water, glucose and electrolytes are necessary to minimize loss of body protein. The following are guidelines for estimating protein requirements:

Adults	Status	Estimated Requirements	
	Normal	0.8 - 1.0 gm/kg/day	
	Moderately stressed	1.0 - 2.0 gm/kg/day)	
	Severely stressed	2.0 - 2.5 gm/kg/day	
	Pediatrics	**Normal (gm/kg/day)**	**Stressed**
	0.0 - 0.5	2.0 gm	2.2 - 3.0 gm
	0.5 - 1.0	1.6 gm	1.6 - 3.0 gm
	1 - 3 years	1.2 gm	1.2 - 3.0 gm
	4 - 6 years	1.1 gm	1.1 - 3.0 gm
	7 - 10 years	1.0 gm	1.0 - 2.5 gm
	11 - 14 years	1.0 gm	1.0 - 2.5 gm
	15 - 24 years	0.85 gm	1.0 - 2.5 gm

Alternatively, 16 to 20 percent of total calories can be provided as protein.

Besides the nutrition and metabolic status of the individual, protein requirements are influenced by energy and nitrogen intake, exercise, the amino acid composition of dietary protein, the digestibility of consumed protein and the reutilization of endogenous protein. Positive nitrogen balance usually does not occur until the acute phase of illness has subsided. Energy administration/consumption of calories reduces nitrogen excretion and therefore improves nitrogen balance.

Nitrogen Intake: Nitrogen balance improves as nitrogen intake increases at any given level of energy intake. Nitrogen needs are based on total energy needs. The suggestion for maintenance is one gram nitrogen (6.25 gm protein) for 200 kcal and for anabolism, the recommendation is one gram nitrogen for 150 kcal.

Amino Acids: Optimal nitrogen balance is achieved when the essential acids are supplemented with a combination of several but not all the nonessential amino acids.

Digestibility: Any increased fecal loss of nitrogen must be accounted for with increased dietary protein.

Reutilization: Reutilization is more efficient during convalescence from a catabolic episode resulting from injury or infection. This results in improved use of dietary amino acids

Protein Requirements of the Critically Ill Obese

Protein requirements are estimated to be 1.0 to 1.7 gm/kg/IBW. At least 150 grams of carbohydrate are needed per day to reduce gluconeogensis. The definitive grams per kg depend on the degree of hypercatabolism. Close monitoring and reassessment is mandatory.

Monitoring

Serial measurement of prealbumin helps determine if adequate amounts of protein and calories are consumed and/or administered. Also a nitrogen balance or protein catabolic rate (PCR) can be determined.

MACRONUTRIENTS

Sodium, chloride, potassium, calcium, magnesium and phosphate are essential to the maintenance of water balance, cardiac function, mineralization of the skeleton, nerve function, muscle and enzyme systems and energy transformation. Protein utilization also is affected by the availability of sodium, potassium and phosphorus intake in the diet. One gram of nitrogen is associated with the retention of 0.08 gm PO_4, 3.1 mEq potassium, 3.5 mEq Na and 2.7 mEq Cl. Those with GI losses > 3000 ml should receive electrolyte replacement.

Sodium, Potassium And Chloride

The recommended electrolyte allowance for a healthy person is 45 to 145 mEq/day of each. The amount needed during illness depends upon the cardiovascular, renal, endocrine status and assessment of gastrointestinal and other losses. Potassium falls during nutritional repletion and is deposited in the newly synthesized cells. Therefore, serum levels may fall abruptly if potassium is not supplied/administered in adequate amounts. Five to six mEq/gm of administered nitrogen and/or 120 to 150 mEq/day are recommended for patients receiving parenteral nutrition.

Phosphorus

Phosphorus is essential to the intermediary metabolism of carbohydrate, protein and fat. Phosphorus moving into the newly synthesized tissue is related to the magnitude of nitrogen retention. The daily allowance of phosphorus should be around 15 mM/1000 nonprotein calories. Patients who are hyperglycemic, requires insulin, have a history of alcoholism, chronic weight loss, chronic antacid or diuretic use and/or are initially deficient will require more. Hypophosphatemia in the critically ill is usually a consequence of nasogastric suction and dextrose (without adequate PO_4) infusions.

Calcium

Calcium requirements are 40 mEq based on 70 to 80 percent of absorption from the gut. Positive calcium balance (5 mg or 0.25 mEq/kg) depends on simultaneous administration of phosphorus, sodium and calcium not nitrogen retention.

Magnesium

The RDA for magnesium is 29 mEq/men and 25 mEq/women. Magnesium plays an important role in protein synthesis. The recommendations are 2 mEq per gram of nitrogen administered.

MICRONUTRIENTS

Prolonged deprivation of various trace elements may unmask clinical manifestations of deficiency. Adult recommendations are listed below. Children and infants needs may vary with age.

Zinc

Zinc is an essential component in the metabolism of lipids, carbohydrates, protein and nucleic acids. Zinc also is involved in bone growth, immunocompetence and maintenance of the special senses (vision, taste and smell). For the normal person, oral supplement of zinc is 10 to 15 mg. Ingestion of zinc in amounts greater than 15 mg/

day orally may aggravate marginal copper deficiency by depressing copper absorption. During parenteral nutrition, the suggested intake is 2.5 to 4.0 mg per day with an additional 2 mg for acutely catabolic patients. Additional amounts are recommended for various losses (see parenteral section).

Copper

Copper is necessary for the proper utilization of iron in hemoglobin synthesis as well as for bone and elastic tissue development and normal function of the central nervous system. Oral recommendations are 1.2 to 3.0 mg per day and 0.5 to 1.5 mg for parenteral nutrition. Intake should be decreased or omitted in patients with hepatobiliary disease because copper is excreted primarily in the bile.

Chromium

Chromium is required to maintain normal glucose tolerance. Oral recommendations are 50 to 290 µg per day, 10 to 15 µg per day parenterally. Chromium is excreted predominately in the urine. Dosage must be adjusted with renal dysfunction.

Manganese

Manganese is involved in protein and energy metabolism. Oral recommendations are 0.7 to 5 mg per day and 0.15 to 0.8 mg per day parenterally. In the presence of biliary tract obstruction, dosage must be adjusted.

Iron

Iron is a constituent of hemoglobin, myoglobin and a number of enzymes. Oral recommendations are 10 mg per day for males and 15 mg per day for females. Normally, patients have substantial stores so parenteral patients are not supplemented. But if the patient requires prolonged or permanent PN, the recommendation is 1.0 to 12.5 mg per day.

Iodine

Iodine is an essential nutrient because it is an integral part of the thyroid hormones. Oral recommendations are 150 µg per day and 1 to 2 µg parenterally.

Selenium

Selenium is a component of glutathione peroxidase and probably provides a means of defense against the accumulation of lipid peroxides and free radicals that damage cell membranes and macronutrients, including DNA. Selenium deficiency has been associated with cardiomyopathy and skeletal myopathy. Oral recommendations are 50 to 70 µg per day and 40 to 120 µg per day parenterally.

Molybdenum

Molybdenum is a constituent of several enzymes, such as aldehyde oxidase, xanthine oxidase and sulfite oxidase. The oral recommendation is 75 to 250 ug per day. Patients on permanent parenteral nutrition may develop tachycardia, tachypnea, neurologic abnormalities and chemical evidence of sulfite oxidase and xanthine oxidase deficiency if it is not added to the solution.

REFEEDING

Refeeding syndrome is a series of metabolic abnormalities occurring as nutrients/calories are provided after a period of starvation. The magnitude of changes is dependent on the degree of starvation and the rate and content of the caloric repletion. Refeeding syndrome involves shifts in glucose metabolism, phosphorus, potassium, magnesium and fluid repletion and development of vitamin deficits.

Chronic PCM results in profound alterations in body composition: diminished lean body mass and body fat increased extracellular fluid space with losses of intracellular phosphorus, potassium and magnesium. The serum levels are not closely correlated with the intracellular and total body stores. These losses impact the functional capacity of the cardiopulmonary, neuromuscular and hematologic systems and every other organ system of the body.

Those at risk for refeeding complications include patients with:

- Classic marasmus and kwashiorkor
- Prolonged intravenous dextrose solutions while remaining NPO
- Absence of any nutrition support (1 - 2 weeks)
- Trauma, sepsis, surgery
- Prolonged fasting
- Morbid obesity with loss of considerable body weight
- Chronic alcoholism
- Anorexia nervosa
- Underlying cardiorespiratory disease

Refeeding can result in many complications if not initiated correctly. The chronically semi-starved patient generally exhibits reduced adipose and lean tissue mass. Visceral proteins are normal or slightly reduced. Slow pulse, low blood pressure, low insulin levels, hypothermia, hypometabolism are common. Thyroid hormone is in the inactive T_3 form and body organs are reduced in mass and when carbohydrate intake is low, the pancreas adapts by having a low insulin secretion rate. Upon refeeding of carbohydrate, the insulin secretion is increased. The amount of CHO fed should not exceed the ability of the pancreas to respond to it.

Refeeding reverses this quiescent state and can be fatal if done rapidly. Excess protein and calories initially may precipitate death by overloading various enzymatic and physiologic functions that may have adapted during malnutrition. As refeeding is initiated, rapid changes occur in thyroid and endocrine function. Oxygen consumption, cardiac output, insulin secretion and energy expenditure all increase. During enteral feeding, organ mass is restored at varying rates: muscle last, kidney gradually, liver quickly and intestinal mucosa within hours to days.

Components of the refeeding syndrome are the metabolic and physiologic consequences of the depletion, repletion, compartmental shifts and interrelationships of phosphorus, potassium, magnesium, glucose metabolism, vitamin deficiency and fluid resuscitation. The following are the effects of each:

Nutrient Involvement	System Affected	Complications
Severe Hypophosphatemia	Cardiac	Altered myocardial function
		Arrhythmia, CHF sudden death
	Hematologic	Altered RBC morphology, hemolysis, WBC dysfunction, depressed platelet function, bleeding
	Hepatic	Liver dysfunction
	Neuromuscular	Acute areflexia, paralysis, confusion, coma, cranial nerve palsy, lethargy, weakness, seizures rhabdomyolysis
	Respiratory	Acute respiratory failure, hyperventilation
	Skeletal	Vitamin D resistant rickets
Severe Hypokalemia	Cardiac	Arrhythmias, cardiac arrest, increased digitalis sensitivity, orthostasis, EKG changes (T flattening, U waves, ST depression)
	Gastrointestinal	Constipation, ileus, worsened encephalopathy
	Renal	Decreased concentrating ability, polyuria, polydipsia, nephropathy
	Neuromuscular	Areflexia, paralysis, nerve palsy, weakness, rhabdomyolysis
	Metabolic	Glucose intolerance, hypokalemic metabolic acidosis
	Respiratory	Acute respiratory depression
Severe Hypomagnesemia	Cardiac	Arrhythmias including torsades de pointes, tachycardia
	Gastrointestinal	Abdominal pain, anorexia, diarrhea, constipation
	Neuromuscular	Hyporelexia, confusion, nerve palsies, fasiculation, lethargy, weakness, seizures, vertigo, tetany, ataxia, irritability, personality changes
Glucose and Fluid Intolerance	Cardiac	CHF, sudden death
	Gastrointestinal	Fatty liver
	Hemodynamic	Dehydration, fluid overload, hypotension
	Metabolic	Hyperglycemia, hypernatremia, ketoacidosis, metabolic acidosis
	Neurologic	HHNK
	Pulmonary	CO_2 retention, respiratory depression
	Renal	Osmotic diuresis, prerenal azotemia
Thiamine Deficiency	Neuromuscular	Atazia, coma, confusion
	Hepatic	Wernickes's encephalopathy

Illustrated below are some complications that may occur with nutritional repletion.

Complication	Prevention
Hyperglycemia	Start slowly . Avoid excess CHO infusion
HHNK	Treat the hyperglycemia
Rebound hypoglycemia	Gradually change infusion rate. Avoid abrupt cessation of glucose infusion
Dehydration	Correct the hyperglycemia
Hypercapnia	Decrease carbohydrate, add fat
Hypokalemia	Add more K (up to 160 mEq/24 hr)
Hyperkalemia	Monitor K; may have underlying renal disease
Hypophosphatemia	Add more (60 mEq intravenous three times a day); does have risks; monitor.
Magnesium deficiency	Add intravenously
Hypocalcemia	Consequence of low magnesium, high phosphorus. May be secondary to low albumin. Sufficient amount should be given. Check ionized calcium.
Refeeding edema	Decrease the CHO load Decrease Na; slow infusion Hypocaloric
Diarrhea	Slow infusion; lactose free
Nausea/vomiting	Slow administration, low fat, low osmolar formula
Cardiopulmonary failure	Decrease rate; lower sodium

These refeeding syndromes are associated more with parenteral nutrition than enteral nutrition but caution and common sense are of key importance in refeeding the semistarved and chronically ill.

CONSEQUENCES OF OVERFEEDING

Overfeeding occurs when a clinical problem arises from administration of more nutrient than the body is prepared to utilize. The problems associated with overfeeding most commonly occur with parenteral nutrition. Liver dysfunction may occur as shown by increased liver function tests (alkaline phosphatase, serum glutamic oxalic transaminase, glutamic pyruvic transaminase, and bilirubin) and increased triglycerides. Fatty liver may result from high glucose loads as a result of excess glucose converting to fat. Increased carbon dioxide production may precipitate respiratory failure or delay weaning from the respirator. Fluid overload and congestive heart failure also have been attributed to overfeeding secondary to excess sodium and increased metabolic activity.

Overfeeding the critically ill patient can be avoided by using a mixed fuel system (i.e., fat and carbohydrate) and avoiding excessive amounts. Fat, which has a lower respiratory quotient, can be substituted for part of the carbohydrate to lower carbon production and maintain normal oxygen consumption.

Some metabolic changes that occur with overfeeding are shown below:

Excess of:	Manifests as:
Protein	Increased nitrogenous waste products Increased BUN - may be a problem in the patient with compromised renal function, a common situation in the critically ill
Fat	Opalescent serum Hyperlipidema GI disturbances Hepatosplenomegaly Anemia Thrombocytopenia Interferes with lab tests: Hgb and serum Na levels
Glucose	Hyperglycemia Hyperosmolarity Fat deposition in the liver Increased carbon dioxide production

SUGGESTIONS FOR REFEEDING

1. Composition of refeeding formulation should be low in sodium with moderate amounts of carbohydrate, fluid and routine vitamin supplementation.
2. Correct phosphorous, potassium, magnesium and give appropriate amounts for restoration, anabolism, and rebuilding of cell mass.
3. Initial feeding slowly: 20 - 25 kcal/kg/day or 1.0 x BEE for 1 - 3 days and increase slowly.
4. Monitor phosphorous, potassium, magnesium, glucose and urinary electrolytes.

Goal is to ensure reasonable rates of repletion while minimizing the side effects of overfeeding. The rate of weight gain should be 120 gm/day of lean tissue with the average weight gain of one kg/week.

The following are estimations of macronutrients:

Macronutrient	Non-ICU patients	ICU patients	Obese	Elderly
Kcal	25 - 30 kcal/kg	20 - 25 kcal/kg	Average of ABW-IBW	20 - 30 kcal/kg
Protein	1.2 - 1.5 gm/kg/IBW	1.5 gm/kg/IBW	1.2 - 1.5 gm/kg/IBW	1.5gm/kg
Carbohydrate	If on TPN 2.5 - 4.0 mg/kg/min	If on TPN 2.5 - 4.0 mg/kg/min	If on TPN 2.5 - 4.0 mg/kg/min average of ABW-IBW	If on TPN 2.5 - 4.0 mg/kg/min
Fat	Remaining Calories	Remaining Calories	Remaining Calories	Remaining Calories
Fluid	30 cc/kg	30 cc/kg	30 cc/kg	30 cc/kg

References

• Bynoe, R et al: Nutrition support in trauma patients. Nutr in Clin Pract 1988; August.

• Butterworth, C and Blackburn, G: Hospital malnutrition. Nutrit Today 1975; 3:8.

• Apelgren, K and Wilmore D: Nutritional care of the critically ill patient. Surg Clin of No Amer 1983; 63:497.

• Abbott, W et al: Nutritional care of the trauma patient. Surg Gyn Obstret 1983; 157:585.

• Long, C: Metabolic response to nonspecific stress. Clin Consult 1983; 3:4.

• Torun, B and Chew, F: Protein Energy Malnutrition. In: Shils, ME, Olson, JA, Shine, M, eds. Philadelphia: Lea and Febiger, 1994.

• Little, RA and Carlson, GL: Insulin Resistance and Tissue Fuel. In: Kinney, JM, Tucker,HN, eds. Organ Metabolism and Nutrition:Ideas for Future Critical Care. New York, Raven Press, 1994.

• Allison, SP: Overview: Substrate and Acute Catabolism. In: Kinney, JM, Tucker,HN, eds. Organ Metabolism and Nutrition:Ideas for Future Critical Care Editors. New York, Raven Press, 1994.

• Hoffer, LJ: Starvation. In: Shils, ME, Olson, JA, Shike, M. eds. Modern Nutrition in Health and Disease. Philadelphia: Lea & Febiger, 1994.

• Levenson, S, Crowley, L and Seifter, E: Starvation. In: Manual of Surgical Nutrition. Philadelphia: W.B. Saunders, 1975.

• Saudek, C and Felig, P: The metabolic events of starvation. The Amer J of Medicine 1976; 60:117.

• Kinney, J: Energy Requirements of The Surgical Patient. In: Manual of Surgical Nutrition. Philadelphia: W.B. Saunders, 1975.

• Kester, D et al: Metabolic response to trauma. Contemp Surg 1997; vol 13.

• Ballinger, W: Surgical Injury: Body Composition, Protein Metabolism and Neuroendocrinology. In: Manual of Surgical Nutrition. Philadelphia: W.B. Saunders, 1975.

• Schultz, Y and Jequier, E: Energy Needs: Assessment and Requirements. In: Shils, ME, Olson, JA, Shine, M, eds. Philadelphia: Lea and Febiger, 1994.

• Crim, MC and Munro, HN: The Proteins and Amino Acids. In: Shils, ME, Olson, JA, Shine, M, eds. Philadelphia: Lea and Febiger, 1994.

• Abbott, W et al: Nutritional care of the trauma patient. Surg Gyn and Obstet 1983; 157-585.

• Kinney, J et al: Tissue fuel and weight loss after injury. J of Clin Path 1970; 23 (suppl 4:64).

• Moore, F and Brennan, M: Surgical Injury: Body Composition, Protein Metabolism and Neuroendocrinology. In: Manual of Surgical Nutrition. Philadelphia: W.B. Saunders, 1975.

• Wilmore, D: The Metabolic Management of the Critically Ill Patient. New York: Plenum Medical Book Company, 1977: 201-3.

• Orme, J and Clemmer, I: Nutrition in the Critical Care Unit. Symposium on Critical Care Medicine. Med Clin of N Amer 1983; 67:1295-1304.

• Oh, MS: Water, Electrolyte and Acid-Base Balance. In: Shils, ME, Olson, JA, Shine, M, eds. Philadelphia: Lea and Febiger, 1994.

• Cluitmans, FH and Meinders, AE: Management of severe hyponatremia: Rapid or slow correction? Am J of Med 1990; 88:161.

• Halpern, ML and Goldstein, MB: Fluid, Electrolyte and Acid-Base Physiology. Philadelphia: WB Saunders 1994.

• Matheny, N: Fluid and Electrolyte Balance. Philadelphia: J.B. Lippincott, 1989.

• Collins, R: Illustrated Manual of Fluid and Electrolyte Disorders. Philadelphia: JB Lippincott, 1983.

• Weinberg, A; Pals JK and Campbell SM: Preventing dehydration in the elderly:the challenge of assessment and treatment. Diet Currents 1994; 21.

• Metheny, N: Fluid and Electrolyte Balance: Nursing Considerations. Philadelphia: J.B. Lippincott Co, 1987.

• Zaloga, GP: Nutrition in Critical Care. St. Louis: Mosby, 1994.

• Albina, JE: Nutrition and wound healing: JPEN 1994; Vol 18.

• Winkler, MF and Mandry, MK: Nutrition and wound healing. Support Line 1992; No 3.

• Albert, J et al: Chronic Submaximal Exercise an Adjunct to Intravenous Feeding in Man. Surg Forum 36:32-34, 1985.

• Lacey, JA: Immune function and nutrition support. RD 1993; No 3.

• Shronts, EP: Basic concepts of immunology and its application to clinical nutrition. Nutrit in Clin Pract 1993; 8:177.

• Twomey, P: Skin tests in nutritional assessment - a critical review. JPEN 1982; 6:50.

• Bates, S et al: Immunological skin testing and interpretation. A plea for uniformity. Cancer 1979; 43:2206.

• National Academy of Sciences. Recommended Dietary Allowances. Wash. D.C., 1989.

• Harris, J and Benedict, F: A Biometric Study of Basal Metabolism in Man. Wash, D.C.: Carnegie Institute of Wash, 1919. Pub. No. 279.

• Amato, P et al: Formulaic methods of estimating calorie requirements in mechanically ventilated obese patients: a reappaisal. Nutrit in Clin Pract 1995; 10:229.

• Williams, RR and Fuenning CR: Circulatory indirect calorimetry in the critically ill. JPEN 1991; No 5.

• Garriel, DR, Jobin, N and DeJonge, LHM: Should we still use the Harris and Benedict Equation? Nutrit in Clin Pract 1996; 11:99.

• Bell, SJ and Forse, RA: Nutrition support of the critically ill patient. Nutrit and the MD 1995; No 11.

• Long, C et al: Metabolic response to injury and illness: estimation of energy and protein needs from indirect calorimetry and nitrogen balance, JPEN 1979; 3:452.

• Ferraro, R and Albu, J: Nutrition support of the critically ill obese patient. (editorial). Nutrit in Clin Pract 1989; 4:25.

• Baron, R: Nutrition support of the critically ill obese patient. Topics in Clin Nutrit 1986; 10: 71.

• Pasulka, P and Kohl, D: Nutrition support of the stressed obese patient. Nutrit in Clin Pract 1989; 4:130.

• Abraham, S: Obese and Overweight Adults in the United States. Vital and Health Statistics. Series II, No. 230.

• Forbes, G: Lean body mass in obesity. Int J Obes 1983; 7:99.

• Karkeck, J: Adjustment for Obesity. ADA Renal Practice Group Newsletter, Winter, 1984.

• Naeye, R: The sizes and number of cells in visceral organs of human obesity. Am J Clin Pathol 1970; 34:251.

• Ireton-Jones, C: Evaluation of energy expenditures in obese patients. Nutrit in Clin Pract 1989; 4:127.

• Baxter, J and Bistrian, B: Moderate hypocaloric parenteral nutrition in the critically ill obese patient. Nutrit in Clin Pract 1989; 4:133.

• Kinney, J et al. Tissue composition of weight loss in surgical patients. Ann of Surg 1968; 3:459.

• Heymsfield, S: Metabolic Changes Associated with Refeeding. ASPEN Update 1982; 4:3:1-2.

• Havala, T and Shronts E: Managing the complications of refeeding. Nutrit in Clin Pract 1990; 5:23.

• Eliam, M: Changing concepts of nutrient requirements in disease; implications for artificial nutritional support. Lancet 1995.

• Solomon, SM and Kirby, DF: The refeeding syndrome: a review. JPEN 1990; No 1.

• Apovian, CM, McMahon, MM and Bistrain, BR: Guideline for refeeding the marasmic patient. Crit Care Med 1990; No 9.

• Olson, EA: Refeeding in the setting of chronic protein-calorie malnutrition. Nutrit and the MD 1991; No 3.

Tables and Figures

Table 1 Available Energy Stores of a 65 kg Man

Table 2 Response to Starvation and Trauma

Table 3 Characteristics of Water and Salt Deficits

Table 4 Signs of Fluid and Electrolyte Imbalance

Table 5 Arterial Blood Gases

. Table 6 Differential Diagnosis of Single Electrolyte Changes

NUTRITION SUPPORT THERAPY

The optimal method of nutrition support depends upon the degree of stress, functional capability of the gastrointestinal tract, the severity of preexisting malnutrition and the risk of refeeding/feeding complications. Inability or refusal to eat may have single or multiple causes. These may include neuromuscular abnormalities, psychosocial disorders, obstructive lesions or organic disease. In children, activity level, feeding history, food allergies, developmental delay in feeding, abnormal eating habits and difficulties in chewing and swallowing have to be evaluated. The preferred way to meet a patient's nutrition need is orally. If oral nutrition is not an option then enteral nutrition should be initiated.

ENTERAL / TUBE FEEDING

The GI tract is an important immunologic organ serving as a barrier to the intestinal toxins and organisms colonizing it. Enteral nutrition appears to reduce infectious complications in the critically ill/injured patient. The GI tract usually can be used immediately after trauma or surgery. Clinical studies show that prompt enteral feeding and the use of special nutrients enhance gut barrier function, prevents microbial translocation, reduces the hypermetabolic response to injury and improves clinical outcomes. The small intestinal motility is usually adequate for enteral nutrition. It is suggested the feedings start within 24 hours of the injury.

During severe stress, intestinal blood flow tends to decrease as blood is shunted to support metabolic processes needed for tissue repair. This can lead to mucosal damage and loss of intestinal barrier function, which in turn leads to alterations in the GI tracts permeability to bacteria or toxins. Nutrients have been shown to increase intestinal blood flow. Early enteral nutrition after metabolic stress may assist in preserving gut mucosal integrity and prevents bacterial translocation. Through maintenance of mucosal blood flow, gastric and colonic motility is impaired following stress and injury.

Early enteral feeding preserves intestinal integrity and function, reduces hepatic protein response and can reduce the rate of infectious complications. The benefits of early enteral nutrition include decreased weight loss, increased nitrogen intake and balance, decreased REE, decreased catabolic hormones, increased jejunal mucosal weight, improved wound healing, decreased bacterial infections and decreased hospital stay and as a result, decrease costs.

Postplyoric feeding makes early feeding more feasible. Post-op return of GI function is as follows:

Stomach: 24 hours. Normal propulsive functions return in 48 - 72 hours. Myoelectric activity is apparent within hours of surgery but not coordinated sufficiently to produce gastric emptying.

Small Intestines: 2 to 5 hours. Relatively normal propulsive function is seen within 12 hours of surgery, making it the best site for early enteral nutrition.

Colon: 3 to 4 days 72 hours post-op there is a sufficient activity of electrical control (slow waves) and electrical response (spike waves) inducing sustained contractions to move gas and bowel contents.

A major argument against early post-op enteral nutrition has been the occurrence of post-op ileus. Clinical signs of an ileus include abdominal distention and lack of bowel sounds and passing gas. Factors prolonging ileus are sympathetic hyperactivity; abdominal distention; intraperitoneal irritation; autonomic, cardiac and pschotropic drugs; electrolyte imbalances; and concomitant diseases.

Optimize early enteral nutrition support into the small bowel by observing the following should be observed:
- Select the formula most appropriate for the clinical condition
- Initiate the support slowly (25 - 40 cc/hour)
- Advance the feeding to meet the desired goal rate within 48 - 72 hours
- Monitor for signs of intolerance

The feasibility of tube feeding is dependent on a functional small bowel allowing absorption of essential nutrients. The patient should be able to tolerate adequate formula without experiencing distress. If the gut works and can be used safely, it should be used.

PATIENT EVALUATION FOR ENTERAL FEEDING

Patient evaluation should include digestive and absorptive capacity, renal function, electrolyte balance, nutritional status, medical therapy, route of administration and drug therapy. Patient acceptance of the tube feeding also is important because psychological problems can alter tolerance. For example, fear can slow down peristaltic action while anger and hostility can increase it. In an ICU, consideration should be given to conscious state and patient position, vent dependent and disease state and/or injury (e.g., diabetes, head injury).

Aborptive site of nutrients:

Duodenum

Vitamins A, B complex
Fe, Ca
Glycerol, fatty acids
Monoglycerides
Amino acids
Mono and Disaccharides

Transverse Colon
Water and biotin

Ileum

Entire – Chloride, Na
Distal – B12 and intrinsic factor
Proximal – Disaccharides

Jejunum (proximal)

Glucose, galactose
Vit C, amino acids
Glycerol, fatty acids
Monoglycerides, biotin
Folic acid, Cu, Zn
K, Pantothenic acid

(Proximal)

Vitamin A, B and Folic acid
Iron, lactose

Jejunum (Distal)

Isomaltose
Maltose
Sucrose, dipeptides

Polymeric formulas contain micornutrients in the form of isolates of intact protein, triglycerides and carbohydrate polymers. They are usually 12 - 18% protein, 40 - 60% carbohydrate and 30 - 40% fat. Monomeric formulas require less digestion than food polymers. Protein in is the form of peptides, carbohydrates in the hydrolyzed state and fat is MCT/LCT. Monomeric formulas are used for severe malabsorption.

Indications for each are shown below:

Polymeric	Monomeric
Coma	Preoperative bowel prep
Impairment of swallowing	Post op transitional feeding
Surgery of the upper GI Tract,	Chronic bowel disease
Chemotherapy/radiation	GI cutaneous fistulas
Protein-calorie malnutrition (mild)	Malabsorption
Hypermetabolism, burns	Infants with small bowel disease
Central nervous system disorders	
Anorexia nervosa, depression	
Head and neck surgery	

CONTRAINDICATIONS FOR TUBE FEEDING

Enteral feedings should not be given to patients with:

- Severe malabsorption
- Severe protein-calorie malnutrition
- Intestinal obstruction
- Peritonitis
- Paralytic ileus
- GI hemorrhage
- Shock
- Intractable vomiting and diarrhea
- Early stages of short bowel syndrome
- Severe pancreatitis
- High risk of aspiration
- High output (> 500 ml/hr)
- External fistula
- Prognosis that does not warrant aggressive nutritional support
- Nutrition support is not desired by the patient or the patient's family
- Inability to obtain enteral access

Enteral feeding is an efficient, safe and cost-effective method of meeting the nutrient needs of the stressed patient. Enteral feedings should fulfill three basic requirements:

- Provide adequate protein and calories
- Maintain electrolyte and mineral balance
- Maintain adequate hydration

FORMULARY

Formularies are cost effective. In developing an enteral formulary, both the specific needs of the patient population and the method of purchasing must be considered. The formulas selected should meet the nutrition needs of 95 - 98 percent of a facility's patients. Prior to establishing a formulary, a needs assessment may be necessary. The assessment should address the patient population needs, trends in medicine, financial constraints and personnel resources. The needs assessment of the patient includes routes of feeding, diagnosis, history of tolerance to the products and a facility assessment. The facility assessment includes space issues: inventory, formula preparation and storage area; personnel issues: available personnel for ordering, receiving and issuing products and preparation and delivering the products to the nursing units.

The goal of a well-designed formulary is to improve the nutritional status of the patients receiving the products; eliminate product duplication and increase effective use of products; decrease inventory and waste costs; and decrease potential complications.

Specialized formulas (off the formulary) should be justified by accounting for the extenuating circumstances that would necessitate using them. Questions such as how long has the patients GI tract been without stimulation, the frequency, consistency and volume of the diarrhea, what nutrition intervention has the patient been receiving and what other enteral formulas has the patient received should be asked prior to implementing a specialized formula. The outcome anticipated from using the specialized formula should be well defined.

Formula characteristics to consider are the digestibility of the nutrients, osmolality, viscosity, nutritional adequacy, ease of use and cost. Digestive and absorptive capacity, renal function, electrolyte balance, nutritional status, medical therapy, route of administration and drug therapy of the patient also must be evaluated. Palatability and acceptability have an important role if the formula is to be consumed orally. Formulas with intact nutrients are better tolerated than formulas with protein hydrolysates and/or amino acids.

Nutritional Characteristics

Nutritional adequacy must be assessed for individual needs. Most tube feedings meet the RDA at approximately 1100cc to 1500cc, depending on the specific formula. If the patient's fluid and /or calorie needs are less, a liquid vitamin supplement should be considered/recommended.

Physical Characteristics

Not only are nutritional requirements and gastrointestinal function important but certain physical characteristics of the formula have to be considered for tolerance. Gastric retention, diarrhea or constipation may indicate tube feeding intolerance. The intolerance may be related to the osmolality, nutrient density, caloric density, pH or residue content.

Osmolality

- Gastric emptying is slowed by solutions with higher mOsms. The higher osmolality causes a greater inhibitory effect. Osmolality may cause gastric retention, nausea and vomiting.

- Hypertonic formulas can cause severe diarrhea, electrolyte depletion and dehydration. Solutions are adjusted to isotonic levels in the duodenum by increasing or decreasing their water content. Hypertonic formulas can cause large fluid shifts into the small bowel.

- Osmolality may affect the solute load and water requirements. Formulas that cause a large renal solute load may cause clinical dehydration. Rehydration needs to occur over a period of a few days to prevent water intoxication.

Calorie-Nutrient Density

- May effect gastric emptying. The greater the nutrient density the slower the emptying rate. Specific nutrients can have an effect – i.e., high fat formulas can cause significant delay in gastric emptying.

- Administration must be gradual if the GI tract has not been used for a period of time. This allows the intestinal enzymes to hydrolyze the nutrients.

pH

- The pH of most commercial formulas is > 3.5. Formulas with a pH of less than 3.5 reduce gastric motility.

Residue

- Low residue formulas may cause constipation in some patients.

Characteristics of the ideal enteral formula are:

- Lactose free
- Low osmolarity
- Suitable viscosity
- Appropriate nitrogen:calorie ratio
- Nutritionally complete
- Readily digestible
- Metabolically tolerated
- Easily administered
- Economical

Types of Formulae

Enteral formulas may be categorized as general, defined/elemental, high nitrogen, high calorie, modified fiber, high calorie/nitrogen, modular and specialized.

The following can be used to describe the type and criteria for selecting a product for the formulary.

General Formula	Designed for patients with intact digestion and absorption. May be used intragastrically and intraduodenally. Many patients can begin on a full strength formula thus more quickly in meeting their desired goals. 30 - 40 gm pro/L 1 cal/cc Lactose free 300 - 400 mOsm/L Low viscosity
Defined / Elemental	Designed for patients with malabsorption or short bowel syndrome. Contains nutrients in elemental form: protein as amino acid and/or peptides and carbohydrates as glucose oligosaccharides. The viscosity is low but osmolarity is high. Start slowly, intragastrically or intraduodenally at half strength. Patient tolerance needs close monitoring. 30 - 40 gm pro/L 1 cal/cc Lactose free 500 mOsm/L Low viscosity

High Nitrogen	Designed for patients requiring higher protein needs. Designed for patients with intact digestion and absorption. May be used intragastrically and intraduodenally. May need to increase water to offset the obligatory renal water loss. 1 cal/cc Lactose free 300 - 400 mOsm/L Low viscosity 40 - 50 gm protein/L
High Calorie	Designed for patients with intact digestive and absorptive capacity requiring higher calorie needs or with a fluid restriction. May be used intragastrically and intraduodenally. 1.5 - 2.0 cal/cc Lactose free 400 - 500 mOsm/L Low viscosity 40 - 50 gm protein/L
High Calorie / N₂	Designed for patients needing higher calories and protein who have intact digestion and absorption. May be used intragastrically and intraduodenally. May need increased water to offset the obligatory renal water loss. 1.5 - 2.0 cal/cc 50 - 60 gm protein/L Lactose free 400 - 500 mOsm/L Low viscosity
Modified Fiber	Designed for patients needing increased fiber (glucose intolerance, constipation, diarrhea) who have full digestive capabilities. Fiber formulas should be carefully selected. In critically ill patients with PCM, insoluble fiber may slow intestinal absorption and further delay motility. Intake should be sufficient to affect bowel function without interfering with absorption of other nutrients. Fiber source, length of use and presence of other mineral-binding agents are factors to consider. 1.0 - 1.2 cal/cc Lactose free 300 - 400 mOsm/L 30 - 40 gm protein/L 7 - 10 gms fiber/L
Peptide Based	Designed for patients who cannot tolerate the hyper-osmotic load presented by elemental diets of amino acids. May be used in cases of hypoalbuminemia-induced diarrhea along with exogenous albumin infusion.
Specialized	Designed for specific organ dysfunction. **Renal** formulas are designed to provide mainly essential amino acids. Some are low in minerals (Mg, PO_4) and some vitamins. Calories are 2.0/cc and some are not nutritionally complete. The osmolarity is high (> 450 mOsm/L) **Hepatic** formulas contain both essential and nonessential amino acids. They contain higher amounts of branched chain amino acids and less aromatic amino acids. The osmolarity is high and they are not nutritionally complete.

Trauma solutions also contain higher amounts of branch chain amino acids. The osmolarity is higher (350 - 950 mOsm/L) and they are nutritionally complete when given in sufficient amounts. Lactose free.

Diabetic formulas are designed to meet the needs of patients with abnormal glucose tolerance (diabetes or stress-induced hyperglycemia). They are nutritionally complete when given in sufficient amounts. Lactose free; fiber supplemented.

Pulmonary formulas are designed to decrease CO_2 production. Low in carbohydrate and high in fat (50 - 60%). Lactose free. The osmolarity is ~ 450 mOsm/L. Nutritionally complete when given in sufficient amounts.

Immune formulas are designed to meet the needs of the critically ill patient. They have glutamine, arginine, omega-3 fatty acids and nucleotides added. Calories range from 1.0 - 1.5 kcal/L and protein 50 - 60 gm/L. Lactose free. Their true clinical efficacy is unknown.

Modular	Designed with single or multiple nutrients (i.e. protein, fat and carbohydrate supplemented with vitamins and minerals). The nutrients can be combined to produce a nutritionally complete formula or used individually to enhance an existing formula. Most patients can tolerate standard formulas, so this type of formula is used infrequently.
Supplements	Supplements are exactly what they state. They are intended to supplement oral intake. They are not designed to be nutritionally complete. Any of the above mentioned formulas can be used as supplements.

Potential risks of modular components given separately include the following:

Protein	The three main sources of protein are intact protein, hydrolyzed protein and crystalline amino acids. The nutritional value varies with the protein source as does osmolality and palatability. They are relatively insoluble; digestibility varies and they are expensive. Available in powder form (insoluble). They do not contribute significantly to osmolarity. **Complications:** Excessive protein used alone can precipitate an osmotic diarrhea. Prerenal azotemia can occur with an inadequate amount of fluid.
Fat	Liquid fat emulsions: butterfat and vegetable oils are the major sources of fat. There are long chain triglycerides and medium chain triglycerides (MCT) modules. MCT does not provide essential fatty acids (EFA) and deficiencies may develop when MCT is used as the only source of fat. Fat is relatively insoluble, digestibility varies, contributes little to osmolality and they are relatively low cost. **Complications:** Possible EFA deficiency. Excess fat can delay the gastric emptying time and cause diarrhea if maldigested.
Carbohydrates	Four sources of CHO are: polysaccharides and oligosaccharides; disaccharides; glucose polymers; and monosaccharides. They come in liquid and powder form, combine easily with liquid formulas and are easily digested. Caloric density varies. Contribution to osmolality varies. Carbohydrate modules are fairly inexpensive. **Complications:** High CHO can cause osmotic diarrhea and dehydration. Overfeeding CHO can cause a fatty liver and increase risk of ventilatory failure secondary to increased carbon dioxide production.

A wide variety of enteral products are on the market. Many have only subtle differences in composition.

DELIVERY

Feeding tubes may be introduced into the gastrointestinal tract at various points. Factors to consider when placing a feeding tube are: the length of time tube feeding is needed, the site of any obstruction, any pending surgery, potential for reflux, the degree of consciousness and the volume needed. The disease state may also determine the location for the tube placement.

Nonsurgical approaches include nasogastric (NG) and nasoduodenal (ND) intubation, while esophagostomy, pharyngotomy, gastrostomy, percutaneous gastrostomy and jejunostomy tubes require surgical insertion.

Nasogastric: Tube Extends to Stomach

Indications	Short term coma Severe diarrhea Major burns Hypermetabolic states Refusal to eat (anorexia nervosa) Nocturnal feeding
Type of Patient	Alert, unrestrained Intact gag and cough reflexes Normal gastric emptying
Contraindications	Gastroesophageal reflux Intractable vomiting, gastric ileus, GI obstruction
Complications	Risk of aspiration Intestinal perforation Lactobezoar Nasal colonization
Administration	Isotonic – can start at full strength Strength is increased before volume

Nasoduodenal / Nasojejunal: Tube Extends Through The Pylorus

Indications	Short-term coma Severe diarrhea Major burns Hypermetabolic states Refusal to eat (anorexia nervosa) Esophageal reflux Nocturnal feeding High risk of pulmonary aspiration Gastroparises Period of gastric dysfunction
Type of patient	Alert, unrestrained Intact gag and cough reflexes Normal gastric emptying High risk of aspiration
Contraindications	Gastroesophageal reflux Intractable vomiting
Complications	Risk of aspiration Intestinal perforation Lactobezoar Nasal colonization Potential GI intolerance at goal rate (bloating, cramping, diarrhea)
Administration	Volume increased before strength, if dilute, increase strength prior to volume

Jejunostomy: Tube Surgically Placed

Indications	Congenital gastrointestinal anomalies Impaired gastric motility Post upper GI surgery Proximal obstruction Total gastrectomy
Type of patient	Long-term feeding High risk of aspiration Esophageal reflux
Contraindications	Low birth weight infant
Complications	Bowel perforation Bacterial overgrowth Malabsorption, GI intolerance
Administration	Volume and mOsm may be limited secondary to dumping, cramps and diarrhea. Infuse dilute formula Increase volume prior to strength

Gastrostomy: Tube Surgically Placed In Stomach

Indications	Post surgery Extensive prolonged tube feeding Inability to suck or swallow Esophageal atresia Tracheoesophageal fistula Esophageal injury with obstruction Severe respiratory disease Home tube feeding
Type of Patient	Intact gag refux No esophageal reflux Stomach uninvolved NG route unavailable
Contraindications	Severe gastroesophageal reflux Intractable vomiting Inadequate emptying
Complications	Tube obstructing pyloric outlet. Potential risk of aspiration
Administration	Strength is dependent upon mOsm of the formula Increase volume before strength

Percutaneous Endoscopic Gastrostomy (PEG)

Indications	Neoplastic obstruction Swallowing difficulties Home tube feeding
Contraindications	Gastric outlet obstruction Active peptic ulcer Ascities Coagulopathy Inability to perform endoscopy Complete esophageal or pharyngeal obstruction Gastroesophageal reflux
Complications	Catheter clogging Wound infections Peristomal leaks Cellulitis Dislodgment Aspiration

Percutaneous Endoscopic Jejunostomy (PEJ)

Indications	Neoplastic obstruction Swallowing difficulties Risk of aspiration Long-term feeding

Contraindications	Gastric Outlet Obstruction
	Inability to perform endoscopy
	Complete esophageal or pharyngeal obstruction
	Gastroesophageal reflux

Complications	Catheter clogging, kinking and knotting
	Dislodgment of the tube
	Duodenogastric reflux
	Aspiration can occur

Administration

Tube placement should be checked prior to initiating a tube feeding. Individual patient differences and tolerances determine the infused rate. A slow initial delivery rate is recommended to prevent cramps, nausea, distention and diarrhea. Tube feeding can begin at full strength if gastrointestinal function is adequate. Additional water assures adequate fluid balance for metabolic processes. The initial rate is usually 40 - 50 cc per hour.

The feeding should be administered for two to four hours and then checked for residuals. If the residuals are less than 150 cc, the feeding can continue. Increase the feeding in increments of 25 cc per hour every twelve hours until the predetermined volume attained. A residual volume greater than 1.5 to 2.0 times the previous hour's infusion volume suggests delayed gastric emptying. Example: at 50 cc per hour residuals should not exceed 100 cc or at 75 cc per hour residuals should not exceed 150 cc. If residuals are greater than 150 cc per hour, either return to the previously tolerated rate or discontinue the tube feeding. No residuals could mean the feeding tube is above fluid level or the tube had collapsed on itself. Residuals cannot be checked in the duodenum or jejunum. If residuals are present, then the tube is in the stomach.

To maintain tube patency, feeding tubes should be irrigated with 40 - 50 ccs sterile water every six to eight hours or whenever the tube feeding is stopped.

Enteral feedings can be administered three ways:

Bolus	50 - 400 cc of feeding over 30 minutes every 4 to 6 hours. Additional water is given after each feeding to rinse the tube and prevent clogging. Bolus feedings can be poorly tolerated (nausea, distention, cramps, diarrhea) if the administration is too rapid. Usually given by gravity method, with the rate controlled by a clamp.
Gravity Feeding	Can be continuous or intermittent. Intermittent feedings of 200 - 400 cc are given over 30 minutes every 2 to 4 hours. Additional water is needed and tolerance may be poor. Continuous infusions occur at a constant rate over 16 - 24 hrs. If infusion is planned for 24 hours the hourly rate should be calculated for 22 hours. This allows for necessary interruptions for equipment changes or administration of medications. Residuals should be checked every 2 to 4 hours. If the residuals exceed 150 cc either stop the feeding or return to the previous tolerated rate. Rates of 100 - 150 ml/hour are usually well tolerated.
Pump	Has the advantage of delivering precise volumes. Pump ensures constant rate and reduces the amount of residuals. Incidence of osmotic diarrhea is reduced. Reduces the potential for gastric retention and vomiting. A wide variety of fluids, including highly viscous solutions, can be used. Some units provide safeguards and alarm systems.

DRUG THERAPY

Enteral medication is a complex issue. Potential problems include drug nutrient interactions, altered nutrient absorption and with concomitantly drug administration, altered drug efficacy.

Commonly prescribed opiates decrease gastric and small intestinal secretions. Morphine decreases gastric motility, delaying emptying and small intestinal motility. The duodenum is affected to a greater extent than the ileum. Effects of these medications on the GI tract may be dose related and have not prevented feeding initiation into the small bowel.

Considerations

- Drug formulation: Slow release and enteric coated drugs should not be crushed. Crushing destroys the integrity of the drug and may alter the desired absorption rate and site. Alternative liquid preparations should be used where possible.

- Crushed drugs given through small-bore feeding tubes or those with small delivery holes may induce clogging. To prevent occlusions, consider the tube diameter, drug viscosity and compatibility of other drugs.

- Osmolality: Medications and electrolyte replacements are hypertonic. This can be resolved if the medications and/or electrolyte replacements can be added to the formula. If incompatibility is a problem, the medications/electrolyte replacements can be diluted with water and administered slowly. Stop the feeding for 15 minute, flush with 90 ml of water prior to administration of the drug and flush again after the drug; and/or give it intravenously.

- Tube placement: Site of absorption and site of action may be affected. The stomach prepares drugs for delivery to the absorptive sites of the small intestines by dissolution. When tube feedings are administered beyond the stomach, a liquid form of the drug may be needed, accounting for the viscosity, pH and osmolality of the drug and the tube diameter.

Administration

Medications in solution, syrup, elixir, suspension or emulsion sometimes are safely administered in bolus through the tube. Flushing dilutes the medication, thus decreasing toxicity and possibly preventing gastric irritation or osmotic diarrhea. GI intolerance may be ameliorated by diluting liquid drugs with 15 to 20 cc of lukewarm water. Another way is to mix the drug with the enteral formula or administ it when the formula is still in the GI tract. The drug and formula will have to have physical and chemical compatibility. The drug should not destroy the emulsion characteristics or decrease the pH of the final solutions causing changes in viscosity, consistency and particle size of the formula. If the medication is added to the formula, the drug should be added slowly while the mixture is vigorously stirred. Flushing the tube with 30 cc of lukewarm water before and after giving the drug can clear the tube and indicate whether the tube has been obstructed. Each medication should be administered separately. Hypertonic medications should be diluted with water. Smaller volumes of tube feeding may promote more rapid absorption and utilization of the drug. Larger-bore tubes may be needed to administer large drug particles.

Hyperosmolar liquid preparations require additional dilution to prevent osmotic diarrhea. These medications must be diluted before entering the small bowel. Failure to do so may cause loss of electrolytes secondary to the osmotic diarrhea. If an undiluted hyperosmolar solution is administered into the stomach, distention, cramping, nausea, vomiting and/or diarrhea may occur.

Extended-release and enteric coated drugs should not be crushed. Extended-release medications are designed to release the outerlayer when in contact with GI fluids. A gradual shredding of multiple layers then occurs over a period of time. Crushing destroys the integrity of the drug and may alter the desired absorption rate and site. Crushing may increase the risk of side effects and the potential for drug toxicity by releasing all the drug at the same time. If the drug has to be crushed, the medication should be diluted in 60 ml of water when given.

Alternative liquid preparations should be used where possible. In case of a fluid restriction, the undiluted drug might be added directly to the tube feeding but only if it is compatible with the feeding.

The parenteral form may be the only liquid formulation available. The problems with parenteral formulation are cost and high osmolality due to the drug concentration. This high osmiolality could result in cramping and diarrhea.

Many drugs are better absorbed in the fasted state and should be given one hour before and two hours after meals. For patients on continuous tube feeding, drugs may need to be given prior to hanging each feeding where possible. The infusion rate can be adjusted during the post-medication period to compensate for the lost infusion/ nutrients.

Biochemical abnormalities associated with medications can be reviewed in the drug section of this book. The common abnormalities effect serum glucose, potassium, sodium, magnesium, phosphorus and lipids.

Incompatibilities

Pharmacokinetic Alterations – This occurs when enteral nutrition alters the bioavailabilty, distribution, metabolism, or elimination of the medications, or the reverse – the medication alters nutrient function.

Drugs can produce side effects such as nausea, vomiting, diarrhea, decreased appetite and electrolytes and metabolic abnormalities. This is not a result of the tube feeding but of the drug. Nutrition therapy should not be changed, but the delivery of the drug can be modified.

The formula can have an effect on the drug's bioavailability. The solution can affect the rate and extent of drug absorption. Diarrhea also can affect drug absorption. The decreased gastrointestinal transit time can result in subtherapeutic drug levels.

Physical – This occurs when mixing a medication and enteral formula results in a change in formula texture (granulation or gel formation), flow rate, viscosity, separation, precipitation, or broken emulsion. A major complication is the clogging of tubes.

Pharmaceutical – This incompatibility is a change in medication dosage form resulting in altered enteral formula or drug potency, efficacy or tolerance. A classic example is crushing enteric-coated tablets or opening slow-release capsules in an effort to reduce the risk of clogging the tube.

Pharmacologic – This is the most frequently encountered drug-nutrient interaction. It involves a medication's mechanism of action leading to enteral feeding intolerance, as manifested by diarrhea, GI distention, nausea, emesis, altered taste perception, altered biochemical levels, or antagonistic activity.

Physiologic – This involves the nonpharmacologic actions of a medication that alters tolerance to nutrition support. Diarrhea related to increased osmolarity is the most common. The majority of diarrhea is caused by medications, especially antibiotics, GI stimulants and prokenetic agents (erythromycin, quindine, digoxin, beta blockers and stimulant laxatives). These incompatibilities can be avoided by changing the route of administration (oral to IM or IV).

Common biochemical abnormalities associated with medications prescribed for tube fed patients are hyperglycemia, hyper/hypokalemia, hyper/hyponatremia, hyper/hypomagnesiumia, hyper/hypophosphatemia, calcium losses and hypertriglyceridemia.

Most incompatibilities are easily treated and can be prevented with proper monitoring. Complications can be resolved by altering the dose or route, changing the feeding schedule, bolusing the drug, diluting the drug with maximum amount of water or, if appropriate, admixing it with the tube feeding.

COMPLICATIONS

Enteral feeding complications can be gastrointestinal, metabolic or mechanical in nature. Gastrointestinal complications include nausea, vomiting, diarrhea, constipation and abdominal distention. Diarrhea may be defined as an increase in the fluidity, volume, or frequency of stool relative to the usual pattern of the patient. Criteria may include an increase in frequency (3 - 4 loose stools per day), an increase in weight (> 200 gms), or a change in the consistency or volume of the stool (> 300ml/liquid stool).

Diarrhea may be osmotic – a reduction in water absorption, caused by sorbitol, enteral formulas, antibiotics, antacids, laxatives, H_2 Blockers and stool softeners. Or it may be secretory – an increase in water secretion by the colon. Secretory diarrhea should be suspected when diarrhea persists for more than 24 hours after the tube feeding is stopped. Conditions/substances causing secretory diarrhea include clostridium difficle, partial bowel obstruction, enteric pathogens, metastatic carcinoid tumors, vasoactive intestinal peptides, lactulose, secreting adenomas and intestinal motility disorders. Differentiation of the two types is made by calculating the osmotic gap between the concentration of sodium and potassium ions in the colonic fluid and the fecal osmolality. Fecal osmolality is between 280 (secretory diarrhea) and 330 (osmotic diarrhea) mOsm. The formula for calculating osmotic gap is:

$$\text{Stool Osmotic Gap} - \text{Measured Stool Osmolality} - 2 \times (\text{Stool Na} + \text{Stool K})$$

Osmotic diarrhea has a greater osmotic gap (160 mOsm/L or more) than secretory diarrhea (usually small to negative osmotic gap). It is important to determine which type of diarrhea is occurring and treat it accordingly.

Metabolic complications include electrolyte and mineral imbalances, dehydration and glucose intolerance. The refeeding syndrome can cause intracellular requirements for phosphorus, potassium and magnesium to rapidly increase as cells are replenished. During this repletion, there is a potential for rapid serum decreases in these elements.

Mechanical complications include tube displacement, tube clogging and pulmonary aspiration which is the most serious. Causes of aspiration can include compromised lower esophageal sphincter, vomiting, altered gag reflux, swallowing dysfunction, delayed gastric emptying, improper position of the feeding tube, head of bed not elevated and decreased mental status.

Each type of complication is presented in **Table 1** along with symptoms, possible causes and prevention/therapy.

Table 1: Complications – Enteral Nutrition

Complication	Symptoms	Cause	Prevention / Therapy
Gastrointestinal	Diarrhea > 3 large stools > 200 gm/stool > 300 ml/liquid stool/day	Medications	Change the type and time Eliminate sorbitol. Adjust for hyperosmolar medications. Give proper antidiarrheal agent. Determine the type and treat accordingly.
		Bolus feeding	Change to continuous feeding.
		Volume overload	Decrease the amount or use a more concentrated tube feeding.
		Rapid administration	Decrease the rate; advance more slowly.
		Hyperosmolar formula (osmotic overload)	Change to isotonic solution. Dilute the formula initially. Start at a lower rate (25 - 30 cc per hour) with increase every 12 - 24 hours.
		Lactose intolerance	Use lactose free formula.
		Fat malabsorption	Use a low fat formula. Use pancreatic enzym supplement if necessary
		Protein calorie malnutrition	Use isotonic solution. Start at a lower rate (25 cc) with increase every 12 to 24 hours.
		Albumin < 2.5gm/dL	Use a peptide based, low fat formula with infusion of salt poor exogenous albumin.
		Cold feedings	Warm to room temperature. Start at a lower rate.
		Impaction	Rectal exam prior to feeding. Adequate water intake. Appropriate motility agent.
		Fear/anxiety	Discontinue feeding. Educate patient. Resume at a lower rate. Add antidiarrheal or bulk forming agent (liquid form).
		Contaminated formula	Discard current formula and bag. Decrease hang time. Sterile techniques for solution additives.
		Decreased bulk	Use a bulk agent diluted with adequate water. Change to fiber containing formula.

Complication	Symptoms	Cause	Prevention / Therapy
	Nausea/vomiting	Patient position	Position patient with head elevated at least 30 to 45 degrees. Position patient on right side to facilitate passage of gastric contents through pylorus.
		Improper tube placement	Check the tube for placement by Xray. Aspirate for contents.
		Fast delivery rate	Lower rate to previously tolerated rate; then advance over 12 to 24 hours.
		Hypertonic solution	Change to isotonic formula. Dilute current feeding and increase over several days.
		Delayed gastric emptying	Stop feeding 2 hours and check residuals. R/O obstruction. Ambulation may help.
		Lactose intolerance	Use lactose free formula.
		Excessive fat	Change to lower fat formula.
		Smell	Add flavorings that do not change mOsm.
	Constipation (no stool x 3 - 4 days)	Dehydration	Monitor intake and output. Add free water if intake is not greater than output by 500 - 1000 ccs.
		Decreased fiber	Use high fiber formula. Administer bulking agent.
		Obstruction	Stop the tube feeding.
	Abdominal distension	Impaction	Rectal exam. Add free water.
		Large gastric residuals (> 150 ml)	Decrease the rate. Confirm the position of tube. R/O obstruction/ paralytic ileus.
		Cold feedings	Warm the formula.
		Rapid infusions	Decrease the rate.
		Hyper-osmolarity	Change to isotonic formula.
		Lactose intolerance	Lactose free formula.
Metabolic	Overhydration	Intestinal Atrophy	Isotonic feeding. Start at 1/2 strength. Decrease volume.
		PCM and Refeeding	Decrease the rate. Restrict free water. Change formula to a calorically dense one. Administer diuretics. Replace Na losses.

Complication	Symptoms	Cause	Prevention / Therapy
	Hyponatremia < 135mEq Na	Excessive free water; fluid overload; excessive GI fluid losses; syndrome of inappropriate SIADH; cardiac, hepatic or renal insufficiency	Assess fluid and electrolyte status; restrict water; use loop diuretics if necessary; provide fluids with appropriate composition; use a calorically dense formula.
	Dehydration	High osmolarity	Change to isotonic formula.
	Hypernatremia > 145 mEq Na	Diabetes Insipidus; inadequate free water; increased fluid losses	Administer free water; assess fluid and electrolyte status; administer appropiate electrolytes.
	Diarrhea	High protein	Decrease the protein content.
		Lack of free water	Add free water. Monitor I&O and labs. Intake should not be greater than output by more than 500 - 1000 ccs.
	Hyperglycemia > 160 mg/dL	Insulin deficiency DM; steroids; sepsis; pancreatitis	Give insulin or oral agent. Discontinue feeding until blood sugar is controlled. Slow rate. Monitor blood sugar. Change formula to a lower CHO; increase fiber content.
	Hypoglycemia < 70 mg/dL	Stop feeding	Add IV glucose; monitor blood sugar. Taper feedings.
	HHNK	Hyperglycemia	Stop the feeding until blood sugar is under control.
	Hyperkalemia > 5 mEq/L	High K feeding GI bleed; Acute dehydration; Renal insufficiency IV potassium Acidosis	Change to lower K formula Give kayexalate, insulin and glucose, adequate fluid. Stop IV potassium. Correct the acidosis.
	Hypokalemia < 3.5 mEq/L	PCM, refeeding syndrome Diarrhea. Diuretics, Insulin administration	Replete potassium. Supplement IV potassium. Monitor labs.
	Hypophosphatemia < 2.5 mg/dL	PCM, refeeding syndrome; anabolism; Insulin administration	Give intravenous phosphorus. Monitor labs.
	Hyperphosphatemia > 4.5 mEq/L	Renal insufficiency; poor perfusion; use of PO_4 antacids	Change the formula. Use a PO_4 binder. Treat cause of poor perfusion. Consider other antacids

Complication	Symptoms	Cause	Prevention / Therapy
	Hypomagnesemia < 1.6 mg/dL	Refeeding syndrome, alcoholism	Replete with IV Mg. Monitor labs.
	Hypermagnesima > 2.7 mg/dL	Renal insufficiency; Mg containing antacids	Change formula to half strength; dc all forms of Mg intake.
	Hypocalcemia < 8.5 mg/dL	Muscle cramps; abdominal cramps; tetany; low albumin; positive Chvostek sign; convulsions; drug therapy	Adequate Ca; repletion of PO4 with Ca; adjust to albumin fluctation.
	Hypercalcemia > 10.5	Renal insufficiency; calcium containing antacids	Decrease the amount of total calcium; use a therapeutically equivalent drug.
	Hypercapnia	Respiratory dysfunctionn; excessive CHO load	Avoid overfeeding; change to a ↑ CHO, ↓ Fat formula.
	Essential fatty acid deficiency	Low linoleic acid formula	Change the formula. Add 5 ml of safflower oil. Use modular fat.
	Abnormal liver function	Increased transaminases secondary to elemental formula	May need to change and/or stop the formula.
	Rapid excessive weight gain > .5 kg/day	Excessive calories and fluid Electrolyte imbalance	Decrease concentration or amount of formula. Evaluate electrolyte balance; adjust formula accordingly.
	Insufficient weight gain < 25 gm/day	Inadequate calories; malabsorption	Use calorically dense formula; increase the rate; change the type for better absorption.
Mechanical	Tubes	Improper size	Change size.
		Improper placement	Check placement.
		Insufficient irrigation	Flush tube with warm water prior to or after each feeding.
	Pulmonary Aspiration	Patient is flat	Elevate head of patient 30 degrees.
		Absent gag reflex	Change site of feeding.
		Gastric reflux	Change to a smaller feeding tube; infuse feedings into duodenum or jejunum.
		Mental obtundation	

MONITORING

Monitoring varies according to patient acuity and duration of the tube feeding. Monitoring techniques may be individualized by institutions, but the areas to monitor remain the same: hydration status, nutrition status and mechanical checks.

Hydration Status

Provision of adequate fluid can prevent dehydration. In ideal hydration status fluid intake equals total fluid output. Monitoring of hydration status includes observing for the following: decreased skin turgor, confusion, serum sodium levels of 145 - 150 mEq/L, thirst, elevated temperature, diminished urine output (less than 500 ml/day), elevated BUN and HCT, decreased body weight (1kg = 2L fluid), increased blood pressure and pulse, dry tongue, urine specific gravity > 1.010, serum osmolality > 280 mOsm and edema. These are signs of inadequate hydration. No formula provides enough free water to meet a patient's fluid requirements. The recommended daily allowance is 1 ml/calorie. On the average, 1 cal/cc formulas contain about 80% water. Patients without water restrictions should receive enough free water to equal at least 20% of total formula volume. Daily I&Os and weights are essential to monitoring hydration status. Conditions that increase fluid needs are infection, fever, vomiting, diarrhea, fistula or wound drainage and concentrated or high protein formulas.

Nutritional Status

Nutritional status can be monitored by assessing albumin and prealbumin, weight, nitrogen balance, mineral status (K, PO_4, Mg and Ca), serum glucose, vitamin status, nutrient intake analysis and I&Os.

Mechanical Checks

Includes x-ray confirmation of the tube position, elevation of the head of the patient (30 degrees), checking for gastric residuals, changing the external tubing and feeding bag daily and irrigation of the tube if the feeding is stopped.

TRANSITIONAL FEEDING

The goals of transitional feeding are to maintain and/or improve current nutritional status and return to normal oral intake. Transitional feeding has to be individualized. The ability to swallow consistently must be established along with any carbohydrate, fat or lactose intolerance's. The type of formula the patient has been on also influences transition. For example, if a patient has been on an elemental tube feeding, a formula containing intact protein, carbohydrate and fat could be administered before the regular diet. Transition to an oral diet should start with six small feedings and progress as tolerated. The diet may require a fat restriction (20 - 40 gms if steatorrhea is present), decreased lactose, low fiber and elimination of simple sugars. In the beginning of the transition, nutritional adequacy should not be of concern. The tube should not removed, allowing for adequacy of nutrients.

To achieve the above goals, a combination of methods may be used. First, stop the tube feeding for one hour before and after each meal, allowing the patient a chance to demonstrate appetite, oral intake and tolerance to food. The daily oral intake should be recorded and evaluated. When the intake is consistently 500 - 750 calories, tube feeding can be stopped during the day. This allows the patient to increase oral intake as confirmed by Nutrient Intake Analysis (calorie count). Second, tube feeding can be given overnight (e.g., 9:00 p.m. - 6:00 a.m.). The amount depends upon the patient's total needs and calculated oral intake. Once the patient consistently orally consumes 2/3 of nutrient needs (for one to three days), the feeding tube can be removed.

The need for creativity, patience and persistence in transitional feeding is well recognized. Consistent nutrition support, slow progression, individualization and regular monitoring of nutritional status are needed during the transitional stage. Consideration also must be given to the discharge status. Patients are discharged much sooner so this transition must occur quickly.

FEEDING EQUIPMENT

Tremendous improvements are being made to the equipment available for enteral feeding. The intention here is not to discuss all available equipment but only to give some guidelines for equipment selection.

Tubes

For nasogastric feeding, soft, small-bore weighted tubes are the most desirable. Most are made of polyurethane or silicone. They cause the least amount of patient discomfort and allow the patient to swallow more easily. Since they do not rapidly disintegrate, they do not need frequent replacement. Polyurethane is stronger and has thinner walls, thus has a larger internal diameter. Silicone provides more flexibility that may be more comfortable but the flexibility and smaller internal diameter may lead to kinking or clogging. Larger tubes are used for nasoduodenal or nasojejunal feeding. **Table 2** provides information on tube and formula compatibility.

Table 2: Tube and Formula Compatibility

Formula Type	Size (Fr) Gravity	Size (Fr) Pump
General	7.3 - 8	6 - 10
Elemental	6.0	6
High density	8.0 - 10	8 - 10
High protein	7.3 - 8	6 - 10
High pro/cal	8.0 - 10	8 - 10
High fiber	8.0 - 10	8 - 10

Flushing needs to done prior to and following the tube feeding and medications.

Containers

Many types of containers are available and should be selected based on meeting the institution's and/or individual's needs. Consideration should be given to capacity, ease of opening, closing and hanging, requirements for special tubing and adaptability to the infusion method. The container should be leakproof, have easy to read calibrations and directions for use, ease of filling and hanging, adaptable tubing port, be disposable or easy to clean, be compatible with enteral pumps and made from non leaching materials. Currently, containers are available in 500 - 2000 ml sizes. They should be designed to minimize the risk of bacterial contamination. Equipment can be adapted, but consideration should be given to the time spent doing so as it may not be cost-effective.

Prepackaged (closed system) feeding formulas are used to decrease nursing time and counter contamination. These products come in rigid containers and ready to hang. Cons for this type of system are limited product availability and inability to change the concentration of the formula and waste if there are frequent changes in the formula. Plastic irrigating bags and rigid plastic containers are being used. Containers (made from medical-grade vinyl or polyvinyl chloride) are disposable to avoid cross-contamination.

Volume Pumps

Pumps should be used for patients who need controlled formula delivery. Conditions requiring pumps are the use of small caliber tube; delivery to small intestine to reduce potential for GI intolerance and minimization of gastric pooling to reduce gastric reflux and pulmonary aspiration. Volumetric pumps (calibrated to infuse a specific volume of fluid at a specific rate - ml/hr) are more accurate than pumps that rely on measurement by drops per minute. Drop size varies with the viscosity of the solution and rate of administration. They usually require jejunal access.

The ideal pump is portable, inexpensive, quiet, volumetric, battery operated (lasting a minimum of eight hours) and easy to use with an alarm system, a suitable range for rate and increment changes, automatic flush features and accuracy to within 10% of prescribed flow. There are many different pumps, some of which are so small they can be carried in a backpack.

HOME ENTERAL NUTRITION

As with hospital enteral support, consideration must be given to the goal of nutritional support, extent of malnutrition, gastrointestinal function, route of delivery, organ dysfunction and appetite. If adequate oral intake is not attainable, home enteral nutrition is a viable option, especially in this era of cost-containment.

One has to be cognizant of the cost of hospitalization. A home enteral nutrition program can improve the quality of life, lower medical costs through shortened length of stay, allow possible return to work and perhaps enhance the years of productivity.

Eligibility Requirements
- Resolution of medical complications/stable clinical status
- Unwarranted continued hospitalization
- Unable to meet nutritional requirements orally
- Documented tolerance of the home feeding
- Need for enteral feeding for three to four weeks or more
- The physical, psychological and socioeconomic status of patient and patient's family should be assessed

Prior to discharge, the monitoring plans must be established as should the type of delivery (e.g., bolus vs gravity) and the rate and volume to be achieved or in force. This enhances a smooth progression to home. Patient and family education must be done in simple and understandable language. Teaching materials can include an audiovisual program reviewing good nutrition, reasons for tube feeding, formula preparation and administration and a discussion of potential problems and how to handle them. Also, written material should be provided. A social worker may be needed to evaluate emotional status and economic situation prior to discharge. A patient may have problems with cash flow upon discharge; therefore, a two to four week supply of formula, supplies and equipment should be sent home with the patient. These articles can be added to the patient's hospital bill and usually are paid by the insurance company. A well-designed home enteral program is safe and cost-effective.

Reimbursement factors consider the duration of the feeding (> 90 days), the formula comprises total nutrition support and documented medical necessity. Cost reimbursement may be essential and some health care plans reimburse for home enteral nutrition. Special formulas can cost up to 100 dollars per day.

Treatment Plan

The design of the treatment plan addresses the nutrition care processes and includes the following elements: nutrition goals, prescribed enteral feeding, preparation and administration of the feeding, infusion times and rates, care of access device, equipment and formula, monitoring plans and methods for communication and documentation including follow-up plans.

The discharge summary should include the disease state(s), height, weight, weight patterns (for the past six months), pertinent labs and drugs, nutritional needs, type of formula, volume and rate per day, fluid requirements, tube feeding system (pump, drip or bolus) and desired goal(s).

The equipment selection considerations are compatibility with access route and feeding formulation; simple operation and maintenance; durability; high performance; quietness and cost-effectiveness.

A home enteral company may be considered for monitoring the patient at home. In selecting a company, the following should be considered: flexibility to meet the patient's/family needs; home delivery capacity/capability (24 hour, year-round service, national versus local service for traveling/vacations); reliability/service record;

personnel with expertise to meet the patients needs (availability of consultative services); QI and a feedback process to the referring facility; and cost effectiveness.

SPECIAL CONSIDERATIONS

Hypoalbuminemic and Malnourished

Malnourished and/or hypoalbuminemic patients may develop diarrhea. Severe protein-calorie malnutrition (PCM) is associated with the loss of intestinal microvilli, villous brush border enzymes and a reduction of intestinal absorptive surface area. These patients may lack the intravascular osmotic force required to draw substrate across the intestinal epithelial cell. A significant decline in serum albumin (1.0 to 1.5 gm/dl) can occur within three to seven days as a result of severe catabolism.

Albumin and oncotic pressure markedly affect gastric emptying and the tolerance, absorption and motility of the gut. One of the main functions of albumin is to maintain oncotic pressure.

A "critical" level of serum albumin can be used to predict disease outcome. The degree of hypoalbuminemia is a prognostic indicator of morbidity and mortality. It is also a strong predictor of the cost of hospitalization.

Protein in the form of small peptides (dipeptides and tripeptides) is more rapidly and efficiently absorbed than in the form of free amino acids. Many studies suggest that the enhanced absorption of protein in the form of a protein hydrolysate and its effect on ureagensis have many clinical applications. This involves patients with impaired digestion or absorption that may limit protein absorption, excessive losses of albumin resulting in both diarrhea and hypoalbuminemia and hypermetabolism in which nitrogen utilization (and decreased ureagensis) is most critical.

Findings suggest that peptide-based formulas may affect albumin turnover in the GI tract directly by affecting mucosal permeability. This may explain partially the rapid recovery in serum albumin.

Patient Selection

Peptide-based formulas and parenteral nutrition are expensive. Suggested patient criteria for these is an albumin below 2.5 gm/dL, significant GI malabsorption, implementation of full medical support on a full code status. Criteria for "critical" albumin needs to be standardized for individual institutions.

Solutions

Either parenteral nutrition (PN) and/or a peptide based formula (PBF) is used with this patient population. In fact, many patients do not need the PN but could tolerate the enteral formula with the exogenous albumin infusion. A PBF should not be used routinely because of its high cost which are yet significantly lower as compared to PN.

Administration

One solution consists of the administration of exogenous albumin and the provision of sufficient nutrients. Using a peptide-based formula and exogenous albumin remarkably improves the clinical symptoms of diarrhea and low albumin. The best solution is a 25% salt poor albumin because it provides the most concentrated source of protein. The concept of albumin replacement therapy continues to be controversial.

A simple equation estimates albumin deficit in hypoalbuminemic patients. The formula for albumin replacement is 3.5g/dL minus the patient's serum albumin, times the patient's weight in kg times three. The factor three is based upon an assumed albumin distribution volume of three deciliters per kg per total body weight.

$$AD\ (gm) = Wt\ (kg) \times 3\ dl/kg \times (3.5 - initial\ SAC\ gm/dl)$$

OR

$$AD = (DSA - PSA)\ (10)\ (\ kg)\ (0.3)$$

where:
AD	=	Albumin Deficit
SAC	=	Serum Albumin Concentration
3 dL	=	30% distribution
DSA	=	Desired Serum Albumin

> **Example:** $(3.5 - 2.5) \times 75\ kg \times 3\ dl/kg = 225\ g$
> Delivery – 3 infusions over 4 to 6 hours

Patients can be corrected at approximately one-third their deficiency per day for three days. Approximately 100 gms (8 units) are required to raise the plasma concentration by 1.0 gm/dlL. Maximum of 150 grams of albumin is infused over a 24 hour period. The goal is a serum albumin of ~ 3.0 gm/dL. Therefore, decrease or discontinue exogenous albumin when serum albumin is ~ 2.5 gm/dL. The nutrient formulation should be reevaluated at this time. According to Page, when you give albumin you give colloid volume; therefore, for each ml of 25% albumin given, decrease the free water by 3 ml, if the patient is in good fluid balance.

Conclusions

- Hypoalbuminemia directly correlates with GI tolerance to enteral formulas.
- Albumin deficit can be calculated and replaced accurately.
- Replacement of albumin leads to enhanced GI tolerance to enteral nutrition.
- Albumin levels remain in the normal range at least one week after replacement unless the patient is newly stressed.
- Restoration of normal serum albumin level can permit enteral nutrition in lieu of more costly parenteral nutrition.

Critically Ill Obese

Obesity has a significant effect in terms of morbidity, mortality, diminished productivity and cost. As weight increases, the prevalence of illnesses increase disportionately. Surgical morbidity is prevalent. Wound complications, thromboembolic disease, myocardial infarction; respiratory failure requiring mechanical ventilatory support and sepsis may be seen even after minor operative procedures.

The critically ill obese patient should be nourished adequately. Hypermetaboslism and hypercatabolism in the critically ill obese quickly deplete even abundant nutrient stores. Once the obese patient is hemodynically stable, enteral nutrition should be initiated.

Problems associated with enteral feeding of the obese include: volume overload and glucose intolerance and risk of myocardial infarction, pulmonary edema and congestive heart failure secondary to fluid retention. The glucose load can cause hyperglycemia in both glucose-intolerant and "normal" stressed patients. The obese are more prone to problems with tube placement. Endoscopy carries a greater risk. Lying flat may exacerbate respiratory disorders. Potential complications of enteral access are:

Nasogastric

- Tube misplacement
- Respiratory insufficiency
- Gastroesophageal reflux and aspiration pneumonia
- Sinusitis
- Inability to achieve postpyloric positioning

Endoscopic

- Aspiration, esophageal or gastric bleeding or perforation, respiratory insuffience
- Superficial skin or soft tissue infection
- Necrotizing fasciitis
- Gastric or intestinal bleeding
- Gastric or intestinal leakage with peritonitis
- Colonic injury
- Fistulization

Surgical Placement

- Thromboembolism
- Respiratory insufficiency
- Cardiac events
- Superficial skin or soft tissue infection
- Necrotizing faciititis

Laparoscopy

- Hypercarbia
- Decreased venous return

Gastric Versus Small Bowel Placement

Obese patients are at greater risk for aspiration pneumonia. The stomach of overweight patients have a larger than normal gastric fluid volume and a lower pH. They have an abnormally high intraabdominal pressure secondary to the large panniculus and increased intraabdominal fat. This problem is exacerbated in the supine position. The potential for gastroesophageal reflux and of aspiration pneumonia is caused by the increase in pressure, coupled with voluminous acidic acid contents.

In the critically ill obese, increased difficulties with positioning, abnormalities of the oropharynx and impaired ability to clear secretions may increase the risk of aspiration. These patients have increased adiposity of the soft tissues of the palate and pharynx.

Patients unable to sit at a 45° angle and unable to have adequate protection of their airway should be fed distal to the pylorus or initially fed parenterally. Percutaneous gastrostomies are not recommended in the obese.

Hypocaloric feeding may be beneficial in this population because this method of feeding promotes use of endogenous fat for energy while maintaining nitrogen homoestatis. The modular formula selected should supply 1.5 to 2.0 grams protein per kilogram of ideal or adjusted body weight without supplying excessive calories. It is still controversial whether the stressed obese patient can mobilize endogenous fat adequately for oxidation when receiving hypocaloric feeding.

The selection of appropriate techniques and nutritional formulation can maximize benefits and minimize complications for the critically ill obese.

Elderly

The needs of older persons have needs that vary depending on whether they are middle-aged (58 - 68), aging (69 - 77), elderly (77 - 85) or aged (86 and up). Gastrointestinal function may alter with advancing age. The loss of LBM contributes to decreased bowel motility. Maldigestion and malabsorption may occur if there is a decrease in digestive enzyme production. A minor insult of relatively short duration can lead to PCM. Lack of attention to nutritional status and inadequate treatment is accompanied by significant increases in morbidity, mortality and health resource utilization.

Indications for enteral feeding in the elderly include mechanical problems such as oral or esophageal obstruction; degenerative chronic diseases with the inability to sustain adequate intake of food and fluids; and acute trauma or diseases with a predicted inadequate po intake for greater than five days. Indications for complications are the same as in the adult population.

Sites

A PEG is preferred for the confused patients requiring extended support for an indefinite period of time. Nasogastric feedings can be used for patients who are cooperative and not confused.

Formulas

The following formula selection and nutrient criteria must be considered:

- **Water:** Adequate water has to be supplied. The elderly experience a reduction in total body water. Patients may dehydrate rapidly under conditions of inadequate fluid intake. A major complication of enteral nutrition among older persons is hypernatremia caused by a formula high in protein and salt. A suggested treatment is to add four percent of the body weight (in kg) for each 10 mEq/L increase in serum sodium above normal as water. Half the fluid deficit should be replaced in 24 hours. Too rapid replacement of water may lead to cerebral edema. The usual fluid recommendation is 30ml/kg. or 1 ml/kcal ingested. In conditions requiring increased fluid intake, the goal is to provide approximately 1000 - 1500 ml of extra fluids per day to meet the increased needs.

- **Calories:** BMR begins to decline after age 30. The average energy allowance for the elderly is 30 Kcal/kg/IBW. Levels may be higher to promote weight gain in the underweight patient or to prevent further weight loss. With decreased energy requirements, there can be inadequate vitamins and minerals needed to maintain health, heal wounds, repair fractured bones, fight infection and make new tissue.

- **Carbohydrate:** Carbohydrate tolerance diminishes with age. The goal is to use more complex carbohydrates to produce a lower osmotic load. Constant carbohydrate ingestion reduces insulin requirements in diabetes, reduces cholesterol concentrations and induces greater nitrogen retention. Increasing the amount of fiber contributes to enhanced bowel motility.

- **Fat:** Fats provide calories, EFAs and needed fat soluble vitamins. Absorption capabilities need to be evaluated first.

- **Protein:** Protein must be adjusted to meet individual needs. Normally 1 gm/kg IBW is adequate. With pressure sores, 1.2 - 1.5 gm/kg may be required. Renal and liver function must be evaluated.

- **Mineral and Trace Elements:** Many factors are involved in minerals and trace element supplementation.

Vitamins: some increases in D, B_6 and B_{12}; decrease in Vit A and folic acid; others do not change. Each person, must be evaluated individually. Each formula must be considered with respect to administration, ingestion and metabolization.

The minerals that need close monitoring are:

- **Calcium/phosphorus:** The Ca:PO$_4$ ratio should be maintained at one or higher.

- **Magnesium:** Factors contributing to magnesium deficiency include certain diuretic and antibiotics, excessive enemas, abuse of alcohol, malabsorption and the syndrome of inappropriate secretion of antidiuretic hormone.

- **Potassium:** The elderly may be on potassium losing diuretics. In persons whose renal tubules fail to secrete enough potassium, hyperkalemia may result.

- **Sodium:** To determine needs requires careful estimation of total body water as well as the serum sodium concentration.

Administration

It is suggested that the rate of enteral nutrition be started at 25 cc per hour and the rate should be increased gradually over 36 - 48 hours until the desired volume is attained.

Monitoring

Physical signs must be monitored including oral hygiene, odor of breath, presence of pulmonary congestion or dependent edema, abdominal ascites, clarity of sensorium, tongue color, body weight, fluid intake and output, nutrient intake, frequency and consistency of bowel movements, presence of diarrhea or constipation, bowel sounds and bladder size.

Dehydration is the most common fluid/electrolyte disturbance in the elderly. Physiologically elderly have altered thirst perception; inability to concentrate urine in response to fluid deficit; constriction of blood vessels supplying vital organs such as the heart, brain and kidneys. A fluid deficit can result in organ ischemia and permanent reduction in organ function. The long-term consequences of fluid deficit can include renal failure and stroke, confusion, lethargy and reduced mental status and decreased skin turgor and skin breakdown.

Medical conditions and therapies causing fluid deficits are fever and infection, diarrhea and vomiting, cardiovascular and renal disease, reduced levels of consciousness and medications.

Hydration status should be carefully monitored by assessing I&O's, urine production and weight and labs during rehydration therapy. Rehydration therapy should continue as long as fluid losses continue or until urine SG returns to normal.

In institutionalized elderly, a common problem is skin breakdown in the form of decubitus ulcers or pressure sores. Pressure sores are classified by stages:

- Stage 1 – Skin is persistently red.
- Stage 2 – A blister or superficial break in the skin.
- Stage 3 – Full thickness of the skin is lost, exposing subcutaneous tissue.
- Stage 4 – Full thickness of the skin is lost, exposing muscle and/or bone.

Depending on the stage, calorie and protein requirements need to be adjusted to promote wound healing.

Hyperemesis Gravidarium

Hyperemesis Gravidarium is an antepartum disorder characterized by severe nausea and vomiting. It usually occurs between the sixth and twelfth week of gestation.

The use of enteral nutrition in this group can be controversial and depends on the cooperation of the patient and a highly skilled and motivated nursing staff. Enteral nutrition can be managed through use of antiemetic drug therapy; a carefully tailored, individualized enteral delivery regimen; and close monitoring. It has been successful in women whose nausea and vomiting are closely linked to the consumption of food. In the postacute stage, a continous low rate infusion of isotonic formula is usually tolerated. Increasing the rate depends on the abdominal comfort of the patient. If nausea and vomiting are persistent, it may be necessary to use parenteral nutrition. See the parenteral nutrition specialty section for more information on the nutrition needs of this patient population.

CLINICAL NUTRITION PATHWAY FOR ENTERAL NUTRITION

Objective: to provide optimal nutrition care compatible with medical treatment for patients who are hypermetabolic and hypercatabolic through planning, implementation and monitoring/evaluating.

System/ Diagnosis	Potential Problems/ Indicators	Assessment	Intervention Monitoring/ Education	Possible Desired Outcome(s)
NGs PEGs ICU Patient	Malnutrition Fever Infection Fluid balance Catabolism/ depletion of LBM Hypermetabolism Hyper- or hypo- glycemia Overfeeding Adequate nutrients for wound healing and protein synthesis Electrolyte imbalances, abnormal ABGs Ongoing medical treatment modalities	History: medical, social, diet, drug, weight patterns Medical goals Biochemical/ABGs Vent settings/vitals Clinical status/GI function Functional status Degree of malnutrition Outcomes/goals Calorie Needs: Kcal 30 - 35/kg/IBW Pro needs: 1.2 - 1.8 gm/kg adjusted for renal and liver function CHO: 50 -60% Kcal Fat: ~ 30% Kcal Fluid: 35 cc/kg; adjust for losses, hydration and organ function Electrolytes: standard adjust per labs/organ function Vitamins: RDAs; extra Vit C if appropriate Minerals: RDAs; adjust per labs	**Phase 1 and 2** Formulate care plan Implement TF Recommend baseline nutrition labs Document/communicate care plan **Phase 3** Progress TF to desired goal rate. Monitor change for elevated LFT's, azotemia, hyperglycemia, lipemic serum, decreased respiratory function, failure to wean form ventilator. Evaluate lab changes pertaining to nutrition and hydration status Monitor residuals Review weights, vital signs, labs, I&Os Evaluate efficacy for po intake Change plan as medical condition necessitates **Phase 4** Transfer/discharge summary/referral for continuum of care	Optimize nutrition status: • Maintain/improve weight • Maintain/improve protein status Improve electrolyte balance Prevent excess CO_2 production if vented Prevent overfeeding Decrease catabolic response to stress Decrease complications Transition to oral feeding when appropriate Education: statement of needs, if appropriate

QUALITY IMPROVEMENT

Quality improvement and/or a process indicator (see section on "Nutrition Support Planning") can be designed for those patients placed on tube feeding. The goal for patients initiated on tube feeding is to receive the tube feeding within 24 hours of the written order and receive 80 - 90% of recommended needs by day two. (**Figure 1**)

Figure 1: Process Flow Diagram of the Existing Process

Figure 2: Cause and Effect of Enteral Nutrition

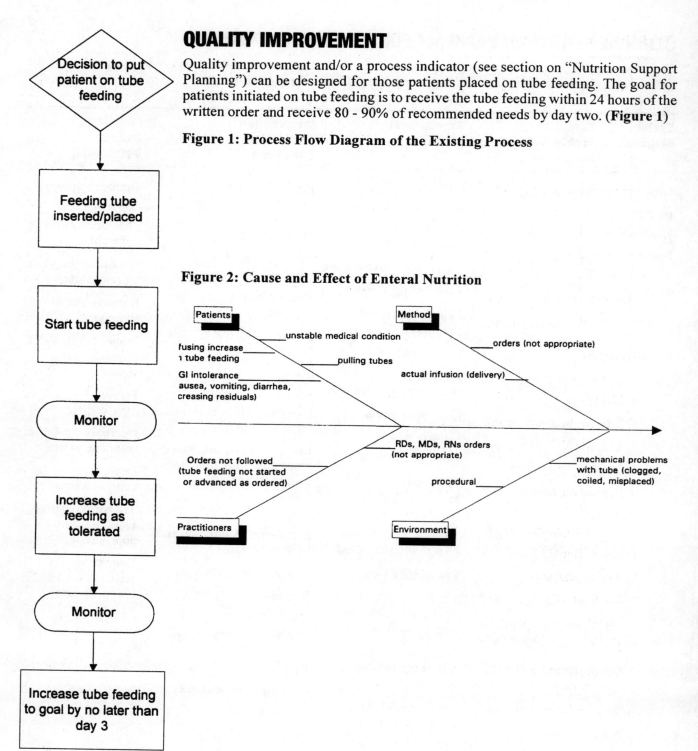

Table 3: QI Monitor for Tube Feeding

Pt	Med Svc	TF Type	Order Date	Start Date	Amt Recommend	Amt Received	Variance	Action	Out-comes

Directions:

1. List all new patients on TF receiving > 50% of needs.

2. List the medical service the patient is on.

3. Record the admit date and the date of the TF order.

4. Record the start date of the TF.

5. Identify type of feeding.

6. Record the amount of TF recommended (i.e. protein and calories).

7. Record the amount of TF received by day 2 of TF (i.e., protein and calories) (data collection is from 12 mn to 12 mn).

8. List variances by definitions below.

9. Record variances by the following definitions.

    Medical – Change in status/surgery/procedural tests.

    Metabolic – Hyperglycemia, hypoglycemia, hypernatremia, risk of aspiration, etc.

    Mechanical – Tube dislodgment, improper placement, administration, clogged tube, broken tube.

    GI Intolerance – Nausea, vomiting, cramping, distention, fullness, diarrhea, constipation, medication intolerance, refeeding syndrome, decreased gastric motility.

10. Record for one month

11. **EXCEPTION:** No code/DNAR

The results of the QI will demonstrate any problems and/or complications associated with advancing tube feeding. The problems become the next QI monitor(s).

PARENTERAL NUTRITION

Parenteral nutrition (PN) is the administration of nutrients (i.e., glucose, amino acids, fats, vitamins and minerals) intravenously by central or peripheral vein. Parenteral nutrition is appropriate only when oral or enteral feeding is inadequate or contraindicated. If the gut works, and can be used safely, it should be used. It also is recommended that patients who have been or will be without adequate enteral nutrition for greater than five days and resumption of an adequate intake is not imminent, receive parenteral nutrition. Nutrition support needs to be initiated to avoid compromising physiologic function in catabolic patients. In critically ill patients, deficits occur after seven days of no nutrition support. Essential nutrients required for normal mucosal growth are usually not found with prolonged use of PN. Prolonged PN leads to mucosal atrophy, enterocyte hypoplasia and decreased intestinal activity. PN often is associated with iatrogenic bowel malnutrition that impairs intestinal epithelial cell proliferation and mucosal repair. The goal of parenteral nutrition is to maintain an adequate nutritional state or improve a poor one.

When initial evaluation discloses ongoing GI dysfunction parenteral nutrition should be started immediately. The solution should be administered within 24 hours of the order.

INDICATIONS

GI Tract Abnormality
- Obstruction
- Severe diarrhea
- Peritonitis
- Persistentvomiting secondary to obstruction
- Fistula
- Short bowel syndrome
- Intestinal motility disorders
- Acute severe pancreatitis
- Acute regional enteritis (Crohn's)
- Severe IBD
- Severe chronic radiation enteritis with obstructive symptoms

Surgery
- Presurgery with severe PCM
- Massive bowel resection
- Congenital abnormalities in the neonate
- Post surgery with prolonged ileus
- Trauma, burns
- Sepsis

Other
- Hyperemesis gravidarum
- Nutritionally depleted patient unable to use GI tract
- Chemotherapy

Criteria for being on parenteral nutrition should include at least one of the following:
- Inadequate calorie and/or protein intake to meet needs
- Inadequate protein intake to meet needs
- OR anticipated inability to eat more than 10 days
- OR chronic illness or three-week acute illness
- OR GI tract not available for use

Contraindications

Parenteral nutrition should not be givenunder the following conditions:
- Patient with a functional GI tract
- PN is anticipated for less than five days
- Inability to access a venous vein
- To delay an urgent surgery
- Minimal stress and trauma
- The GI tract can be used within a week
- The prognosis does not warrant aggressive nutrition support
- Nutrition support is not desired by the patient or the patient's family
- The risks exceed the potential benefits

NUTRIENT REQUIREMENTS

Protein and Energy

The specific disease state and nutritional status have to be considered and calories and protein prescribed accordingly to the patient's need. To paraphrase Stan Dudrick, MD, it is essential for the physician to recognize that no single intravenous nutrient solution can be ideal for all conditions and all patients at all times, or for the same patient during various phases of his/her pathologic process.

Protein requirements must be calculated individually for each patient. 1.0 to 1.5 grams protein per kilogram IBW per day for anabolism and 1.5 to 2.0 for severe stress is suggested. Increasing protein above optimum levels decreases net protein utilization, even when calories are adequate or excessive. Calorie requirements are approximately 28 - 30 kcal/kg/IBW for maintenance, 30 - 35 kcal/kg/IBW post surgery and 35+ kcal/kg/IBW for the septic patient.

Studies have shown that when parenteral nutrition solutions are given orally rather than parenterally, a significantly greater weight gain is experienced. In actual practice it has been found that a patient receiving an intravenous calorie intake equal to his/her measured caloric expenditure along with adequate nitrogen often does not achieve weight gain or nitrogen equilibrium. This calorie inefficiency is attributed to the alternate route of entry (central vein rather than portal) and to the obligatory lipogenesis occurring in response to the hyperinsulinemia which results from a constant dextrose infusion.

Vitamins

Vitamin requirements for parenteral nutrition are not well understood and the altered requirements with specific diseases are ill defined. Research in the area has been limited. The Nutritional Advisory Group on Total Parenteral Nutrition of the American Medical Association has made some recommendations for adult and pediatric TPN patients. These are summarized along with the 1989 Recommended Daily Allowances (RDA) in **Table 4**.

Minerals

Mineral requirements in parenteral nutrition vary greatly depending upon the status of the patient. During catabolism body tissues are metabolized for energy and releasing nitrogen and other minerals. During this time deficiency can develop quickly as intracellular ions, especially potassium, magnesium, calcium and phosphate are rapidly excreted. These minerals, along with sodium and chloride, are essential for cardiac function, water balance, skeletal mineralization and energy transformation as well as nerve, muscle and enzyme function.

Fluid Needs

Fluid needs should be based upon preexisting excess or deficiency states, ongoing losses and cardiac and renal function. Patients with a normal fluid balance and without cardiorenal dysfunction can receive up to 4000 cc or more per day. Restrictions may be necessary for renal, liver, cardiac and pulmonary diseases.

When determining fluid balance consideration must be given to drugs and medications. The total volume of fluid needed to deliver drugs intravenously is often substantial (one liter is the average). This can limit the volume of the nutrient solution. Drugs, when compatible, should be administered in the parenteral solution or through the parenteral nutrition infusion apparatus.

Daily weight, Specific Gravity, hematocrit and input and outputs are adjunctive indexes in the assessment of fluid status.

SOLUTION FORMULATIONS

In a substrate formulation, it is important to provide calories that can be utilized efficiently. The formulation of parenteral solutions is highly individualized. Their composition is dependent upon the individual's calorie, protein, mineral, vitamin and fluid requirements. Almost any solution needed can be formulated from the nutrient sources available. Requirements depend upon the nutritional status and underlying disease process of the patient. Solutions can be designed to be administered either by central or peripheral vein.

Nutrient adequacy is affected by the solution's nutrient content, volume of solution administered, the individual's physical condition, other forms of nutrient intake and use of medications or therapy.

Glucose

At the present time, Dextrose is used almost exclusively as the carbohydrate source. Its caloric density is 3.48 calories per gram and is available in concentrations of 5 to 70 per cent. Ten percent dextrose solutions may be given peripherally, but more concentrated solutions must be given through a central or major vein.

Hyperglycemia is the most common metabolic complication associated with parenteral nutrition. The complication can be controlled by limiting the dextrose infusion rate.

The rate of glucose metabolism varies. Normally adults can utilize about 0.5 gms/kg/hr. Hypermetabolic patients can tolerate even higher amounts, about 1.2 gms/kg/hr. Diabetic patients use 4 mg/kg/min and the severly malnourished patients use 2mg/kg/min. When hypertonic dextrose solutions are infused, insulin demand increases.

Example: Maximum CHO tolerance for a 50 kg patient:

5 mg x (wt in kg) x (60 min/hr x 24 hrs) = 5 x 50 x 1440 = 360 gm CHO
1000 mg/gram 1000

When the infusion rate exceeds the capacity of the pancreas to produce insulin, blood glucose levels may rise uncontrollably. Coma and neurogenic dysfunction may occur with glucose levels of 1000 mg/ml or higher. When the renal threshold for glucose is exceeded, an osmotic diuresis occurs which produces glycosuria, water depletion and possible electrolyte imbalance. Many who experience these problems are undiagnosed maturity-onset diabetics.

At least 100 to 150 gm of glucose should be infused to achieve maximum impact on nitrogen balance and provide the energy substrate for certain key tissues requiring glucose as the sole or major energy source. Glucose should be infused together with the nitrogen source. Simultaneous infusion is associated with an improvement in nitrogen balance.

Starvation, stress, major trauma, pain, infection and shock decrease pancreatic response to a glucose load. Along with a decreased insulin production, peripheral insulin resistance occurs as a result of the high circulating levels of glucocorticoids and catecholamines released in response to stress. The following guidelines have been suggested for the addition of insulin depending on the morning serum glucose levels.

Serum Glucose mg/dl)	Units Of Insulin Added
200 - 249	10
250 - 299	15
300 - 349	20
350 - 399	25
400 - 499	30

Carbon dioxide production and oxygen consumption may be increased by high carbohydrate loads thus leading to respiratory distress. Replacing part of the carbohydrate calories with fat can decrease carbon dioxide production by lowering the respiratory quotient. Provide 40 to 60 percent of calories as fat in the final solution to decrease this risk. For further information, refer to the case study on respiratory management in the appendix.

Amino Acids

The protein component must meet essential amino acid requirements as well as total nitrogen needs. Mixtures of essential and nonessential amino acids are available in concentrations from 3 to 15 percent. Amino acid solutions are formulated to meet the amino acid needs of both adults and children and are based on the amino acid profiles proven to be of high biological value when taken orally. When amino acids are given intravenously, some go directly into circulation and are metabolized by other body tissues before reaching the liver. For this reason, it is important to monitor serum transport proteins to ensure adequate protein intake. Each gram of protein yields 3.4 calories.

Amino acid solutions are recommended over protein hydrolysates for several reasons. The protein utilization of hydrolysates is somewhat uncertain as up to 50 percent may be excreted in the urine because the hydrolysis of the protein is incomplete and unpredictable. The ammonia content of these solutions also can present a risk as hyperammonemia has been documented and is especially dangerous in infants and those with hepatic or renal dysfunction. High levels of ammonia may also promote acidosis. Amino acids normally are mixed with dextrose to produce a final concentration of 50% amino acids and 50% dextrose.

Fat

Fat solutions are calorically dense, isotonic solutions. Two intravenous fat sources are currently available: One is an emulsion of soybean oil, phospholipids and glycerol, the other is an emulsion of safflower oil, egg phosphatides and glycerol. They are available in either 10 or 20 percent solutions yielding 1.1 or 2.0 calories per milliliter, respectively. They may be given through central or peripheral veins as they are isotonic. They also can lower the osmolarity of parenteral solutions given peripherally at the same time. For best utilization, lipids should be infused along with carbohydrates and protein.

Fat particles are approximately the size of chylomicrons and are metabolized and utilized the same way. Normally they are rapidly metabolized by lipoprotein lipase at a rate of 3 to 4 grams/kg/24 hours. This rate, however, depends on the serum concentration. Metabolism is faster initially when the serum concentration is lower. As the serum concentration increases, the rate of fat metabolism slows. If the infusion rate exceeds the maximum metabolic capacity, "overload syndrome" and other adverse reactions can occur. Symptoms include marked hyperlipidemia, gastrointestinal disturbances, hepatosplenomegaly with impaired hepatic function, anemia, thrombocytopenia, prolonged clotting time, elevated prothrombin time and spontaneous bleeding. This syndrome has occurred mainly in children. Other potential reactions include wheezing, erythema, wheals and urticaria, tachycardia, tachypnea, hepatomegaly and elevated liver function tests (SGOT and LDH). A test dose should be given at a rate of 0.1 ml/min for the first 15 minutes. If no adverse reactions occur, the rate can be increased. Usually 500 cc is given over six to eight hours for 10% and 8 - 12 hours for 20% but 12 - 24 hour infusion may be better tolerated.

Utilization of fat emulsions also depends on carbohydrate metabolism. If sufficient carbohydrate is not provided simultaneously, optimal fat utilization does not occur and hyperlipidemia and other complications may result. To provide maximum utilization and prevent complications, it is recommended that no more than 60 percent of total calories be supplied as lipid.

When fat-free isocaloric or hypercaloric diets are given, fatty acid deficiency can develop within 10 to 14 days. This does not occur when the intake is hypocaloric and fat stores are catabolized for energy releasing essential fatty acids in the process. Furthermore, the high insulin levels induced by the infusion of concentrated glucose solutions also inhibits lipolysis and the release of EFA.

Several advantages exist to using a fat emulsion instead of glucose. Lipids provide a near iso-osmolar intravenous solution, do not cause sustained hyperglycemia or hyperosmolar diuresis and maintain normal levels of fatty acids, insulin and ketones, protect against fatty infiltration of the liver, do not cause profound respiratory compromise as glucose does and provide a more concentrated source of calories.

Tolerance to fat emulsions can be determined by administering a 10% solution at a rate of one ml/min for 15 - 30 min. If no adverse reactions, the rate may be increased to 80 - 100 ml/hour. With the 20% solution the administration should be 0.5 ml/min for 15 - 30 minutes. If no adverse reactions occur, the rate can be increased to 60 ml/hour.

Indications for the use of fat are: 1) to treat or prevent essential fatty acid deficiency (EFAD); 2) to avoid carbohydrate intolerance; and 3) to provide a concentrated source of calories. When used to prevent EFAD, fatty acid solutions should provide a minimum of 3 to 4 percent of the total daily calories as linoleic acid. Total fat should not exceed 2.5 gm/kg/day or 60% of calories. Fat can constitute 25 - 30% of calories in hypermetabolic patients.

Lipid clearance: Baseline serum TG level needs to be established prior to starting the fat emulsions. The use of fat emulsions can be limited to providing EFAs only if the TG concentration (adult) is greater than 400 mg/dL six hours after infusion. Acceptable TG levels can vary with different facilities and philosophies.

Contraindication for use is abnormal lipid metabolism: hyperlipidemia; lipid nephrosis or acute pancreatitis accompanied or caused by hyperlipidemia; moderate to severe liver disease; compromised pulmonary function; hematopoietic malfunction; and severe egg allergy.

Vitamins

Adult vitamin preparations for parenteral use contain approximately twice the RDA for the water soluble vitamins thiamin, riboflavin, niacin, vitamin B_{12} and ascorbic acid. When water soluble vitamins are administered too rapidly, serum levels may temporarily exceed the renal threshold and some are excreted in the urine. Giving twice the RDA provides a safety factor for covering these losses as well as meeting the increased needs for hypermetabolism, prior deficiencies and formation of new tissue.

Increased amounts of biotin may be needed when the intestinal tract is not used or when normal intestinal flora has been altered by drugs, disease or bowel resection. The recommendation for 60 mgs of biotin is based on preliminary data showing that adults on prolonged parenteral nutrition maintain normal blood levels with this amount. Vitamin K is not included in intravenous vitamin preparations, as it may alter prothrombin time in individuals receiving anticoagulants. Two to four milligrams per week should be given parenterally depending upon the prothrombin time.

Deficiencies of water soluble vitamins can develop quickly in patients receiving parenteral nutrition, so it is important to begin supplementation early. Vitamins should be infused daily over a number of hours to prevent excessive renal excretion of those that are water soluble. The common procedure is to add the vitamins to the first liter/bag of solution each day. Fat soluble vitamins are stored so deficiencies take longer to develop. Excess intravenous supplementation has led to toxic levels in some patients. The recommendation for fat soluble vitamins is equal to the RDA. Multiples of the AMA recommendations are suggested for two or more days for patients with multiple vitamin deficiencies or markedly increased requirements.

Table 4: Recommendations For Parenteral Vitamin Supplementation

AMA Recommendations

Vitamin	RDA (1989)	Adults	11 years	< 11 years
A (IU)	4000	3300	3300	3300
D (IU)	200	200	200	400
E (IU)	10	10	10	7
Thiamin (mg)	1.0 - 1.5	3	3	1.2
Riboflavin (mg)	1 .1 - 1.8	3.6	3.6	1.4
Niacin (mg)	15	40	40	17
Pantothenic Acid (mg)	5 - 10	15	5	5
Folate (µg)	180 - 200	400 µg	400 µg	140 µg
B_{12} (µg)	2.0	5	5	1.0
Biotin (µg)	100 - 200	60 µg	60 µg	20 µg
Ascorbic Acid (µg)	60	100	100	80

Minerals

Mineral needs should be reviewed and adjusted on the basis of laboratory values and hydration. Suggested levels of supplementation are shown in **Table 5**. As mentioned in the "Medical Nutrition Therapy" section, requirements for potassium, magnesium and phosphorus bear a significant relationship to nitrogen intake, caloric needs and nutritional status. Deficiencies develop when insufficient amounts are provided. Commercial solutions are available and are intended to meet the normal range of requirements.

Table 5: Parenteral Mineral Supplementation for Adults

Amount per Kilogram Body Weight

Mineral	Basal	Mild To Moderate Depletion	Severe Catabolism	Comment
Sodium	1- 4 mEq	2 - 3 mEq	3 - 4 mEq	
Potassium	0.7 - 0.9 mEq	2 mEq	3 - 4 mEq	Give 5 to 6 mEq/gm N infused.
Calcium	0.22 mEq	0.3 mEq	0.4 mEq	0.25 mEq/kg needed for Ca equilibrium. Dependent on simultaneous administration of PO_4 & Na, not N retention

Magnesium	0.3 mEq	0.3 - 0.4 mEq	0.6 - 0.8 mEq	Give 2 mEq per gm N infused.
Phosphorus	0.3 mEq	0.8 mEq	1.2 - 2 mEq	Needs related to nitrogen retention which is related to calorie intake. Give 15 to 25 mEq PO_4 per 1000 glucose calories. Available as $NaPO_4$ or KPO_4.

Table 6 can approximate mineral needs based on biochemical data.

Table 6: Daily Mineral Requirements

	Lab Value	Daily Needs
Potassium	Above 4.8 4.0 - 4.8 3.5 - 3.9 < 3.5	None 20 - 30 mEq 40 - 50 mEq 80 - 90 mEq
Sodium	Above 142 136 - 142 < 136	None 25 - 50 mEq 50 - 100 mEq
Calcium (ionized)	> 2.58 2.32 - 2.58 < 2.32	None 5 - 10 mEq 10 - 20 mEq
Phosphorus	Above 4.5 3.0 - 4.5 < 3.0 < 2.0	None 20 mM 40 - 80 mM 80 mM
Magnesium	Above 2.0 1.5 - 2.0 < 1.5	None 16 - 24 mEq 24 - 32 mEq
Chloride	Above 104 101 - 104 98 - 100 < 98	None 20 - 25 mEq 40 - 50 mEq 90 - 100 mEq

Trace Elements

Requirements for trace minerals should be met on the basis of serum levels. Iron, copper and zinc are of the most concern.

Indications for parenteral **iron** use are limited. Patients with iron deficiency anemia are candidates, assuming an inability to absorb or tolerate oral iron. Iron is generally given in milligram doses intramuscularly when needed but should not be given until serum levels are known. Dosing guidelines: In determining the amount of iron to administer, distinction has to be made between the need to replace a deficient state and replete stores, to replace iron loss resulting from significant or ongoing blood loss or to provide normal maintenance requirements. Iron dextran injection is available for IV and IM use.

Adverse effects are localized or systemic reactions. Local reactions include pain, brown staining of the skin, sterile abscesses, necrosis, atrophy, sarcoma formation and phlebitis. An immediate reaction is hypersensitivity, which ranges from mild (malaise, itching, urticaria, sweating, myalgia, arthralgia and febrile episode) and transient to life-threatening, anaphylactic reactions (respiratory difficulty and cardiovascular collapse). Systemic reactions (may be delayed 24 - 48 hours post injection) include lymphadenopathy, myalgia, arthialgia, backache, fever, headache, nausea, vomiting and dizziness.

Iron is contraindicated in any type of anemia other than iron-deficiency secondary to risk of developing iron overload. When transferrin levels are too low to bind iron sufficiently, serum levels of circulating free iron rise. Serum transferrin levels are commonly low in patients receiving parenteral nutrition, making them more susceptible to bacterial and fungal infections. Critically ill or malnourished patients often have no bone marrow response to iron and increased levels may increase their susceptibility to infection also.

Copper may be given intravenously at a rate of one milligram per day to one milligram per week. Because of the risk of toxicity, Copper should not be given unless serum levels have been checked.

Zinc should be given parenterally at the rate of two to four milligrams per day. More may be needed when wound healing is poor or serum levels are low. Requirements are increased with diarrhea or intestinal losses.

Chromium, Manganese and **Iodine** also are added to parenteral solutions. Occasionally **Molybdenum** and **Selenium** are added for patients requiring prolonged parenteral therapy.

Recommendations for daily supplementation of trace minerals are given as shown in **Table 7**.

Table 7: Recommendations for Daily Supplementation of Trace Elements

Minerals	Oral	Parenteral	Comments
Zinc (mg)	10 - 15	2.5 - 4.0	May need to add more if severely catabolic Significant intestinal fluid loss Excessive stool or ileostomy output.
Copper (mg)	1.5 - 3.0	0.5 - 1.5	May need to add more if excessive fistula loss or diarrhea.
Iron (mg) – Men	10	1	Need to be cautious.
Iron (mg) – Women	15	1	
Chromium (µg)	50 - 290	10 - 15	
Manganese (mg)	2 - 5	0.15 - 0.8	
Iodine (µg)	150	1 - 2	
Selenium (µg)	55 - 70	40 - 120	
Molybdenum (µg)	75 - 250		Is present in water.

Parenteral Nutrition Solutions

Solutions can be designed to meet the needs of the individual patient. Total nutrient admixtures contain the patients daily carbohydrate, protein, fat, electrolytes, minerals, vitamins, trace elements and water needs in an all-in-one solution. This method has been shown to be very cost-effective, safe and simple to administer.

ADMINISTRATION

Prior to initiating PN, any serious potassium, phosphorus and volume imbalances need to be corrected. Infusion of parenteral nutrition solutions should begin gradually secondary to the high concentration of glucose. An initial rate of 40 cc per hour or one liter per 24 hours is the suggested rate. Additional fluid needs can be met with a peripheral line in the usual way. If the initial infusion rate is tolerated it can be increased to 80 cc per hour on the second day. The rate is increased continually until the required volume and/or calorie level is achieved. Blood glucose levels should be monitored daily and urine glucose every six hours. Blood sugar levels should stabilize below 200 mg% and a urine glucose of one to two plus normally does not require insulin. Insulin can be added to each liter of solution for those with a hyperglycemic response or excessive glycosuria. The risks of overfeeding have been discussed previously.

COMPLICATIONS

Many complications are associated with parenteral nutrition; **Table 8** summarizes the more common ones. Cause, symptoms and appropriate therapy are also included.

Tabel 8: Complications of Parenteral Nutrition

Complications	Symptoms	Cause	Prevention / Therapy
	Elevated blood glucose	Carbohydrate intolerance; too rapid infusion; diabetes; stress response infection	Decrease rate and/or CHO; treat infection; give insulin Goal: glucose < 200; dextrose infusion rate not to exceed 4 - 5 mg/kg/min
Hyperglycemia > 160 mg/dL	Hypothermia; somnolence; lethargy; peripheral vasoconstriction	Interruption of infusion or sudden stoppage	Proper infusion rate or restart infusion or start D10W.
	Elevated blood glucose and urine sugars > +2	Hyperglycemia Glucose intolerance	Insulin Drip; Correct free water deficit.
Hypoglycemia < 70 mg/dL	Hyperglycemia: elevated serum sodium and osmolality; seizures; somnolence; coma		
Dehydration (Hyperosmolar Nonketotic)	Weight loss	Inadequate fluid; fluid losses	Adjust fluid to cover losses and needs
	Weight gain	Excess fluid Compromised renal/cardiac function	Limit volume; concentrate solution; consider diuretics
Dehydration Overhydration	Paresthesias; malaise; mental confusion; bone pain; hyperventilation; weakness; decreased red blood cell; function; respiratory arrest	Inadequate phosphate; anabolism; excess losses; refeeding syndrome	Increase phosphate supplementation
Hypophosphatemia < 2.5 mg/dL	Renal failure	Excessive PO_4	Decrease IV PO_4 Stop current PN; Restart with ↓ PO_4
Hyperphosphatemia > 4.5mg/dL Hypokakemia < 3.5 mEq/L	Muscular weakness; cardiac arrhythmia	Excessive K+ loss; diuretics; Mg deficit; Insulin therapy; alkalosis; anabolism; inadequate supplementation	Increase potassium supplementation correct alkalosis

Complications	Symptoms	Cause	Prevention / Therapy
Hyperkalemia > 5.0 mEq/L	DM, RF, K + sparing diuretics, acidosis, K+ containing drugs	Excessive K+ acute dehydration; acidosis; renal insufficiency	Stop PN; change solution; correct acidosis
Hypomagnesemia < 1.6 mg/dL	Vertigo; lethargy; weakness; distention; seizures; tetany	Inadequate Mg; excess losses; anabolism; refeeding syndrome	Increase magnesium supplementation
Hypocalcemia < 8.5 mg/dL	Muscle cramps; abdominal cramps; tetany; positive Chvostek sign; convulsions	Inadequate Ca administration; repletion of phosphorus without attention to the reciprocal change in calcium; low albumin; CRF	Increase Ca supplementation monitor serum Ica, PO_4 and albumin fluctuations
Hyper-ammonemia	Elevated blood ammonia levels; somnolence; lethargy; seizures; coma	Hepatic dysfunction; deficiency in urea cycle amino acids; insufficient arginine binding; excessive protein load; low nonprotein cal to N ratio	Slow infusion rate; discontinue infusion; increase Kcal:N ratio; decrease protein; administer lactulose
Hyponatremia < 130 mEq/L	Lethargy; oliguria; hypotension; weakness; confusion	Water intoxication; excess Na loss, RF, CHF, DM	Restrict free water; increase sodium supplementation
Hypernataremia > 145 mEq/L	Fever, tachycardia, loss of skin turgor	Dehydration; increased Na; excessove hypertonic saline	Increase fluid Decrease/delete Na from solution
Prerenal Azotemia	Lassitude	Dehydration; calorie:N imbalance	Correct calorie:N ratio; insulin if hyperglycemic; correct free water deficit
Hyperchloremic, metabolic acidosis $CO_2 < 25mM/L$ $CL > 110$ mEq/L	Decrease in blood pH; decrease in serum HCO_3; decrease in base excess; increase in serum Cl; increase in serum Na	Excessive renal or GI loss of base; infusion of preformed hydrogen ion; inadequate amount of base-producing substance in PN solution to neutralize acid products of amino acid degradation	Decrease chloride excess in PN by exchanging chloride ion with acetate ion

MONITORING

Individuals on parenteral nutrition require careful monitoring. The intracelluar ions K, PO_4 and Mg should be monitered closely to avoid arrhythmias, paresthesias and seizures during infusion especially as PN is initiated. The Na:Cl ratio should be 1:1 to prevent hyperchloremic metabolic acidosis. Acetate salt can be added to decrease the amount of Cl and correct the acidosis. During the first 5 to 7 days monitoring should occur daily. Once the patient is stable, the schedule in **Table 9** can be followed.

Table 9: Schedule for Monitoring Parenteral Nutrition

Metabolic Parameters	Frequency	Nutrition	Frequency
I & O	Daily	Body Weight	Daily
Urine Glucose	Daily	Serum Albumin	Weekly
CBC	2 - 3 times/wk	Prealbumin	Every 2 - 3 days until increases
*Chemistries	2 - 3 times/week	Zinc, Copper	Weekly
**Liver Indices	2 times/week	N₂ Balance	1 time/week

*glucose, electrolytes, calcium, magnesium, phosphorus, BUN, creatinine, HCT
**bilirubin, SGOT, SGPT, alkaline phosphatase*

The goal of parenteral nutrition is a positive nitrogen balance (4 to 6 grams) and either a weight gain or weight maintenance. Weight gain should not exceed 250 grams per day as excess calories are converted to fat, much of which is deposited in the liver. Fluid retention may occur if solutions provide fluid in excess of needs. A strict intake and output record is essential for fluid management.

PERIPHERAL PARENTERAL NUTRITION

Parenteral nutrition via a peripheral vein can be used for patients who have good peripheral veins and total calorie needs between 2000 and 2500. Possible candidates are those who have normal renal function and lipid metabolism and who are NPO for 7 to 10 days, or have postoperative ileus or limited accessibility to a central vein. Peripheral infusions can also be used to supplement enteral nutrition in the patient who remains hypocaloric and catabolic. The goals of peripheral parenteral nutrition (PPN) are to fulfill energy needs, preserve or restore body tissue, maintain electrolyte, vitamin, mineral and fluid status and prevent essential fatty acid deficiency. This method is safe as long as patients are monitored. Monitoring should be done the same as with central parenteral nutrition.

Solutions for PPN contain dextrose, amino acids, vitamins, minerals and trace elements. Intravenous fat is given simultaneously to protect the vein and to provide about 40 to 50% of total calories. The flow rate of the lipid can be adjusted so that fat infuses the entire time amino acids and dextrose are infused. Peripheral nutrition solutions can be infused up to 125 cc per hour. The final solution is approximately 500 to 600 mOsm/liter when it enters the vein. Daily infusion of PPN can include 20% fat emulsion, D20W and 10% amino acids. Final dextrose concentration should not exceed 12.5% secondary to the risk of phlebitis. A typical day's requirement can be met with one liter of dextrose, one liter of amino acids and one liter of fat. Depending on the concentrations of the nutrient solutions chosen, total energy and protein could be 2000 - 2200 and 70 - 80 grams respectively.

Potential complications include phlebitis and possibly sepsis and all the other complications associated with central line parenteral nutrition.

PICC

A peripheral intravenous catheter (PICC) can be placed to provide ready access to the blood system and avoid repeated needle sticks or intravenous insertions. This indwelling catheter consists of a bundle of at least two and flexible slicone tubes that can be left in place for months. The PICC is inserted after a small incision is made in the neck or upper chest. The PICC is led under the skin several inches and then threaded via one of the major veins into the right atrium of the heart.

The PICC is used to draw blood for tests and infuse medications, nutrients, fluids, blood and platelet transfusions. Multiple tubes make it possible to perform different functions simultaneously.

CYCLIC PARENTERAL NUTRITION

Cyclic parenteral nutrition is the intermittent infusion of nutrients over a specified period of time. It is used most often for patients going home on parenteral nutrition. The length of infusion is determined by the volume required and the maximum toleration rate. It usually occurs overnight with infusion over 12 to 18 hours. Potential advantages include prevention or treatment of the hepatotoxicities induced by continuous PN and improved quality of life through resumption of daytime activities. Consideration must be given to CHO homeostasis during the transition periods to cyclic infusion.

The transition period is begun once the patient's nutritional and fluid requirements are determined. Patients need to be monitored for the development of rebound hyperglycemia. Monitoring involves checking blood sugars one hour after tapering the infusion and any time a patient develops nausea, tremor, sweating, anxiety or lethargy. If hypoglycemia occurs, the one hour taper off period should be extended to two hours or the total time of infusion should be lengthened. If hyperglycemia (> 250mg/dL) occurs, fat calories should be increased in an attempt to control blood glucose. If the hyperglycemia persists, the infusion time should be increased.

TRANSITIONAL FEEDING

Before instituting enteral intake the patient must have adequate intestinal function, including a normal gastric emptying rate. If the bowel has been at rest, the prolonged lack of intraluminal nutrition may have diminished digestive and absorptive function. The control of appetite is thought to be mediated by both peripheral and central systems. PN bypasses some of the peripheral systems which are thought to affect appetite. A long term parenteral nutrition patient usually has very little appetite or desire to eat secondary to the high levels of glucose and amino acids in the blood. These are strong inhibitors of gastric secretion and peristalsis. The patient may experience the sensation of hunger but usually eats only small amounts of food. Approximately five days are needed for the gut to adapt to enteral intake.

Parenteral nutrition solutions should be tapered over 24 to 48 hours before they are stopped to avoid hyperinsulinism. This rate should be reduced to 0.01 gm/kg/hour prior to cessation. During this transition the patient can be given small frequent feedings as tolerated.

Cyclic parenteral nutrition can be done at night to supplement oral intake and avoid the appetite suppression of continuous infusion. When the patient has achieved near normal intake, the infusion catheter can be heparinized and left in place for the next 24 to 48 hours. Nutrient intake should be recorded at this time to substantiate oral intake. If oral intake remains adequate, the catheter can be removed.

HOME PARENTERAL NUTRITION

Considerations must be given to the goal of nutrition support, extent of malnutrition and any gastrointestinal function. The inability to sustain life through the GI tract mandates home parenteral nutrition (HPN). The same guidelines as home enteral nutrition can be followed.

One has to be cognizant of the cost of hospitalization. A home parenteral nutrition program can improve the quality of life, lower medical costs through shortened length of stay, allow possible return to work and perhaps enhance the years of productivity.

Suggested criteria for home parenteral nutrition include the resolution of medical complications, unwarranted continued hospitalization, patient cooperation, family support and a need for parenteral nutrition for three to four weeks or more. Not all patients are candidates for home parenteral nutrition. The physical, psychological and socioeconomic status of each patient and patient's family should be assessed.

Eligibility

The treatment plan and selection of a home parenteral company should follow the same guidelines as described in the enteral part of this section.

Cyclic PN (intermittent infusion over a specific period of time) is most often used for patients going home on PN. The length of infusion is determined by the volume required and the maximum toleration rate.

Prior to discharge, the delivery rate and volume should be established and in force. This enhances a smooth progression to home. Patient and family education needs to be done in simple and understandable language. Teaching materials can include an audiovisual program reviewing good nutrition, reasons for parenteral nutrition, solution administration and a discussion of potential problems and how to handle them. Written material should be provided. A social worker is necessary to evaluate emotional status and economic situation prior to discharge. A home parenteral company may be considered for monitoring the patient at home. Cost reimbursement may be essential and some health care plans reimburse for home parenteral nutrition. A patient may have problems with cash flow upon discharge, therefore, a two to four week supply of supplies and equipment should be sent home with the patient. These articles can be added to the patient's hospital bill and are usually paid by the insurance company. A well-designed home parenteral program is safe and cost effective.

Long Term Complications

Long term complications include essential fatty acid deficiency, impaired wound healing and possible mild diarrhea if there is no oral intake. The incidence of cholelithiasis is increased with long-term PN. Cases of chronic liver disease, metabolic bone disease and steatohepatitis have been reported. Development of metabolic bone disease may involve the following: excessive protein intake producing a negative calcium balance, cyclic infusions causing a calciuretic effect, and D-lactate accumulation causing metabolic acidosis and osteomalacia. Muscle weakness, cardiomyopathy and death have been associated with inadequate levels of selenium. Hepatic steatosis, muscle weakness and myopathy have been associated with carnitine deficiency.

SPECIAL CONSIDERATIONS

Critically Ill Obese

Peripheral and central venous access is more difficult because of the anatomic changes caused by excess adipose tissue. It is likely that obese patients have a greater risk of mechanical complications from central line placement.

In the critically ill obese patient, it is beneficial to avoid infusion of large quantities of glucose to reduce the chance of insulin resistance, carbohydrate intolerance and frank diabetes mellitus. Hypocaloric infusions could be considered for this patient population. Hypocaloric feedings may facilitate weaning from the ventilator. Some studies suggest that amino acid infusion may improve the hypoxic and hypercarbic ventilatory responses (compared with hypocaloric dextrose infusions). Also, CO_2 production is minimized.

Energy needs can be determined on a resting energy expenditure of 8 - 10 kcal/lb for females and 10 - 12 kcal/lb for males based on actual body weight for the significantly obese (> 150% IBW) and morbidly obese (greater than 100 lbs IBW). For feeding to remain hypocaloric and protein sparing, calories should be provided at a level of about 300 - 500 less than the estimated needs.

Protein can be provided at 1.5 to 2.0 gm/kg/IBW secondary to increased lean body mass in the extremely obese. A 24 hour urinary creatinine determination could estimate the magnitude of the increased LBM.

Essential fatty acid deficiency is avoided by mobilization of endogenous stores of essential fatty acids as fats oxidize to supply the energy deficits (300 - 500 kcal). Lipids should be added to meet the high energy requirements of the severely catabolic obese patient and/or minimize the impact on the glucose metabolism of the extremely glucose intolerant patient.

Elderly

Reduced and slowed physical activity and a fall in basal metabolism and basal heat production occur with aging. The nutritional requirements must be adjusted for the physiologic and metabolic changes that occur during aging and modifiations must be made for chronic and critical illnesses. The elderly person with gastrointestinal dysfunction may be a candidate for parenteral nutrition.

Before initiating parenteral nutrition, cardiac, pulmonary and renal function must be evaluated. Indications for parenteral nutrition in the elderly are predicted intolerance of enteral nutrition greater than five days, severe hypotension, GUT failure and enteroabdominal fistulas.

Formula Composition Considerations

Calories	A calorie requirement of 38 kcal/m2/hr at age 30 falls to 30 kcal/m2/hr; at age 80 - approximately a 20% reduction. Therefore, calorie needs for the elderly must be calculated with caution.
Protein	The rate of protein synthesis and turnover is modestly reduced in older persons. A protein intake of 1gm/kg/IBW, with adjustments to accommodate losses, should be appropriate. Renal and liver function must be evaluated. A careful balance must be established to meet needs, replace losses and not overload the system.
Carbohydrate	Glucose tolerance deteriorates with age. Hypertonic glucose should be infused slowly to avoid hyperglycemia. Infusing insulin is a common practice in patients with impaired glucose tolerance.
Fat	Serum lipids increase in concentration with age. Lipid clearance needs to be monitored at regular intervals in older persons. Lipid clearance rates decrease in the elderly. Fat emulsions are contraindicated in patients who have impaired ability to clear lipids.
Vitamins	There is no evidence that absorption of vitamins is impaired with aging. But absorption may be affected by a variety of diseases that are common in the elderly. The dosages prescribed by the AMA are probably adequate unless there is a frank deficiency of one or more.
Minerals	Mineral requirements depend upon renal status, chronic medical problems, restricted sodium intake, medications, state of bone mineralization and soft-tissue calcification. All minerals should be provided in the amounts dictated by individual medical and nutritional status. Electrolyte balance needs to be monitored for renal or pulmonary insufficiency.
Fluid Balance	Water balance may be affected by diminished renal function. Cardiac output also decreases with age. Several liters of fluid a day via the circulatory system may cause stress of its own. Fluid balance must be carefully estimated and monitored. The elderly are prone to rapid shifts in fluid compartments and must be monitored for overhydration leading to pulmonary edema or renal insufficiency.
Acid-base Balance	The diffusion capacity of the lung changes with age. There is a decrement of about eight per cent per decade, thus indicating a less efficient acid-base control mechanism. The kidneys eliminate fixed acids. Also there is impaired renal function, the kidney's response is less effective.

Patients must be monitored regularly and frequently. The effect of multiple drug therapies on nutrient utilization, the effects of parenteral nutrition on subsequent GI function, the renal response to large infusion volumes and the electrolyte changes all need constant attention.

Hyperemesis Gravidarium

Parenteral nutrition is recommended for severe hyperemeis patients who are unable to eat or tolerate enteral feeding to such a degree that maternal weight gain and fetal growth and development are impaired.

Indications for use are as follows:

- Inaccessible or inadequate GI route
- Maternal malnutrition (prepregnancy malnutrition)
- Weight loss > 1kg/week x four consecutive weeks
- Total weight loss of 6 kg
- Failure to gain weight
- Chronic disease
- Hypoalbuminemia (albumin < 2.0 gm/dL)
- Prolonged dysfunction of GI tract (hyperemesis gravidarum)
- Chronic underlying diseases: IBD, Crohns, diabetic gastroenteropathy

Adequate nutrition is important. PN should be provided early to minimize the effects of malnutrition on fetal and maternal outcome. Poor nutrition in the first trimester can lead to a prematuare birth, perinatal mortality and congenital malformation of the CNS. **Table 10** addresses nutrition needs and weight gain during preganacy.

Labs and weights should be monitored frequently and glucose tolerance should be assessed. The renal threshold for glucose is lowered during pregnancy, resulting in increased urinary glucose. To determine adequacy of protein intake, urea nitrogen should be monitored. Appropriate changes in weight indicate adequate maternal nutrition and fetal development.

Table 10: Nutrition Needs and Weight Gain During Pregnancy

Weight Gain	Calories	Protein	Fat	Electrolytes	Trace Minerals	Vitamins
Singleton						
Weight gain 10.9 - 12.3 kg	Normal weight 30 - 35 kcal/kg	1 - 1.2 gm/kg/IBW	Need to prevent EFA deficiency; no clinical evidence to show induced premature labor, fatty infiltration of the placenta or any pulmonary complication in neonates	1200 mg Ca 30 mg Iron 1200 PO₄ 320 mg Mg	400 µg folic acid; 17 mg niacin; 1.6 mg Riboflavin; 1.5 mg Thiamin; 2.2 mg B₆; 2.2 µg B₁₂; 800 µg RE A; 70 mg C; 10 µg D; 10 mg E	175 µg Iodine 15 mg Zinc 65 µg Selenium
12.5 - 18 kg	Underweight 35 - 40 kcal/kg	Moderate to severe stress 1.5 - 2.0 gm/IBW				
7.0 - 11.5 kg	Overweight 25 - 30 kcal/kg					
Twin						
Weight gain 18.2 - 36.4 kg or ~ 20 kg	38 kcal/kg/ IBW	1.5 gm/ kg/IBW		2000 mg Ca; 60 mg Iron; 2000 mg PO₄; 500 mg Mg;	800 mcg Folic acid; 25 mg Niacin; 3.0 mg Riboflavin; 3.0 mg Thiamin; 4.4 mg B₆; 3.0 mg B₁₂; 1000 µg RE A; 150 mg C; 20 µg D; 14 mg E.	300 µg Iodine; 30 mg Zinc; 75 µg Selenium
Triplet or Quad						
Weight gain 20 - 40 kg	40 kcal/kg/ IBW	1.7 gm/ kg/IBW		3000 mg Ca; 90 mg Iron 3000 mg PO₄; 750 mg Mg;	1200 mcg Folic acid; 35 mg Niacin; 4.0 mg Riboflavin; 4.0 mg Thiamin; 6.0 mg B₆; 4.0 mg B₁₂; 1200 µg RE A; 200 mg C; 20 µg D; 16 mg E.	400 µg Iodine; 45 mg Zinc; 90 µg Selenium

PN complications are similar to those listed previously. Metabolic complications usually consist of problems with glucose control and electrolyte and fluid imbalance.

CLINICAL NUTRITION PATHWAY FOR PARENTERAL NUTRITION

Objective: to provide optimal nutritional care compatible with medical treatment for parenteral patients who are hypermetabolic and hypercatabolic through planning, implementation and monitoring/evaluating.

System/ Diagnosis	Potential Problems/ Indicators	Assessment	Intervention Monitoring/ Education	Possible Desired Outcome(s)
GI Dysfunction	Malnutrition Overfeeding Fever Infection Fluid balance Catabolism/ depletion of LBM Hyper-metabolism Excess CHO Hyper/hypo glycemia Rapid lipid infusion Adequate nutrients for wound healing and protein synthesis Electrolyte imbalances Abnormal ABGs Ongoing medical treatment modalities	History: medical, social, diet, drug and weight patterns Medical goals Biochemical/ABGs Vent settings/vitals Clinical status/GI function Functional status Outcomes/goals Determine needs: Kcal 25 - 30 /kg/IBW Pro 1.2 - 1.8 gm/kg; adjust for renal & liver function CHO no > 5.0 gm/kg/d no > 3.5 gm/kg/min Fat: 1 - 1.5 gm/kg/day over 12 - 24 hr adjust for sedation with Propofol Fluid: 35 cc/kg; adjust for losses, hydration and organ function Electrolytes: standard; adjust per labs/organ function Vitamins: RDAs; extra Vit C if appropriate Minerals: RDAs; adjust for PCM	**Phase 1 and 2** Formulate care plan Implement PN Recommend baseline nutrition labs Document/communicate **Phase 3** Progress PN to desired rate Monitor for elevated LFT's, azotemia, hyperglycemia, lipemic serum, decreased respiratory function, failure to wean (if in ICU and vented) Evaluate lab changes pertaining to nutrition and hydration status Monitor I&O's, bowel function Evaluate efficacy for po/ enteral intake Change plan as medical condition necessitates **Phase 4** Transfer/discharge summary referral for continuum of care	Optimize nutrition status: maintain/ improve wt; maintain/ improve protein status Improve electrolyte balance Prevent/ correct excess CO_2 production Prevent overfeeding Decrease catabolic response to stress Maintain GI mucosal integrity, if appropriate Decrease complications Transition to oral feeding, when appropriate Education: statement of needs, if appropriate

QUALITY IMPROVEMENT

Quality improvement and/or a process indicator can be designed for patients placed on parenteral nutrition or initiated on parenteral nutrition should be started within 24 hours of the written order and receive 80 - 90% of recommended needs by day two. A patient will not experience the following:

BS < 100 mg/dl or > 250 mg/dl; **Serum: Na** >145; **K:** < 3.5 or > 5.0; **Mg** < 1.6 or > 2.7 and **PO₄**, 2.5 or > 5.0.

Table 11: Clinical QI Monitor for Parenteral Nutrition

Pt	Med Svc	PN Type	Order Date	Start Date	Amt Recommend	Amt Received	Variance	Action	Out-comes

Directions:

1. List all new patients receiving > 50% of needs from PN.

2. List the medical service of the patient.

3. Record the admit date and the date of the PN order.

4. Record the start date of the PN.

5. Identify type of PN (central or peripheral).

6. Record the amount of PN by protein and calories recommended.

7. Record the amount of PN by protein and calories received by day 2 of PN.

    (data collection is from 12 mn to 12 mn).

8. List variances by definitions below.

9. Record variances by the following definitions.

    Medical – Change in status/surgery/procedural tests.

    Metabolic – Hyperglycemia, hypoglycemia, hypernatremia, risk of aspiration, etc.

    Mechanical – Line dislodgment, improper placement, administration.

    GI – Nausea, vomiting, cramping, distention, fullness, diarrhea, constipation, medication intolerance, refeeding syndrome.

10. Record for one month.

11. **EXCEPTION:** No code/DNAR.

The results of the QI demonstrates any problems and/or complications associated with advancing parenteral nutrition. The problems become the next QI monitor(s).

References

- Tougher-Decker, R: Enteral formulary design. Support Line 1992; Vol 14: No 2.

- Kudsk, KA: Clinical application of enteral nutrition. Nutr in Clin Pract 1994; 9:165.

- Rombeau, J and Rolandelli, RH: Enteral and Tube Feeding. Philadelphia: W.B. Saunders, 1996.

- Shike, M: Enteral Nutrition Support. In: Shils, ME, Olson, JA, Shike, M, eds. Philadelphia: Lea and Febiger, 1994.

- ASPEN Board of Directors. Guidelines for the use of parenteral and enteral nutrition in adult and pediatric patients. JPEN 1993; 17 (supl):7SA.

- Chicago Dietetic Association. Manual of Clinical Dietetics. Chicago: American Dietetic Assosciation, 1996.

- Campbell, SM: Maintaining hydration status in the elderly persons: problems and solutions. Support Line 1992; No 3.

- Page, CP: Overview enteral feeding: The past and the future. RD 1994; No 2.

- Akexander, JW: Early enteral nutrition: RD 1994; No 2.

- Palmer, RM: Acute hospital care of the elderly: minimizing the risk of functional decline. Clev Clin J of Med 1995; Mar/Apr.

- Clevenger, FW and Rodriques, DJ: Decision making for enteral feeding administration: the why behind where and how. Nutr in Clin Pract 10:104-113, June 1995.

- Eisenberg, PG: Causes of diarrhea in tube-fed patients:a comprehensive approach to diagnosis and management: Nutr in Clin Pract 1993; 8:119.

- Charney, P and Martindale, R: Early enteral nutrition support in metabolic stress. RD 1994; No 1.

- Charney, P and Martindale, R: Early postoperative enteral nutrition; feasibility and recommendations. RD 1993; No l.

- The 1995 ASPEN standards for nutrition support in hospitalized patients: Nutr in Clin Pract 1995; 10:206.

- National Research Council. Recommended Daily Allowances. Washington, DC:National Academy Press, 1989.

- Multivitamin preparations for parenteral use: a statement by the nutrition advisory group. JPEN 1979; 3:258.

- Egging, P: Enteral nutrition from a pharmacist's perspective. Nutr Supp Serv 1987; No 4.

- Speerhas, RA: Administering medications with enteral feedings. Support Line 1994; No 5.

- Diarrhea in tube-fed patients does not require cessation of enteral feeding. Pharm Pract News 1995; Feb.

- Kohn, C: Techniques for evaluation and managing diarrhea in the tube fed patient. Nutr in Clin Pract 1987.

- Silberman, H: Parenteral and Enteral Nutrition. Norwalk: Appleton and Lange, 1989.

- Andrassy, R and Durr, E: Albumin: use in nutrition support. Nutr Clin Pract 1988; 3:226.

- Tayek, J: Albumin synthesis and nutritional assessment. Nutr in Clin Pract 1988; Dec.

- Albira, J et al: Nitrogen utilization from elemental diets. JPEN 1985; No 4.

- Silk, D et al: Use of peptides rather than free amino acid nitrogen source in chemically defined "elemental" diets. JPEN 1980; No 4.

- Brinson, R and Kilts, B: Hypoalbuminemia as an indicator of diarrheal incidence in critically ill patients. Crit Care Med 1987; 15:506.

- Wolfe, B: Ongoing controversies regarding albumin and nutrition support. Nutr in Clin Pract 1988; No 3.

• Brinson, R, Curtis, W and Singh, M: Diarrhea in the intensive care unit: the role of hypoalbuminemia and the response to peptide-based chemically defined diet. J Am Coll Nutr 1987; No 6.

• Andrassey, R: Gut Barrier/Immune Response. Contemp Surg 1989; No 2A.

• Chernoff, R: Physiologic aging and nutritional status. Nutr in Clin Pract 1990; 5:8.

• Lipschitz, DA: Approaches to the nutritional support of the older patient. Clin in Geriat Med 1995; No 4.

• Shikora, SA: Enteral feeding tube placement in obese patients: considerations for sion support: Nutr in Clin Pract 1997; 12:S9.

• Karkeck, JM: Nutrition support for the elderly. Nutr in Clin Pract 1993; 8:211.

• Barclay, BA: Experience with enteral nutrition in the treatment of hyperemesis gravidarum. Nutr in Clin Pract 1990; 5:153.

• Boyce, RA: Enteral nutrition in hyperemesis gravidarum: a new development. J Am Diet Assoc 1992; No 6.

• Gulley, RM, VanderPleog, N and Gulley, JM: Treatment of hyperemesis gravidarum with nasogastric feeding. Nutr in Clin Pract 1993; 8:33.

• Pederson, AL, Worthington-Roberts, B and Hicker, DE: Weight gain patterns during twin gestation. J Am Diet Assoc 1989; No 5.

• Hyltander, A: Intravenous feeding and its effect on energy and nitrogen metabolism. Nutr in Clin Pract 1994; 9:51.

• Rombeau, J and Lew, JI: Nutrition and the Gut. In: Kinney, JM, Tucker, HN, eds. Organ Metabolism and Nutrition: Ideas for Future Critical Care. New York: Raven Press 1994.

• Shils, ME: Parenteral Nutrition. In: Shils, ME, Olson, JA, Shike, M, eds. Philadelphia: Lea and Febiger, 1994.

• Nussbaum, MS and Fischer, JE: Parenteral Nutrition. In: Zaloga, GP, ed. Nutrition In Critical Care. St Louis: Mosby, 1994.

• Kumpf, VJ: Parenteral iron supplementation. Nutr in Clin Pract 1996; 11:139

• Rosmarin DK, Wardlaw, GM and Mirtallo, J: Hyperglycemia associated with high, continuous infusion rates of total parenteral nutrition dextrose. Nutr in Clin Pract 1996; 11:151.

• Barr, L et al: Essential fatty acid deficiency during total parenteral nutrition. Abstr Ann of Surg 1981; 193:304.

• Practical Aspects of PV TPN. A Clinical Guide to Peripheral Vein Total Parenteral Nutrition. Chicago: Abbott Laboratories, 1983.

• Hardin, T, Page, C and Schwesinger, W: Rapid replacement of serum albumin in patients receiving total parenteral nutrition. Surg Gyn and Obst 1986; Oct.

• Baxter, J and Bistrian, B: Moderate hypocaloric parenteral nutrition in the critically ill obese oatient. Nutr In Clin Pract 1989; Aug.

• MCCrae, JD, O'Shea, R and Udine, LM: Parenteral nutrition: hospital to home. J Am Diet Assoc 1993; No 6.

• Wolk, RA and Rayburn, W: Parenteral nutrition in the obstetric patient. Nutr in Clin Pract 1990; 5:139.

• Amato, P and Quercia, RA: A historical perspective and review of the safety of lipid emulsion In pregnancy. Nutr in Clin Pract 1991; 6:189.

• Roqriquez, M: Effects of TPN on appetite. Support Line 1992; No 3.

• Luke, B: Univ. Mich. Med. Cent, Ob/Gyn. Personal communication.

Tables and Figures

CLINICAL PATHWAYS FOR NUTRITION INTERVENTION

Coordinated care is a multidisciplinary clinical process that describes, tracks, and monitors patient care to achieve cost and quality outcomes. The care process organizes and sequences the desired outcomes and anticipated health care team interventions. The process can be described as a pathway/care map to track patient's interventions and outcomes throughout their hospital stay. Each day of hospitalization has interventions and outcomes depicted. The pathways are established to ensure processes are standardized and result in a defined positive outcome(s). The pathways should be flexible working models designed for the use of all health care team members and provide guidelines to ensure a uniform level of care is provided to all patients.

The goals of coordinated care are to:
- Improve coordination of patient care activities among providers and between departments
- Provide clinical data that is used to identify opportunities for improving care
- Improve patient satisfaction
- Improve staff efficiency and effectiveness
- Enhance staff satisfaction
- Improve productivity

Clinical pathways are part of the Clinical Outcomes Management model which is based on the following framework:
- Patient-centered care
- Established patient outcomes
- Parameters for objectively measuring outcomes
- Effective and prudent use of resources
- Multidisciplinary collaborative practice environment
- Continuity of care across the continuum of health care delivery (pre-admission and post discharge)

The benefits of coordinated care are:
- Ability to define outcomes and costs of care to patients, payers, and referring physicians/health care providers
- Improvement in the process and coordination of care
- Long term cost savings

Nutrition is part of the clinical pathway. The nutrition care process needs to be implemented in each clinical pathway and/or care map that follows the hospital course of the patient.

Clinical nutrition pathways promote efficient, cost-effective quality nutrition care through measurable outcomes.

The primary purpose of the clinical nutrition pathways is to provide pertinent nutrition care to the appropriate patient(s). Pathways can be realistically written after nutrition assessment and nutrition care programs are established, and patients at high nutritional risk are identified. They must be explicit, measurable and reflect the optimal level of care that should be achieved. Pathways can be established by medical service (i.e., surgery, gastroenterology, etc.), by feeding modality (tube feeding and/or parenteral nutrition), or by disease state or a combination of all three. Pathways can be written in stages and/or phases.

Phase 1 -	Identification	Day 1
Phase 2 -	Decision making	Day 1 - 2
Phase 3 -	Treatment	Day 2 - 3 until discharge
Phase 4 -	Discharge/continuum of care	

Pathways mandate that individual nutrition care plans be documented and reviewed. Quality Improvement programs should be implemented around these pathways. Nutrition outcomes are observed throughout the hospitalization and are based on medical intervention goals for the patient.

The following are guidelines for specific disease states. They are written with current knowledge of the top DRG's and specific disease states, average length of stay, and current nutrition intervention recommendations. The indicators serve as a screen or flag to identify potential problem areas.

System/ Diagnosis	Potential Problems/ Indicators	Assessment	Intervention/ Monitoring/ Education	Possible Desired Outcome(s)
Cancer Gastric LOS 10 - 13 days	Anorexia Decreased appetite, early satiety Nausea/vomiting Weight loss/muscle wasting Poor nutritional status Dumping syndrome Weakness Low cellular immunity Visceral protein depletion Malabsorption (fat soluble vits, minerals, protein, fat) Possible lactose intolerance Hypoglycemia • Nausea • Hunger • Anxiety • Tremors Diarrhea Decreased gastric motility Loss of bile salts Fluid imbalance Sodium imbalance Pernicious anemia	Medical intervention goals Histories: medical, social, dietary, drug Weight/weight patterns Biochemical Clinical symptoms GI function/vital signs Functional status/ ADLs Hydration status Goals of therapy Education / discharge needs Determine needs: Kcal: 30 - 35/kg IBW Protein: 1.3 - 1.5 gm/kg IBW Fat: evaluate for malabsorption Fluid: 35 ccs/kg + losses Electrolytes: standard plus losses Vitamins: RDAs Minerals: standard recommendations	**Phase 1 and 2** Formulate care plan Implement feeding modality Recommend baseline nutrition labs Recommend multivitamins Document/comm-unicate care plan **Phase 3** Monitor medical progress; change care plan if condition warrants Achieve desired goals of feeding modalilty. If po: small feeding, low lactose, fiber, fat as appropriate Document / communicate any concerns Review labs, I&Os, wt, drugs, vital signs, medical plan Education process **Phase 4** Discharge summary and referral	Maintain and/or minimize wt loss Preserve/restore LBM Prevent dumping syndrome Adequate nutrient intake to perform ADLs Normal fluid and electrolyte status Prevent/control steatorrhea Prevent calcium malabsorption Prevent infection Prevent sepsis Prevent cachexia Correct anemia Comprehension and adherence to any dietary recommendations If patient is determined to have inadequate nutrition knowledge, plan for continuum of care

System/ Diagnosis	Potential Problems/ Indicators	Assessment	Intervention/ Monitoring/ Education	Possible Desired Outcome(s)
Cancer **Breast** **LOS 8 days**	Weight loss/muscle wasting Treatments Fluid imbalance Mineral depletion (Mg, PO_4) Alternative herbal or medical therapy Anorexia Preexisting diseases Anemia Decreased appetite Early satiety Nausea Vomiting Visceral protein depletion	Medical intervention goals Histories: medical, social, dietary, drug Weight/weight patterns Biochemical Drug/nutrient interactions Clinical symptoms GI function/vital signs Functional status Hydration status Goals of therapy Education/discharge needs Determine needs: Kcal: 30 - 35/kg IBW Protein: 1.3 - 1.5 gm/kg IBW; adjust for ARF/RI CHO: 50 - 60% Fat: 25 - 30% Fluid: 35 ccs/kg + losses Electrolytes: standard plus losses Vitamins: RDAs + 500 Vit C post chemotherapy Minerals: standard	**Phase 1 and 2** Formulate care plan Implement feeding modality Recommend baseline nutrition labs Recommend multivitamins Document/communicate care plan **Phase 3** Monitor medical progress; change care plan if condition warrants Achieve desired goals of feeding modalilty If po: small feedings, low fat (meeting 75% of needs) Document/ communicate any concerns Review labs, I&Os, wt, drugs, vital signs, medical plan Education process **Phase 4** Discharge summary and referral	Maintain and/or minimize wt loss Preserve/restore LBM Adequate nutrient intake to perform ADLs Normal fluid and electrolyte status Prevent cachexia Correct anemia Comprehension and adherence to any dietary recommendations If patient is determined to have inadequate nutrition knowledge, plan for continuum of care

System/ Diagnosis	Potential Problems/ Indicators	Assessment	Intervention/ Monitoring/ Education	Possible Desired Outcome(s)
Cancer **Solid Tumor** **Adenocarcinoma** **Sarcoma** **LOS 7 - 17 days**	Weight loss/muscle wasting Treatment related atrophy, stenosis Chemo and/or XRT related nausea, vomiting, diarrhea Fluid imbalance Mineral depletion (Mg, PO_4) Alternative herbal or medical therapy Anorexia Preexisting diseases Anemia Decreased appetite Early satiety Visceral protein depletion Wound healing if surgery is performed Possibility of PEG/ PEJ feeding Decreased immune function	Medical intervention goals Histories: medical, social, dietary, drug Weight/weight patterns Biochemical Drug/nutrient interactions Clinical symptoms GI function/vital signs Functional status Hydration status Goals of therapy Education needs Discharge needs Determine needs: Kcal: 30 - 35/kg IBW adjust for obesity Protein: 1.3 - 1.5 gm/kg IBW adjust for obesity Fat: 25 - 30% Fluid: 35 ccs/kg + losses or protocol Electrolytes: standard plus losses Vitamins: RDAs + 500 Vit C post chemotherapy Minerals: standard	**Phase 1 and 2** Formulate care plan Implement feeding modality Recommend baseline nutrition labs Recommend multivitamins Document/ communicate care plan **Phase 3** Monitor medical progress; change care plan if condition warrants Achieve desired goals of feeding modalilty If po: small feeding low fat (meeting 75% of needs) Document/ communicate any concerns Review labs, I&Os, wt, drugs, vital signs, medical plan Education process **Phase 4** Discharge summary and referral	Maintain and/or minimize wt loss Preserve/restore LBM Adequate nutrient intake to perform ADLs Normal fluid and electrolyte status Prevent cachexia Correct anemia Comprehension and adherence to any dietary recommendations If patient is determined to have inadequate nutrition knowledge, plan for continuum of care

System/ Diagnosis	Potential Problems/ Indicators	Assessment	Intervention/ Monitoring/ Education	Possible Desired Outcome(s)
Cancer **Liquid tumor** **Leukemia, lymphoma, nonhodgkin multiple myleoma** **LOS 5 - 7 days**	Weight loss/muscle wasting Treatment related atrophy, stenosis Chemo and/or XRT related nausea, vomiting, diarrhea Fluid imbalance Mineral depletion (Mg, PO_4) Alternative herbal or medical therapy Anorexia Preexisting diseases Anemia Decreased appetite Early satiety Visceral protein depletion Decreased immune function	Medical intervention goals Histories: medical, social, dietary, drug Weight/weight patterns Biochemical Drug/nutrient interactions Clinical symptoms GI function/vital signs Functional status Hydration status Goals of therapy Education needs Discharge needs Determine needs: Kcal: 30 - 35/kg IBW adjust for obesity Protein: 1.3 - 1.5 gm/kg IBW Fat: 25 - 30% Fluid: 35 ccs/kg + losses or protocol Electrolytes: standard plus losses Vitamins: RDAs + 500 Vit C post chemotherapy Minerals: standard	**Phase 1 and 2** Formulate care plan Implement feeding modality Recommend nutrition labs Recommend multivitamins Document/ communicate care plan **Phase 3** Monitor medical progress Achieve desired goals of feeding If po: small feeding low fat (meeting 75% of needs) HD #4: if intake is < 50% of needs → cyclic TPN Document/ communicate Review labs, I&Os, wt, drugs, vital signs, medical plan Change plan if medical condition necessitates it Education process **Phase 4** Discharge summary and referral	Maintain and/or minimize wt loss Preserve/restore LBM Maintain and/or prevent decline in nutrition status Adequate nutrient intake to perform ADLs Normal fluid and electrolyte status Prevent cachexia Correct anemia Help support tolerance to medical therapy Comprehension and adherence to any dietary recommendations If patient is determined to have inadequate nutrition knowledge, plan for continuum of care

System/ Diagnosis	Potential Problems/ Indicators	Assessment	Intervention/ Monitoring/ Education	Possible Desired Outcome(s)
Cancer Prostate **Radical Cystopros–tactecomy** **LOS 7 days**	Prolonged ileus Metabolic acidosis Fluid imbalance Nausea Vomiting Loss of appetite Wound healing Weight loss/muscle wasting/visceral protein depletion Chemotherapy • Oral ulcerations • Glossitis • Stomatitis • Nausea • Vomiting • Diarrhea • Anorexia • Electrolyte imbalance Radiation • Nausea, vomiting • Diarrhea Anemia Early satiety Wound healing	Medical intervention goals Histories: medical, social, dietary, drug weight/weight patterns Biochemical Drug/nutrient interactions Clinical symptoms GI function/vital signs Functional status Hydration status Goals of therapy Education/discharge needs Determine needs: Kcal: 30 - 35/kg IBW adjust for obesity Protein: 1.3 - 1.5 gm/kg IBW adjust for renal fx CHO: calculate utilization if on TPN Fluid: 35 ccs/kg + losses Electolytes: standard plus losses Vitamins: RDAs + 500 Vit C post chemotherapy Minerals: standard	**Phase 1 and 2** Formulate care plan Implement feeding modality Recommend nutrition labs Recommend multivitamins Document/ communicate care plan **Phase 3** Monitor medical progress Achieve desired goals of feeding If po: small feedings, low fat (meeting 75% of needs); if still NPO or < 50% of needs → cyclic TPN Document/ communicate Review labs, I&Os, wt, drugs, vital signs, medical plan Change plan if medical condition necessitates it Education process **Phase 4** Discharge summary and referral	Maintain and/or minimize wt loss Preserve/restore LBM Maintain and/or prevent decline in nutrition status Adequate nutrient intake to perform ADLs Normal fluid and electrolyte status Prevent cachexia Correct anemia Support tolerance to medical therapy Comprehension and adherence to any dietary recommendations If patient is determined to have inadequate nutrition knowledge, plan for continuum of care

System/ Diagnosis	Potential Problems/ Indicators	Assessment	Intervention/ Monitoring/ Education	Possible Desired Outcome(s)
Cancer **Ovarian** **Stage III or IV** **LOS 7 - 10 days**	Prolonged ileus Bowel obstruction Fluid imbalance Nausea Vomiting Diarrhea Loss of appetite Early satiety Wound healing Weight loss/muscle wasting/visceral protein depletion Refeeding syndrome Chemo and/or XRT related nausea, vomiting, diarrhea Anemia	Medical goals Histories: medical, social, dietary, drug weight/weight patterns Biochemical Drug/nutrient interactions Clinical symptoms GI function/vital signs Functional status Hydration status Goals of therapy Education/ discharge needs Determine needs: Kcal: 30 - 35/kg IBW 20 - 25/kg ABW if chronic starvation Protein: 1.3 - 1.5 gm/kg IBW 1.5 -1.75 kg ABW if malnourished CHO: calculate utilization if on TPN Fluid: 35 ccs/kg + losses Electolytes: standard plus losses Vitamins: RDAs + 500 Vit C post chemotherapy Minerals: standard	**Phase 1 and 2** Formulate care plan Implement feeding modality Recommend nutrition labs Recommend multivitamins Document/ communicate care plan **Phase 3** Monitor medical progress Achieve desired goals of feeding Document / communicate Review labs, I&Os, wt, drugs, vital signs, medical plan Change plan if medical condition necessitates it Education process **Phase 4** Discharge summary and referral	Maintain and/or minimize wt loss Preserve /restore LBM Maintain and/or prevent decline in nutrition status Adequate nutrient intake to perform ADLs Normal fluid and electrolyte status Correct anemia Support tolerance to medical therapy Comprehension and adherence to any dietary recommendations If patient is determined to have inadequate nutrition knowledge, plan for continuum of care

System/ Diagnosis	Potential Problems/ Indicators	Assessment	Intervention/ Monitoring/ Education	Possible Desired Outcome(s)
Cancer **Head and Neck** **Surgical** **LOS 7 - 14 days**	Dysphagia - pre and post op Acute weight loss Odynophagia Obstruction ETOH abuse Tobacco abuse Aspiration risk Taste alteration Anorexia Nausea Vomiting Oral mucositis Decreased sense of smell Altered CHO/ Energy metabolism Cancer cachexia Chewing/ swallowing problems Postop: stomatitis and mucositits Diarrhea Constipation	Histories: medical, social, dietary, drug, medical treatments Medical intervention goals Weight/weight patterns Biochemical Drug/ nutrient interactions Functional Status GI function/clinical status/vital signs Education needs, home referral if on tube feeding Goals of therapy Discharge needs Determine needs: Kcal: 30 - 35/kg IBW Protein: 1.3 - 1.5/kg Fluid: 35 ccs/kg Electrolytes: standard; replace losses Vitamins: RDA + C, thiamin, folate Minerals: standard plus Zn as needed	**Phase 1 and 2** Initiate continous enteral support Recommend vitamins Recommend baseline nutrition labs Formulate document, and communicate plan **Phase 3** Achieve ~ 80% of desired goals of EN Monitor I&Os, vitals Change to intermittent gravity drip feeds, when appropriate POD #4 Recommend wound healing labs Monitor I&Os, wts POD #7 Inititate oral diet in nonirradiated pt; total laryngectomy-zero aspiration risk, liquids or mech soft diet. Aspiration risk- speech consult, dysphagia diet Monitor I&Os, wts POD #12 In irradiated patient monitor Cu if still on Zn supplement **Phase 4** Discharge summary and referral	Wound healing Maintain/minimize weight loss Restore/maintain LBM Adequate calorie and protein intake Maximize benefits of therapy Prevent/reverse immunosuppression Achieve optimal nutrition status Comprehension of and adherence to any dietary recommendations If patient is determined to have inadequate nutrition knowledge, plan for continuum of care

System/ Diagnosis	Potential Problems/ Indicators	Assessment	Intervention/ Monitoring/ Education	Possible Desired Outcome(s)
Cancer **Head and Neck** **Radiation** **LOS 6 - 7 days**	Dyshpagia Acute weight loss Taste alteration Odynophagia Obstruction ETOH abuse Tobacco use Anorexia Nausea Vomiting Oral Mucositis Mouth dryness Increased saliva viscosity Decreased sense of smell Esophageal inflammation Esophageal stricture or perforation Depressed immune function	Histories: medical, social, dietary, drug, medical treatments Medical intervention goals Weight/weight patterns Biochemical Drug/ nutrient interactions Functional Status GI Function/clinical status/vital signs Education needs, home referral if PEG placement Goals of therapy Discharge needs Determine needs: Kcal: 30 - 35/kg IBW Protein: 1.3 - 1.5/kg Fluid: 35 ccs/kg Electrolytes: RDAs Vitamins: RDA + Vit C after XRT is completed Minerals: standard plus Zn as needed	**Phase 1 and 2** Determine modality of feeding - usually a dysphagia diet Recommend vitamin Recommend baseline nutrition labs Formulate care plan Document/ communicate plan **Phase 3** Monitor adequacy of po intake and severity of dysphagia/mouth pain Monitor medical condition and change care plan as appropriate Education process Referral process Monitor labs, wts, I&Os, vital signs, po intake Document and communicate **Phase 4** Discharge summary to home health care agency	Maintain/restore LBM Maintain adequate po to perform ADLs Maintain/minimize weight loss Maintain/improve hydration status Cessation of alcohol and tobacco Comprehension and adherence to any dietary recommendation If patient is determined to have inadequate nutrition knowledge, plan for continuum of care

System/ Diagnosis	Potential Problems/ Indicators	Assessment	Intervention/ Monitoring/ Education	Possible Desired Outcome(s)
Cancer **Cervical with TPE** **LOS 8 days**	Prolonged ileus Metablic acidosis Fluid Imbalance Nausea Vomiting Loss of appetite Wound healing Weight loss/muscle wasting/ visceral protein depletion Refeeding syndrome Chemo and/or XRT related nausea, vomiting, diarrhea Anemia Decreased appetite Early satiety	Medical intervention goals Histories: medical, social, dietary, drug, weight/weight patterns Biochemical Drug/nutrient interactions Clinical symptoms GI function/vital signs Functional status Hydration status Goals of therapy Education/discharge needs Determine needs: Kcal: 30 - 35/kg IBW 20 - 25/kg ABW if malnourished Protein: 1.3 - 1.5 gm/kg IBW 1.5 - 1.75 kg ABW if malnourished CHO: calculate utilization if on TPN Fluid: 35 ccs/kg + losses Electrolytes: standard plus losses Vitamins: RDAs + 500 Vit C post chemotherapy Minerals: standard	**Phase 1 and 2** Formulate care plan Implement feeding modality Recommend nutrition labs Recommend multivitamins Document/ communicate care plan **Phase 3** Monitor medical progress Achieve desired goals of feeding Document / communicate Review labs, I&Os, wt, drugs, vital signs, medical plan Change plan if medical condition necessitates it Education process Communicate plan **Phase 4** Discharge summary and referral	Maintain and/or minimize wt loss Preserve/ restore LBM Maintain and/or prevent decline in nutrition status Adequate nutrient intake to perform ADLs Normal fluid and electrolyte status Correct anemia Support tolerance to medical therapy Comprehension and adherence to any dietary recommendations If patient is determined to have inadequate nutrition knowledge, plan for continuum of care

System/ Diagnosis	Potential Problems/ Indicators	Assessment	Intervention/ Monitoring/ Education	Possible Desired Outcome(s)
Cardiac **CHF** **LOS 6 days**	Cardiac cachexia Loss of LBM Poor intake Early Satiety Gastroparesis Taste & smell Dyspnea/SOB Decreased cardiac output impairing delivery of cellular nultrients Hypermetabolism secondary to high E requirements and low cardiac & pulmonary function Malabsorption secondary to bowel edema & interstitital cellular effects of hypoxia Renal insufficiency secondary to cardiac drugs	Histories: medical, social, diet drug Weight and weight patterns Drug/nutrient interaction Functional status/ ADLs Clinical status/GI function/vital signs Discharge planning needs Goals of therapy Determine needs: Kcal: 30 - 35/kg IBW or dry wt; adjust accordingly for the elderly and obese; use FICK equation if Swans Ganz is utiliized Protein: 1.0 - 1.5 gm IBW or dry weight Fluid: 35 ccs/kg Electroytes: standard with supplemental K, additional Mg, PO_4, Ca as needed Vitamins: RDAs Minerals: standard	**Phase 1 and 2** Formulate nutrition care plan Determine feeding modality: if po - 2 gm Na with Am. Heart Assoc. recs if hyperlipidemic; small frequent feedings; fluid restriction of free water when indicated (< 120 Na) Document/ communicate care plan Recommend baseline nutrition labs **Phase 3** Monitor effects of cardiac medications on renal status and adjust diet/care plan as approp Nutrient intake analysis as indicated Adjust care plan as medical condition and/or therapy necessitates Document and communicate the nutrition care plan **Phase 4** Discharge summary with referral for follow-up	Improve nutrition status Improve protein status Minimize weight loss Maintain LBM Prevent further depletion Prevent malnutrition and/ or wasting Decrease malabsorption Eliminate or reduce edema Increase intake Comprehension of and adherence to dietary needs Patient assessed with inadequate nutrition knowledge have a plan for continuum of care

System/ Diagnosis	Potential Problems/ Indicators	Assessment	Intervention/ Monitoring/ Education	Possible Desired Outcome(s)
Cardiac **CAD** **Requiring A CABG** **LOS 8 days**	**Pre-op:** Loss of body mass 10 - 15% wt loss Low albumin < 3.2 mg/dL **Post-op:** Anorexia Anemia secondary to blood loss Edema secondary to surgery Hyperglycemia secondary to surgical stress or preexisting DM	Histories: medical, social and dietary, drug Medical intervention goals Weight patterns Biochemical Drug/nutrient interactions Functional status/ ADLs Clinical status/GI function/vital signs Goals of therapy Discharge planning needs Educational needs	**Phase 1 and 2** Formulate the nutrition care plan Implement the nutrition care plan Document the nutrition care plan Communicate the nutrition care plan with the health care team Recommend baseline nutrition labs NPO if extubated, clear liquid. **Phase 3** Active bowel sound, initiate solid foods If intubated - initiate nutrition support with tube feeding Po - monitor intake; If po intake is < 50% of needs - consider tube feeding if patient is at risk Monitor vital signs Initiate education process **Phase 4** Discharge summary and referral for follow-up	Maintain and/or minimize weight loss Preserve LBM Adequate intake of nutrients Optimal nutrition status Provide appropriate nutrition education Comprehension of and adherence to dietary restrictions Patient assessed with inadequate knowledge of nutrition needs have a plan for continuum of care

System/ Diagnosis	Potential Problems/ Indicators	Assessment	Intervention/ Monitoring/ Education	Possible Desired Outcome(s)
Cardiac **Mitral/Aortic Valve Replacement** **LOS 7 - 11 days**	**Pre-op:** Loss of body mass 10 - 15% wt loss Low albumin < 3.2 CHF **Post-op:** Anorexia Anemia secondary to blood loss Edema secondary to surgery Anticoagulant therapy as required	Histories: medical, social, diet drug, weight/ weight patterns Medical goals Biochemical Drug/nutrient interactions Functional status/ ADLs Clinlical status/GI status/vitals signs Education/discharge needs Discharge planning needs Goals of therapy Determine needs: Kcal: 30 - 35/kg IBW or dry weight; adjust for obesity and/or the elderly Protein: 1.3 - 1.5/kg IBW or dry weight; adjust for renal insufficiency Fluid: 30 - 35 ccs/kg Electrolytes: standard replace K as needed Vitamins: RDAs adjust for RI if appropriate Minerals: standard	**Phase 1 and 2** Formulate nutrition care plan Diet: clear liquid if extubated Document care plan Communicate care plan with team Recommend baseline nutrition labs **Phase 3** If still intubated consider TF Evaluate for po intake (active bowel sounds) Evaluate I&Os Review weights, labs, vital signs and po If po intake is inadequate < 50% consider TF Communicate concerns with team Document concerns Start education process surgical nutrition guidelines, coumadin teaching, AHA guidelines **Phase 4** Discharge summary and referral for followup	Adequate oral intake Improved hydration and electrolyte status Weight maintained and/or dry weight gain and/or weight loss minimized post operatively Protein repletion and/or minimize protein depletion Appropriate education is provided and understood If patient is determined to have inadequate nutrition knowledge, a plan for continnum of care

System/ Diagnosis	Potential Problems/ Indicators	Assessment	Intervention/ Monitoring/ Education	Possible Desired Outcome(s)
Endocrine **Diabetes** **Type 1** **Type 2** **LOS 5 - 7 days**	Malnutrition Poor dentition Gastric motility Nephropathy Dialysis Neuropathy CHD/CHF Hypokalemia Refeeding syndrome Acute hypophosphatemia upon initiation of feeding Alcohol abuse Diarrhea Other chronic diseases Hyperglycemia IGT (impaired glucose tolerance) Obesity Ketoacidosis Somogyi effect Osteoporosis Anorexia Hypertension	Medical goals Histories: medical, social, dietary, drug, weight/weight patterns Biochemical Drug/nutrient interactions Clinical symptoms/ GI function/vital signs Functional status/ ADLs/IDALs Hydration status Goals of therapy Determine needs: 25 - 30 kcal/kg Protein: 1.2 - 1.5 gm/kg IBW; adjust for renal/liver dysfunction CHO: 50 - 55%; increased fiber Fat: 30%; cholesterol < 300 mg/day Fluid: 35 ccs/kg + losses; 25 cc/kg for renal/hepatic dysfunction Discharge plans Education evaluation	**Phase 1 and 2** Formulate care plan Implement feeding modality Recommend baseline nutrition labs Recommend multivitamins, if appropriate Document/ communicate plan **Phase 3** Monitor medical progress Achieve desired goals of intake Review labs, I&Os, wt, drugs, vital signs, monitor glucose; additional insulin on sliding scale as necessary; bowel function medical plan Document/ communicate Change plan if medical condition necessitates it Review effectiveness of the care plan **Phase 4** Discharge summary and referral	Maintain and/or prevent decline in nutrition status • Maintain and/or minimize wt loss • Preserve/ restore LBM Improve fluid and electrolyte status Adjust nutrition support to changing medical therapy Improved GT Glycemic control Comprehension and adherence to dietary recommendations, insulin regimen, and possible exercise program Discharge summary: • Current nutrition support • Summary of nutrition therapies • Statement of expected progress • Recommendations for follow-up • Education needs

System/ Diagnosis	Potential Problems/ Indicators	Assessment	Intervention/ Monitoring/ Education	Possible Desired Outcome(s)
Gastrointestinal **Crohns** **Medical** **LOS 5 - 8 days**	Malnutrition Protein losing enteropathy Diarrhea Acute, severe weight loss secondary to diminished food intake and inflammation Nutrient deficiencies Anemia Fluid retention Electrolyte Imbalance Intolerance to po	Hx: medical, social, dietary, drug Weight patterns Biochemical Drug/nutrient interactions Medical goals Clinical symptoms/ GI function/vital signs Functional status/ ADLs Hydration status Feeding modality Education needs, Goals of therapy Discharge plans Determine needs: Kcal: 30 - 35/kg IBW Protein: 1.3 - 1.5 gm/kg Fluid: 35 cc/kg plus losses Electrolytes: standard plus replace losses Vitamins: RDA add for ileum removal Minerals: standard plus Zn, Fe, Folate	**Phase 1 and 2** Determine feeding modality - if po, modify fat, fiber, lactose; avoid gas-producing foods Formulate care plan Recommend baseline labs Document/ communicate plan **Phase 3** Goal: to achieve desired intake via po or EN/PN Review labs, I&Os, medical progress, vital signs Monitor intake, I&Os, albumin and electrolytes, wt, Start education process Communicate any concerns Document progress of care plan and education Adjust care plan as medical condition and/or therapy necessitates **Phase 4** Discharge summary and referral	Preserve/ improve LBM Decrease fecal output Reduce steatorrhea Normalize electrolytes Adequate calorie and protein intake Optimal nutrition status Improve hydration status Comprehension and adherence to dietary recommendations If patient is determilned to have inadequate nutriton knowledge plan for continuum of care

System/ Diagnosis	Potential Problems/ Indicators	Assessment	Intervention/ Monitoring/ Education	Possible Desired Outcome(s)
Gastrointestinal Crohns Surgical LOS 5 - 12 days	Diarrhea, nausea, vomiting, weight loss Fever, fluid imbalance, high output through ostomy Electrolyte losses Diminished po intake Inflammation Impaired immune response Wound healing Anemia, iron, B_{12}, folate secondary to blood loss, poor intake Malabsorption, water soluble vitamins, folate, fat soluble vits Lactose, fat intolerance Hypoalbuminemia secondary to protein loss, ↓ intake and ↑ production Loss of absorptive surface Ileal resection with bile salt deficiency Steatorrhea Blind loop bacterial overgrowth	Hx: medical, social surgical, dietary, drug weight patterns Clinical symptoms/ GI function/vital signs, Hydration status Functional status/ ADLs Drug/nutrient interactions Medical goals Determine goal of therapy/education needs/dc plans Determine needs: Kcal: 30 - 35/kg IBW possibly up to 45 Protein: 1.3 - 1.5/kg IBW Fat: MCT if appropriate; low fat for steatorrhea CHO: low lactose if appropriate Fluid: 35 ccs/kg; replace losses secondary to diarrhea, NG output and drains Vitamins: RDA - if ileum removed - ADEKB_{12} plus water soluble for stearorrhea Minerals: Zn, Ca, Mg for repletion.	**Phase 1 and 2** NPO Determine feeding modality Formulate care plan Recommend vitamins and minerals Recommend baseline nutrition labs Document plan Communicate plan **Phase 3** Review feeding modality and adjust as needed Desired goal of intake achieved Monitor I&Os Review labs, I&Os, wt, drugs, vital signs, medical plan Change plan if medical condition necessitates it Education process Communicate plan **Phase 4** Discharge summary and referral	Maintain/ minimize weight loss Restore/improve LBM Decrease diarrhea Adequate po intake Normalize electrolytes Control lactose intolerance Replace protein/ glycogen stores Prevent infection Promote wound healing Improve hydration status; decrease excessive output Comprehension of and adherence to any dietary recommendations If patient is determined to have inadequate knowledge, plan for continuum of care

System/ Diagnosis	Potential Problems/ Indicators	Assessment	Intervention/ Monitoring/ Education	Possible Desired Outcome(s)
Gastrointestinal **Ulcerative Colitis** **LOS 5 - 10 days** **Ileostomy, (colostomy)** **LOS 5 - 10 days**	Malnutrition Wound healing Protein losing enteopathy Anemia Dehydration Diarrhea Electrolyte imbalance Intolerance to po Decreased absorption Excessive GI loss Nausea Anorexia Fear of eating Decreased transit time	Histories: medical, social, dietary, drug Weight/weight patterns Biochemical Drug/nutrient interactions Clinical symptoms GI function/vital signs Acute stage - bowel rest Functional status Hydration status Goals of therapy Education needs Discharge needs Determine Needs: Kcal: 30 - 35/kg Protein: 1.2 - 1.5 gm/kg IBW Fluid: 35 ccs/kg + losses from diarrhea & ostomy output Electrolytes: standard; replace losses Vitamins: RDA + ADEK B$_{12}$ if ileum is gone Minerals: standard	**Phase 1 and 2** Determine feeding modality If bowel sounds present suggest clear liquid Recommend nutrition labs Formulate/ document care plan **Phase 3** Clear liquids Monitor medical progress and change/implement nutrition intervention accordingly POD #3 If still NPO, recommend alternative nutrition support Review wt, labs, I&Os, vital signs Document / communicate care POD # 4 Achieve desired po - 6 small feedings as tolerated or EN/PN Initiate NIA if po is < 50% of needs Monitor labs, wts, I&Os, vital signs Education process **Phase 4** Discharge summary and referral	Preserve /restore LBM Maintain/ minimize weight loss Decrease diarrhea Correct anemia Improve hydration status Adequate protein and calorie intake Normalize electrolye balance Comprehension of and adherence to any dietary recommendations If patient is determined to have inadequate nutrition knowledge, plan for continuum of care

System/ Diagnosis	Potential Problems/ Indicators	Assessment	Intervention/ Monitoring/ Education	Possible Desired Outcome(s)
Gastrointestinal Pancreatitis (Acute) LOS 5 - 7 days	Stearorrhea Malabsorption Diarrhea Hyperglycemia ETOH abuse Tube placement for early enteral feeding Hypertriglyceridemia Poor intake Weight loss Low albumin	Medical intervention goals Histories: medical, social, dietary, drug Weight patterns Biochemical, lipase, amylase Drug/nutrient interactions Clinical symptoms/ GI function/vital signs Functional status Hydration status Goals of therapy Education needs Discharge needs Determine needs: Kcal: 30 - 35/kg IBW Protein: 1.2 - 1.5 gm/kg Fat: low-mod (30 - 40 gm) CHO: complex Fluids: 35 ccs/kg + losses Electrolytes: standard replace losses Vitamins:RDAs+vit C; thiamin, folate if ETOH abuse Minerals: standard	**Phase 1 and 2** If postop with J-tube, initiate elemental diet Formulate care plan Determine feeding modality if po: low fat, 5 - 6 small meals + pancreatic enzymes if necessary With moderate to severe disease inititate TPN; lipids contraindicated only if disease is secondary to a fasting TG > 500; monitor; chronic pancreatitis: ↓ fat, MCT based Recommend baseline nutrition labs Document/ communicate plan **Phase 3** Review labs, I&Os, wt, drugs,vital signs, medical plan Change plan if medical condition necessitates it Education process **Phase 4** Discharge summary and referral	Decrease diarrhea Maintain/ minimize weight loss Maintian/ improve LBM Maintain adquate flluid/electrolyte balance Prevent malabsorption Control hyperglycemia Chronic: alleviate steatorrhea control/prevent Hyperglycemia, PCM, maldigestion, diarrhea Adequate energy for ADLs Comprehension of and adherence to any dietary recommendations If patient is determined to have inadequate nutrition knowledge, plan for continuum of care

System/ Diagnosis	Potential Problems/ Indicators	Assessment	Intervention/ Monitoring/ Education	Possible Desired Outcome(s)
Gastric surgery Billroth I&II Total gastrectomy Esphago-gastrectomy Whipple's Gastro-enterostomy Gastro-jejunostomy Post gastrectomy Ileal resection LOS 8 - 15 days	**Pre op** • GI involvement • Early satiety • Dysphagia • Weight loss • Nausea, vomiting **Post op** • Wound healing • Dumping • Intestinal damage • Malabsorption • Diarrhea • Steatorrhea • Lactase deficiency • Protein losing enteropathy Obstruction - N/V; leads to electrolyte and protein losses Hypoglycemia • Nausea • Hunger • Anxiety • Tremors Malabsorption Dumping Decreased gastric motility Early satiety Loss of bile salts Fluid imbalance Sodium imbalance Fat malabsorption Diarrhea, steatorrhea Ca and Mg depletion Vit B_{12} malabsorption Fat-soluble vitamin malabsorption	Medical intervention goals Histories: medical, social, dietary, drug Weight/weight patterns Biochemical Drug/nutrient interactions Clinical symptoms/ GI function/vital signs Functional status Hydration status Goals of therapy Education needs Readiness to learn Discharge needs Determine needs: Kcal: 30 - 35/kg IBW Protein: 1.3 - 1.5 gm/kg IBW Fat: evaluate for malabsorption Fluid: 35 ccs/kg + losses Electrolytes: standard plus losses Vitamins: RDAs plus 250 - 500 Vit C Minerals: standard plus Zn if necessary	**Phase 1 and 2** Formulate care plan Implement feeding modality Recommend nutrition labs Recommend multivitamins + C Document/ communicate plan Monitor medical progress; change care plan if condition warrants **Phase 3** Achieve desired goals of feeding modalilty If po: small feeding low lactose, fiber, fat as appropriate Document / communicate any concerns Review labs, I&Os, wt, drugs, vital signs, medical plan Change plan if medical condition necessitates it Education process Communicate plan **Phase 4** Discharge summary and referral	Maintain and/or minimize wt loss Preserve/ restore LBM Wound healing Prevent dumping Adequate nutrient intake to perform ADLs Normal fluid and electrolyte status Prevent steatorrhea Prevent calcium malabsorption Prevent B_{12}, folacin deficiency Prevent sepsis Prevent cachexia Correct anemia Comprehension and adherence to any dietary recommendations If patient is determined to have inadequate nutrition knowledge, plan for continuum of care

System/ Diagnosis	Potential Problems/ Indicators	Assessment	Intervention/ Monitoring/ Education	Possible Desired Outcome(s)
Hepatic **Hepatic disorders** **Biliary cirrhosis** **Hepatic cirrohosis** **Acute Liver disease** **LOS 7 - 8 days**	Malnutrition Muscle wasting Fluid imbalance Pending encephalopathy Nutrient deficiencies Decreased appetitie secondary to disease and ascities Malabsorption (fat and vitamins) Anorexia Albumnin - Ammonia levels Fat maldigestion Steatorrhea Hyperglycemia Hypoglycemia	Medical goals Histories: medical, social, dietary, drug, weight patterns Biochemical Drug/nutrient interactions Clinical symptoms/ GI function/vital signs Functional status Hydration status Goals of therapy Education/discharge needs Determine needs: Kcal: 30 - 40/kg IBW Protein: 0.5 gm/kg if symptoms of encephalopathy or elevated ammonia; 0.5 - 1.5 gms based on encephalopathy Fluid: 35 ccs/kg unless Na decreases Electrolytes: standard; monitor K if on spironolactone Vitamins: RDAs + folic acid, B$_{12}$, thiamin, Vit C, Fe, Zn if ETOH abuse Minerals: standard; monitor Cu for Wilsons disease	**Phase 1 and 2** Formulate care plan Vitamin recommendations Document care plan Communicate plan Recommend baseline nutrition labs **Phase 3** Monitor medical progress; change care plan if condition warrants Achieve desired goals of intake Monitor K if on spirolactone Review labs, I&Os, wt, drugs, vital signs, medical plan Document/ communicate plan Education process **Phase 4** Discharge summary and referral	Dry weight maintenance and/ or improvement Control ascites Corrrect fluid balance Control encephalopathy Adequate protein calorie intake Control diarrhea Prevent fat steatosis and steatorrhea Maintain/improve LBM Support liver regeneration Prevent or correct PCM Improve quality of life Comprehension and adherence to any dietary recommendations If patient is determined to have inadequate nutrition knowledge, plan for continuum of care

System/ Diagnosis	Potential Problems/ Indicators	Assessment	Intervention/ Monitoring/ Education	Possible Desired Outcome(s)
Geriatric **> 70 years** **LOS 5 - 7 days**	Malnutrition Poor dentition Immobility Disruption of GI function Altered mental status Impairment of senses Decreased taste and smell sensations Decreased renal function Cardiovascular or respiratory problems Bowel function Fluid status Arthritis Food fadism Polypharmacy Multiple chronic disease impact on nutritional status	Medical intervention goals Histories: medical, social, dietary, drug, weight/weight patterns Biochemical Drug/nutrient interactions Clinical symptoms GI function/vital signs Functional status/ ADLs/IDALs Hydration status Goals of therapy Determine needs: Kcal: 25 - 30 kcal/kg Protein: 1.0 gm/kg IBW; adjust for renal/liver dysfunction CHO: 50 - 55% Fat: 30% Fluid: 30 ccs/kg + losses Electrolytes: standard; adjust per labs Vitamins: RDAs Minerals: standard recommendations	**Phase 1 and 2** Formulate care plan Implement feeding modality Recommend baseline nutrition labs Recommend multivitamins, if appropriate Document/ communicate care plan **Phase 3** Monitor medical progress Achieve desired goals of intake Document / communicate Review labs, I&Os, wt, drugs, vital signs, medical plan Change plan if medical condition necessitates it Review effectiveness of the care plan Communicate/ document the nutrition progress **Phase 4** Discharge summary and referral	Maintain and/or prevent decline in nutrition status • Maintain and/or minimize wt loss • Preserve /restore LBM Normal fluid and electrolyte status Adjust nutrition support to changing medical therapy Improve glucose tolerance Comprehension and adherence to any dietary recommendations Transfer summary: • Current nutrition support • Summary of nutrition therapies • Statement of expected progress • Recommendations for follow-up Education: statement of needs, if appropriate

System/ Diagnosis	Potential Problems/ Indicators	Assessment	Intervention/ Monitoring/ Education	Possible Desired Outcome(s)
Geriatric **Critically ill elderly** **> 65 years** **LOS 5 - 7 days**	Malnutrition Poor dentition Immobility Disruption of GI function Altered mental status Impairment of senses Decreased taste and smell sensations Decreased renal function Compromised cardiac or pulmonary function Limited reserves Refeeding syndrome Need for early intervention Bowel function Fluid status Arthritis Food fadism Polypharmacy Multiple chronic disease impact on nutritional status	Medical goals Histories: medical, social, dietary, drug, weight/weight patterns Biochemical Drug/nutrient interactions Clinical symptoms GI function/vital signs Functional status/ADLs/IADLs Hydration status Goals of therapy Determine needs: 25 - 30kcal/kg Protein: 1.5 gm/kg IBW; adjust for renal/liver dysfunction if on PN CHO: no > 5.0gm/ kg/day Fat: 1 - 1.5 gm/kg/ day over 12 - 24 hours; adjust for Propofol sedation Fluid: 30 ccs/kg + losses; 25 cc/kg for renal/hepatic dysfunction Electrolytes: standard; adjust per labs Vitamins/minerals: standard	**Phase 1 and 2** Formulate care plan Implement feeding modality Recommend baseline nutrition labs Recommend multivitamins, if appropriate Document/ communicate care plan **Phase 3** Monitor medical progress Achieve desired goals of intake Review labs, I&Os, LFTs, wt, drugs, vital signs, for decreased respiratory function/ failure to wean, bowel function and medical plan Document/ communicate plan Change plan if medical condition necessitates it Review effectiveness of the care plan **Phase 4** Discharge summary and referral	Maintain and/or prevent decline in nutrition status Maintain and/or minimize wt loss preserve/restore LBM Normal fluid and electrolyte status Adjust nutrition support to changing medical therapy Improve glucose tolerance Comprehension and adherence to any dietary recommendations Transfer summary: • Current nutrition support • Summary of nutrition therapies • Statement of expected progress • Recommendations for follow-up Education: statement of needs, if appropriate

System/ Diagnosis	Potential Problems/ Indicators	Assessment	Intervention/ Monitoring/ Education	Possible Desired Outcome(s)
Immune **Sepsis** **ICU –** **LOS 5 - 8 days**	Malnutrition Overfeeding Fever Infection Catabolism/ depletion of LBM Hypermetabolism Excess CHO Rapid lipid infusion Adequate nutrients for wound healing and protein synthesis On-going medical treatment modalities	History: medical, social, diet, drug, wt/wt patterns Medical goals Biochemical/ ABG's Vent settings/vitals Drug/nutrient interactions Clinical status/GI function Functional status Outcomes/goals Determine needs: Kcal: 25 - 30/kg IBW Protein: 1.5 - 2.0 gm/kg adjust for renal/liver function If on TPN: CHO no > 5.0 gm/kg/d no > 3.5 gm/kg/min/d Fat: 11.5 gm/kg/day over 12 - 24 hr, adjust for Propofol sedation Fluid: 35 ccs/kg; adjust for hydration, losses, and organ function Electrolytes: standard; adjust per labs Vitamins: RDAs, extra Vit C if appropriate Minerals: standard recommendations	**Phase 1 and 2** Formulate care plan Implement appropriate feeding modality Recommend baseline nutrition labs Document care plan Communicate the plan **Phase 3** Progress feeding to desired goal rate. Monitor for elevated LFT's, hyperglycemia, azotemia, lipemic serum, decreased respiratory function failure to wean Evaluate lab changes pertaining to nutrition and hydration status. Monitor residuals, I&O's, bowel function if on TF Evaluate efficacy for po intake. **Phase 4** Dc/transfer with summary of weights, vital signs, labs, feeding modality	Optimize nutrition status • Maintain/ improve weight • Maintain/improve protein status • Correct/ improve electrolyte balance, prevent/ correct excess CO_2 Prevent overfeeding Maintain GI muscosal integrity Decrease catabolic response to stress Transition to oral feeding Transfer summary: • Current nutrition support • Summary of nutrition therapies • Statement of expected progress • Recommendations for follow-up • Education needs

System/ Diagnosis	Potential Problems/ Indicators	Assessment	Intervention/ Monitoring/ Education	Possible Desired Outcome(s)
Immune **HIV/Aids** **LOS 6 -10 days**	Asympotomatic infection Fever > 1 month Aids wasting (chronic and acute weight loss) Weight loss > 10% Chronic diarrhea Malabsorption Ability to meet nutritional needs Vitamin/mineral deficit Megadosing of vitamin/mineral/ herbal supplements Fatigue Malabsorption Oral lesions, chewing and swallowing problems Decreased appetite Early satiety Nausea, vomiting Hypermetabolism Renal dysfunction Liver dysfunction Unproved nutrition/ medical treatments	Histories: medical, social, diet, drug Weight patterns Biochemical Drug/nutrient interactions Functional status ADLs Clinical status/GI function/vital signs Discharge needs Ability to meet nutritional needs Safe food handling practice knowledge Goals of therapy Determine Needs: Kcal: 35 - 40/kg Protein: maintenance 1 - 1.4/kg IBW underweight 1.5+ Fluid: 35 ccs/kg plus losses Electrolytes: standard; replace losses Vitamins: RDAs Minerals: standard recommendations	**Phase 1 and 2** Formulate Care Plan Implement appropriate feeding modality. Po - 6 sm feedings as tol Communicate care plan with the health care team Implement discharge planning Recommend baseline nutrition labs **Phase 3** Assess intake Evaluate I&O's. Replace fluid/ nutrients as needed Review labs, weights, I&O, meds, vital signs Adjust care plan as medical condition/ therapy necessitates Document the plan in a timely manner qod Communicate the plan Education: safe food handling and nutrition guidelines **Phase 4** Discharge summary and arrange for home referral, if appropriate	Optimize nutrition status: • Weight maintenance • Maintain LBM • Prevent wasting Correct/ improve fluid, electrolyte status Minimize diarrhea, nausea, vomiting Improve oral lesions Participation in resistance exercise 3 x week Enhance the effectiveness of medical therapy Improve well-being Appropriate nutrition education comprehended If patient assessed to have inadequate nutrition knowledge, a plan for continuum of care

System/ Diagnosis	Potential Problems/ Indicators	Assessment	Intervention/ Monitoring/ Education	Possible Desired Outcome(s)
Immune **MOF** **ICU** **LOS 5 - 10 days**	Malnutrition Overfeeding Liver dysfunction Renal dysfunction GI dysfunction Congestive heart failure ARDS Sepsis	Histories: medical, social, drug and diet Weight/weight patterns Vital signs Biochemical/ABGs Clinical status: GI, renal, hepatic, cardiac, respiratory Drug/nutrient interactions Functional status ADLs Degree of malnutrition Feeding modality Desired goals and outcomes Determine needs: Kcal: 30 - 35/kg IBW 21/kg if obese and ventilated Protein: 1.2 - 1.5 gm dependent upon renal/liver function Fluid: 35 ccs/kg adjust per losses function Vitamins: RDAs adjust per losses Minerals: standard adjust per lab/losses	**Phase 1 and 2** Formulate care plan Implement appropriate feeding modality Recommend baseline nutrition labs Document the plan Communicate the nutrition care plan with the health care team **Phase 3** Evaluate feeding modality Monitor I&Os Monitor labs/ABGs Monitor clinical status Monitor vital signs Evaluate/adjust goals of therapy Adjust care plan as medical condition and/or therapy necessitates Document/ communicate the nutrition care plan **Phase 4** Dc/transfer with summary of weights, vital signs, labs, feeding modality	Appropriate intake of nutrients Weight maintained and/or improved Weight loss minimized Improved hydration status Protein repletion and/or minimize protein depletion Prevent malnutrition Transfer summary: • Current nutrition support • Summary of nutrition therapies • Statement of expected progress • Recommendations for follow-up Education: statement of needs if appropriate

System/ Diagnosis	Potential Problems/ Indicators	Assessment	Intervention/ Monitoring/ Education	Possible Desired Outcome(s)
Pulmonary **Obese, Vented**	CO_2 retention Delayed weaning Refeeding syndrome Liver dysfunction Cardiac dysfunction Malnutrition Hyperglycemia Azotemia Lipemic serum Decreased respiratory function	Medical intervention goals Histories: medical, social, dietary, drug, weight/weight patterns Biochemical Drug/nutrient interactions Clinical symptoms/ GI function/vital signs Functional status Hydration status Goals of therapy Determine needs: Kcal: 21/kg/ABW + 400 kcal Protein: 1.2 - 1.5 gm/kg IBW; adjust for renal/liver dysfunction CHO: calculate utilization if on TPN no > 5.0 gm/ kg/d Fat: 1 - 1.5 gm/kg/d over 12 - 24 hour, adjust for Propofol sedative Fluid: 35 ccs/kg + losses Electrolytes: standard adjust per labs Vitamins: RDAs Minerals: standard	**Phase 1 and 2** Formulate care plan Implement feeding modality Recommend baseline nutrition labs Recommend multivitamins Document/ communicate care plan **Phase 3** Monitor medical progress Achieve desired goals of feeding Document/ communicate the care plan Review labs, I&Os, wt, drugs, vital signs, medical plan, ABGs, vent settings, LFTs Change plan if medical condition necessitates it Review effectiveness of the care plan **Phase 4** Discharge summary and referral	Maintain and/or prevent decline in nutrition status Maintain and/or minimize wt loss Preserve/ restore LBM Normal fluid and electrolyte status Wean from the vent Adjust nutrition support to changing medical therapy Transition to oral intake

System/ Diagnosis	Potential Problems/ Indicators	Assessment	Intervention/ Monitoring/ Education	Possible Desired Outcome(s)
Pulmonary **COPD** **LOS 6 - 7 days**	Malnutrition affects to the ventilatory system Refeeding syndrome Intestinal discomfort SOB ↓ LBM/catabolism of muscle mass Hypermetabolism ↓ Appetite; taste changes; chronic sputum production ↑ Energy expenditure Hydration status Medications Depression, fatigue Infection Pulmonary edema On-going medical treatment modalities Education: knowledge and readiness to learn	History: medical, social, diet, drug, wt/wt patterns, smoking pattern Medical goals Biochemical/ ABG's Vent settings/vitals Drug/nutrient interactions Clinical status/GI function Functional status/ ADLs Outcomes/goals Discharge needs Determine needs: Kcal: 25 - 30/kg IBW Protein: 1.3 - 1.5 gm/kg If on PN: CHO no > 5.0 gm/kg/d; no > 3.5 gm/kg/min/d Fat: 50% Fluid: 35 ccs/kg; adjust if volume sensitive Electrolytes: standard; adjust per labs Vitamins: RDAs Minerals: standard recommendations	**Phase 1 and 2** Formulate care plan Implement appropriate feeding modality Recommend baseline nutrition labs Document care plan Communicate the plan **Phase 3** Progress feeding to desired goal rate. Monitor for elevated LFT's, hyperglycemia, decreased respiratory function, failure to wean Evaluate lab changes pertaining to nutrition and hydration status. Evaluate diet order/ efficacy for po intake. Transition to oral feeding **Phase 4** Dc/transfer with summary of weights, vital signs, labs, feeding modality	Optimize nutrition status • Maintain/ improve weight; maintain/ improve protein status; correct/ improve electrolyte balance; prevent/ correct excess CO_2; prevent overfeeding maintain GI muscosal integrity Decrease catabolic response to stress Promote/improve respiratory muscle function ↓ SOB Reduce gastric distention, bloating Transfer summary: • Current nutrition support • Recommendations for follow-up

System/ Diagnosis	Potential Problems/ Indicators	Assessment	Intervention/ Monitoring/ Education	Possible Desired Outcome(s)
Pulmonary **Respiratory Failure** **LOS 6 - 7 days** **ARDS** **LOS 8 - 9 days**	Malnutrition affects to the ventilatory system SOB ↓ LBM/catabolism of muscle mass Hypermetabolism ↑ Energy expenditure Hydration status Medications Ascities Pulmonary edema Infection Ongoing medical treatment modalities	History: medical, social, diet, drug, wt/wt patterns, Medical goals Biochemical/ ABG's Vent settings/vitals Drug/nutrient interactions Clinical status/GI function Functional status/ ADLs Outcomes/goals Discharge needs Determine needs: Kcal: 25 - 30/kg IBW Protein: 1.3 - 1.5 gm/kg If on PN: CHO no > 5.0 gm/kg/d; no > 3.5 gm/kg/ min/d Fat: 50% Fluid: 35 ccs/kg; adjust if volume sensitive Electrolytes: standard; adjust per labs Vitamins: RDAs Minerals: standard	**Phase 1 and 2** Formulate care plan Implement appropriate feeding modality Recommend baseline nutrition labs Document care plan Communicate the plan **Phase 3** Progress feeding to desired goal rate. Monitor for elevated LFT's, hyperglycemia, decreased respiratory function, failure to wean Evaluate lab changes pertaining to nutrition and hydration status Evaluate diet order/ efficacy for po intake. Transition to oral feeding **Phase 4** Dc/transfer with summary of weights, vital signs, labs, feeding modality	Optimize nutrition status • Maintain/ improve weight • Maintain/ improve protein status • Correct/ improve electrolyte balance • Prevent/ correct excess CO_2 • Prevent overfeeding Maintain GI muscosal integrity; Decrease catabolic response to stress Improve resistance to infection Transfer summary: • Current nutrition support • Summary of nutrition therapies • Statement of expected progress • Recommendations for follow-up • Education needs

System/ Diagnosis	Potential Problems/ Indicators	Assessment	Intervention/ Monitoring/ Education	Possible Desired Outcome(s)
Pulmonary **Cystic Fibrosis** **LOS 5 days**	Weight loss PO intake to meet needs Fat malabsosrption (steatorrhea) Pancreatic insufficiency (glucose intolerance) Anorexia Maldigestion of protein and carbohydrate Vomiting, diarrhea Dehydration Electrolyte disorders (Mg, Cl, Na, K) Vitamin deficits (AEK) Compliance with pancreatic enzymes Infection Ongoing medical treatment modalities	History: medical, social, diet, drug, wt/wt patterns, Medical goals Biochemical/ ABG's Vent settings/vitals Drug/nutrient interactions Clinical status/GI function Functional status/ ADLs Outcomes/goals Discharge needs Education needs Determine needs: Kcal: 30 - 35/kg IBW Protein: 1.3 - 1.7 gm/kg Fat 40 - 50% if on pancreatic enzymes Fluid: 35 ccs/kg; adjust for losses Electrolytes: standard; adjust per labs Vitamins: RDAs plus extra ADE Minerals: standard 5 - 6 small meals	**Phase 1 and 2** Formulate care plan Implement appropriate feeding modality Recommend baseline nutrition labs Recommend multivitamins and pancreatic enzymes Document care plan Communicate the plan **Phase 3** Monitor medical progress Progress feeding to desired goals Monitor lab changes pertaining to nutrition and hydration status Evaluate po intake Education process **Phase 4** Discharge with summary of weights, vital signs, labs, current nutrition support, summary of nutrition therapies, statement of expected progress, and recommendations for follow-up	Optimize nutrition status • Maintain/ improve weight • Maintain/ improve protein status Correct/improve electrolyte balance Optimize pulmonary function; increase muscle strength and endurance Enhance quality of life Prevent diarrhea Prevent anemia Prevent azotorrhea, steatorrhea Improve glucose tolerance Comprehension and adherence to any dietary recommendations

System/ Diagnosis	Potential Problems/ Indicators	Assessment	Intervention/ Monitoring/ Education	Possible Desired Outcome(s)
Renal **Hemodialysis** **LOS 5 - 7 days**	Protein losses Protein intake Fluid imbalance Weight Loss Electrolyte imbalance High Triglycerides Vitamin Status Unstable parameters BUN < 40 or > 90 K < 3.5 or > 5.8 PO4 < 2.4 or > 6.0 Alb < 3.5 gm/dL Unintentional weight loss/gain > 3 kg Interdialytic weight gains exceed threshold more than 3 consecutive times	Histories: medical, social, dietary, drug Medical intervention goals Weight/weight patterns Biochemical Drug/nutrient interactions Nutrition knowledge Clinical Status/GI function/vital signs Functional Status Goals of therapy Determine needs: Kcal: 30 - 35/kg IBW adjust for obesity Protein: 1.2 - 1.5 gm/kg IBW Fluid: 750 ccs+ urine output; desired wt gain between dialysis is 1 - 1.5 kg Electrolytes: restrict NA, K, PO4 as needed Vitamins: nephrocaps + Fe, Vit E Minerals: standard; supplement PRN	**Phase 1 and 2** Formulate care plan Implement po 2 - 3 gm Na, 2 - 3 gm K, 1 - 1.2 gm PO4, fluids as appropriate Recommend renal vitamins Document care plan Communicate plan **Phase 3** Monitor intake Start education process Recommend baseline nutrition labs Review, labs, wts, drugs, I&Os, vital signs **Phase 4** Discharge summary and refer for further follow-up	Restore/maintain LBM Normalize fluid balance Normalize electrolyte balance Adequate energy/ protein intake Comprehension of and adherence to dietary needs/ restrictions If patient assessed with inadequate nutrition knowledge have a plan for continuum of care

System/ Diagnosis	Potential Problems/ Indicators	Assessment	Intervention/ Monitoring/ Education	Possible Desired Outcome(s)
Renal **Acute** **LOS 5 - 7 days**	Oliguria Anuria Glucose intolerance PCM Electrolyte imbalance Fluid imbalance Decreased urine output Protein catabolism Lipid intolerance Uremia	Histories: medical, social, diet, drug, weight patterns Biochemical status, functional status Clinical status/GI function/vital signs Education/discharge Determine needs: Kcal: 30 - 50/kg IBW; adjust for dry weight Protein: non-dialized 0.5 - 1.0 IBW hemodialysis: 1.0 - 1.5 IBW; continous dialysis 1.5 - 2.0 IBW CHO: oral - 60%; TPN: < 5gm/kg includes IV& dialysate Fat: oral 30 - 35%; TPN: 1 gm/kg/ 12 - 24° Fluid: output +750 cc Electrolytes: Na: anuric/oliguric, 500 - 1000 mg; K: anuric/oliguric,1gm Diuretic phase: replace losses depending upon serum levels, edema, and frequency of dialysis and drug therapy Fluid: Daily I&O's Anuric/oliguric replace output plus 500 ml; Diuretic phase: large amount may needed Vitamins: water soluble if dialyzed Minerals: Mg, PO₄	**Phase 1 and 2** Formulate care plan Implement po 2 - 3 gm Na, 2 - 3 gm K, 1 - 1.2 gm PO₄, fluid as appropriate Recommend renal vitamins Recommend baseline nutrition labs Document/ Communicare plan **Phase 3** Monitor intake Review vital signs Start education process, if needed Review, labs, wts, drugs, I&Os Monitor clinical status Adjust care plan as medical condition and/or therapy necessitates Evaluate/adjust goals of therapy **Phase 4** Discharge summary and refer for follow-up	Restore/maintain LBM Prevent/minimize weight loss Optimal intake Control electrolyte abnormalities Achieve fluid balance Maintain electrolyte/ mineral balance Prevent/correct uremia Delay need for maintenance dialysis Comprehension of dietary needs/ restrictions If patient assessed with inadequate nutriton knowledge have a plan for continuum of care

System/ Diagnosis	Potential Problems/ Indicators	Assessment	Intervention/ Monitoring/ Education	Possible Desired Outcome(s)
Renal **Chronic Renal Insufficiency** **LOS 7 days**	Low albumin Weight loss Glucose intolerance Uremic symptoms Electrolyte imbalance Fluid imbalance Decreased urine output Protein catabolism Lipid intolerance	Histories: medical, social, diet, drug, weight patterns Medical goals Biochemical Drug/nutrient interactions Functional status Clinical status/GI function/vital signs Goals of therapy Education/discharge planning Determine needs: Kcal: 30 - 35/kg IBW; if catabolic 45/kg; if obese 20 - 30/kg IBW Protein: 0.6 - 0.8 gm/kg Fluid: output + 750 cc Electrolytes: Na: anuric/oliguric, 500 - 1000 mg; K: anuric/oliguric, 1gm Diuretic phase: replace losses adjust for serum levels, edema Fluid: Daily I&O's Anuric-oliguric: replace output + 500 ml; Diuretic phase: large amount may needed Minerals: Mg, PO_4	**Phase 1 and 2** Formulate care plan Implement po as per labs and I&O's fluid as appropriate; Recommend renal vitamins Request labs as needed Recommend baseline nutrition labs Document/ communicate plan **Phase 3** Monitor intake Review, labs, wts, drugs, I&Os Start education process, if needed Monitor clinical status/vital signs Adjust care plan as medical condition and/or therapy necessitates Evaluate/adjust goals of therapy Finish education **Phase 4** Discharge summary and refer for further follow-up	Slow progression of disease Delay need for maintenance dialysis Decrease weight loss Meet nutrition needs Normalize electrolytes Prevent further catabolism/ maintain LBM Minimize uremic complications Maintain acceptable fluid balance Comprehension of and adherence to any dietary restrictions If patient assessed with inadequate nutrition knowledge have a plan for continuum of care

System/ Diagnosis	Potential Problems/ Indicators	Assessment	Intervention/ Monitoring/ Education	Possible Desired Outcome(s)
Renal **Chronic** **LOS 4 - 6 days**	Low albumin Weight loss Fluid imbalance Uremic symptoms Impaired ability to excrete water, Na, K, Mg, PO$_4$ Decreased Ca absorption < 60 gms protein for women may be deficient in iron, niacin, riboflavin, thiamin, calcium TG/glucose intolerance In DM - gastroparesis and fluctuating blood sugars Anemia Poor appetite Nausea Abdominal pain	Histories: medical, social, diet, drug, weight patterns Medical intervention goals Biochemical Drug/nutrient interactions Functional status/ ADLs Clinical status/GI function/number of days of dialysis/ week/ vital signs Goals of therapy Education/discharge planning Determine needs: Kcal: 30 - 35/kg IBW adjust for obesity Protein: based on GFR ml/min gm/kg 20 - 25 0.8 gm/kg 15 - 20 0.7 gm/kg 10 - 15 0.6 gm/kg 5 - 10 0.5 gm/kg Fluid: 750 ccs + urine output Electrolyte: restrict Na K, PO$_4$ as needed Vitamins: nephrocaps Minerals: standard supplement PRN	**Phase 1 and 2** Formulate care plan Implement diet order Recommend renal vitamins + iron Recommend baseline nutrition labs Document care Communicate care **Phase 3** Monitor intake, I&Os, albumin and electrolytes, vital signs Monitor blood sugars if DM Start education process Communicate any concerns Document progress of care plan and education Adjust care plan as medical condition and/or therapy necessitates Evaluate/adjust goals of therapy **Phase 4** Discharge summary and refer for further follow-up	Decrease uremic symptoms Minimize tissue catabolism/ maintain LBM Retard the progression of renal failure Normalize fluid balance Maintain/ improve weight Minimize tissue catabolism/ maintain LBM Correct anemia Comprehension of and adherence to dietary restrictions If patient assessed with inadequate nurition knowledge have a plan for continuum of care

System/ Diagnosis	Potential Problems/ Indicators	Assessment	Intervention/ Monitoring/ Education	Possible Desired Outcome(s)
Renal Peritoneal Dialysis LOS 1 - 5 days	PCM Anorexia Fluid imbalance Electrolyte imbalance Elevated TG level CHO intolerance Anemia Infection Obesity Minerals - excess or deficiency Protein losses Edema Muscle wasting Hypertension SOB Catabolism	Histories: medical, social, diet, drug, weight patterns Medical goals Biochemical Drug/nutrient interactions Functional status Clinical status/GI function/number of days of dialysis/ week/vital signs Goals of therapy Education needs Discharge planning Determine needs: Kcal/Kg IBW 25 - 35/maintenance 35 - 50/repletion 20 - 25/reduction 35 with DM Protein: 1.2 - 1.3/ maintenance 1.5/repletion Fluid: 750 cc + urine output Electrolytes: K: 2 - 3 gms; Na: 2 - 4 gms; PO_4 1.0 - 1.2 gms Vitamins: nehprocaps + Vit E; supplement as needed	**Phase 1 and 2** Formulate care plan Implement diet order Recommend renal vitamins + iron Document care Communicate care **Phase 3** Monitor intake, I&Os, albumin and electrolytes, vital signs Start education process Communicate any concerns Document progress of care plan and education Adjust care plan as medical condition and/or therapy necessitates Evaluate/adjust goals of therapy **Phase 4** Discharge summary and referral	Opitmal intake for sparing of protein for tissue repair and synthesis Prevent anorexia Compensate for protein losses Maintain blood pressure Maintain acceptable fluid status Normalize electrolyte balance Maintain/improve weight Maintain mineral balance Prevent/correct uremia Comprehension of and adherence to dietary needs/ restrictions If patient assessed with inadequate nutriton knowledge have a plan for continuum of care

System/ Diagnosis	Potential Problems/ Indicators	Assessment	Intervention/ Monitoring/ Education	Possible Desired Outcome(s)
Renal **Nephrotic Syndrome** **LOS 5 - 7 days**	Hyperlipidemia Proteinuria Hypertension Edema Hypotension Catabolism Protein malnutrition Weight loss Poor appetite Low albumin < 2.5 - 2.0 gm/dl	Histories: medical, social, diet, drug, Weight patterns Biochemical Drug/nutrient interactions Functional status/ ADLs Clinical status/GI function/vital signs Goals of therapy Education/ Discharge planning Determine needs: Kcal: 35- 40/kg IBW Protein: 0.6 - 1.0 gm/kg dependent on GFR, plus gm/gm replacement of urinary protein losses Lipids: 30 - 35% Fluid: unrestricted unless output is < 1L Electrolytes: Na: 1 - 3 gm/day K: no restriction Vitamins: if less than 60 gm protein supplement with niacin, riboflavin, thiamin + 1000- 1500 calcium	**Phase 1 and 2** Formulate care plan Implement diet order Recommend B vitamins + Ca Recommend baseline nutrition labs Document/ communicate care **Phase 3** Monitor intake, I&Os, albumin and electrolytes, weight, GFR, urinary protein losses, lipid profile, vital signs Start education process Communicate any concerns Document progress of care plan and education Adjust care plan as medical condition and/or therapy necessitates Evaluate/adjust goals of therapy **Phase 4** Discharge summary and referral	Correct edema Correct proteinuria Control HTN Slow progression of renal disease Prevent muscle catatbolism Provide adequate nutrients Achieve/maintain edema-free IBW Decrease albumin excretion Slow rate of GFR decline Comprehension of and adherence to any dietary recommendations If patient is determined to have inadequate nutrition knowledge, plan for continuum of care

References

- Co-ordinated Care. University of Washington Medical Center, 1996.

- Diagnostic Nutrition Care Plans. University of Washington Medical Center, 1997.

- Bower, KA: Developing and Using Critical Paths. In: Lord, J, ed. The Physician Leader's Guide. Rockville, MD: Quality Letter, 1991.

- Price, J and Crawley, M: Case Management: Impact on Dietitians. CNM 1993; No 4..

- Lykins, TC: Nutrition Support Clinical Pathways. Nutr in Clin Pract 1996; 11:16.

- Palmer, RM: Acute hospital care of the elderly: minimizing the risk of functional decline. Cleveland Clin J of Med 1995; Mar/Apr.

- Ellwood, PM: Outcomes management: a technology of patient experience. N. Eng J Med 1988; 318:1549.

- Zeman, FJ: Clinical Nutrion and Dietetics. New York: McMillan, 1991.

- Manual of Clinical Dietetics. Chicago, IL: American Dietetic Asosciation, 1993.

- St. Anthony's DRG Guidebook. Reston VA, 1997.

NUTRITION ASSESSMENT OF THE PEDIATRIC PATIENT

Substantial changes in growth, body composition and development occur during the period between birth and adolescence. Nutrient needs, nutritional risks, feeding skills and behaviors and growth patterns change as the individual moves from the newborn period into adolescence. **Table 1** lists developmental characteristics for pediatric patients at various stages. Major illness, injury and surgery impose increased metabolic demands on individuals with preexisting high energy/protein needs for growth and, in the case of infants and young children, with little reserve.

Protein-Energy-Malnutrition (PEM) occurs in 20 - 40% of hospitalized pediatric patients with as high as 60% in infants less than three months old. Factors that can affect their nutritional status are psychological stress of being hospitalized, meals withheld secondary to diagnostic tests, rotation of staff at frequent intervals. Metabolic stress, failure to help feed those who requiring assistance, failure to replace spilled meals, inappropriate or lack of use of enteral nutrition, failure to recognize increased needs and inadequate supervision of meal times also contribute to poor nutritional status.

Pediatric patients are at high risk for growth failure and PEM during acute and chronic illness as demonstrated in **Table 2**. This is secondary to the following:

- Decreased reserves
- Increased needs for growth
- Alteration in fuel metabolism during illness or injury
- Hypermetabolism during illness and injury
- Altered intake due to anorexia, fatigue, or intolerance

PEM and growth failure, additionally have been associated with specific disease states (cancer, HIV, liver disease, renal disease, cystic fibrosis/respiratory disease, GI dysfunction) secondary to the following:

- Altered metabolism
- Altered utilization
- Malabsorbtion
- Anorexia
- Decreased intake
- Medical/drug therapies
- Altered needs

Malnutrition may impact recovery negatively and contribute to prolonged hospital stays or rehospitalizations. In providing nutritional support to the pediatric patient, consideration should be given to the following:

- Age/gender
- Disease states
- Developmental stage/needs
- Growth phase/needs

Table 1: Characteristics of Pediatric Patients

Age	Growth	Development	
Birth - 6 months	20 - 25 g/d weight gain. Doubles birthweight by 4 - 5 months of age.	Root, suck-swallow-breath coordination. Transitions: head control, rolling over, sitting, grasping objects, transferring objects, mouthing objects.	Nipples liquids from bottle or breast fed by caregiver.
6 months - 1 year	15 g/d weight gain, Triples birthweight by one year of age.	Mature suck pattern. Disappearance of root reflex by 6 months. Grasps and brings objects to mouth. Transitions: Munching/chewing occurs. Sits alone. Pincer grasp. Tongue can maneuver food and lick off lower lip. Reaches.	Transition to semisolid and solid foods. Voluntary acceptance and rejection of food occurs. Self feeding skills emerge.
1 - 5 years	Average yearly weight gain approximates 2.3 kg/year. Birthweight quadruples by 2 years of age. Height doubles between 3 - 4 years.	Walking, fine motor and language skills emerging and being refined. Socialization skills emerging and being refined.	Participation in family life and socialization relating to food/meals.
School age	Average yearly increments in weight gain approximate 2.3 kg/year until 9 - 10 years.		Asserts independence regarding food choices.
Adolescence	Adolescent growth spurt occurs with a rapid increase in rate of weight gain and height. Changes are accompanied by changes in body proportion and body composition. 3 x birth length by 13 years.		Independence. Changing self/body image. Sexual maturation. Peer acceptance influences food choices and eating patterns. Tendency to skip meals, increased snacking on fast foods, candy, pop. Risk taking behavior may be of concern.

Table 2: Disease States Associated with Growth Failure and Protein Calorie Malnutrition:

Disease States	Comments	Nutrition Implications
Cancer	Severe malnutrition associated with advanced cancer and treatment. Factors include anorexia, taste changes, side effects of treatment and diminished oral intake. Fever, infection and tumor growth may increase metabolic rate and energy needs. If malabsorbtion is present, additional vitamin/mineral deficits may occur.	Protein Energy Additional vitamin/mineral deficits may occur with malabsorbtion and drug-nutrient interactions.
Cystic Fibrosis and respiratory disease.	Increased energy needs secondary to increased work of breathing. Infections further increase energy needs. Anorexia and increased work of breathing may further diminish intake (infants have difficulty coordinating suck-swallow-breathing with increased respiratory rates). Malabsorbtion of fats and fat soluble vitamins occur with CF. Drug-nutrient interactions may impact growth and nutrient needs.	Energy. Fat soluble vitamins. Check individual medications for impact on vitamin/mineral/electrolyte status.
GI dysfunction with malabsorbtion (IBD, Crohn's Disease, Short Bowel Syndrome).	Nutritional issues related to degree of malabsorbtion. Malabsorbtion of carbohydrate, fat, protein and vitamin/minerals may occur. With short bowel syndrome, the site and length of bowel loss will influence specific nutrient issues.	IBD/Crohn's Disease Protein Energy Fat/fat soluble vitamins Folate Iron Zinc Short Bowel Syndrome Fluid/electrolytes CHO/Fat malabsorption Energy Fat soluble vitamins minerals (Ca, Zn) Loss of distal ileum → B_{12} deficiency.
HIV	Failure to thrive is common in HIV infected children. Chronic infections and diarrhea lead to increased needs and malabsorbtion of nutrients.	Energy Vitamins/minerals due to malabsorbtion and diarrhea. Fluid and electrolytes
Liver Disease	Growth failure and PEM are associated with poor intake, malabsorbtion and altered utilization. Alterations in CHO and fat tolerance may occur.	Protein Energy Fat/fat soluble vitamins Calcium Hypo/hyperglycemia Hypertriglyceridemia Fluid/electrolyte imbalance

Table 2: Disease States Associated with Growth Failure and Protein Calorie Malnutrition

Disease States	Comments	Nutrition Implications
Renal Disease	Infants and children with renal failure may be catabolic. Intake may be diminished secondary to fluid intolerance and anorexia.	Energy Protein Fluid and electrolytes Calcium Vitamin D

Adapted from: Pediatric Nutrition Support Guidelines ASPEN Board of Directors Vol 17 No 4 Supplement July-August 1993

MEDICAL NUTRITION CARE PROCESS FOR THE PEDIATRIC PATIENT

Ongoing nutrition assessment is an integral part of the nutritional support of the pediatric patient. An initial assessment/screening provides baseline data and identifies risks in all patients as identified in Pediatric Screening form **Figure 1**. **Figure 2** demonstrates the screening criteria used for acute care pediatrics/adolescence. In addition to identifying specific nutrient alterations, baseline data should be collected on all patients to permit serial monitoring of nutritional status. No single procedure identifies growth failure secondary to malnutrition. Nutrition assessment includes the evaluation of clinica, anthropometric, laboratory and dietary information as demonstrated in **Table 3**.

Figure 1: Pediatric Screening Form

S: _____

Wt. Change   N   V   D   Appetite Change   Dysphagia/chewing difficulty

Yes   No   NA   Yes   No   NA   Yes   No   NA

Vitamin / mineral supplement   Food Allergies

Yes   No   Specify:

Special diet

Drugs: prescription   Over-the-counter

O: _____

Age _____   Wt _____ kg _____ % ile   Wt/Ht _____ % ile

Ht _____ cm _____ % ile   Head Circumference _____ % ile

Labs: Hct: _____ Hbg: _____ Albumin: _____ Others: _____

Diagnosis: _____ Diet Order _____

A: _____

Nutritional Status:

☐ High Risk   ☐ Moderate Risk   ☐ Not Compromised

Comments:

P: _____

☐ Provide Basic Nutrition Services: Reevaluate in 6 days

☐ Screening data not available, please order: _____

☐ Nutrition Assessment

☐ Nutrient Intake Analysis (NIA)

☐ Nutrition Counseling

Other:

R.D./D.T. Signature _____ Date _____

Figure 2: Nutritional Risk Criteria for Pediatrics/Adolescence

Criteria for determining Nutritional Risk	Low s Risk	Moderate Risk	High Risk
Diagnosis	HIV positive Hypertension Cardiac Disease Controlled DM Nutritional anemia	Moderate Risk AIDS Burns < 20 % BA Cancer Cerebral palsy Chronic lung disease DM - new onset or uncontrolled Esophogeal stricture Intestinal obstruction Pica Pneumonia TF or PN dependent Recent hospitalization Pregnancy	High Risk ARF Cystic fibrosis Congential heart disease Crohn's disease Eating disorders Failure to thrive GER Malnutrition Malabsorption/ maldigestion Major abdominal surgery Pancreatitis Prematurity Short bowel syndrome Ulcerative colitis Sepsis Inborn errors of metabolism Multiple trauma Increased nutrient requirements
Weight loss*	None	< 5% in 1 month growth deceleration	> 5% in one month
Weight/height ratio			< 90th percentile of standard
Labs: ++ albumin prealbumin	3.5 gm/dL > 17 mg/dL	2.8 - 3.4 gm/dL 11 - 17 mg/dL	< 2.8 gm/dL < 10 mg/dL
Subjective Factors	Good/fair appetite Chewing problems Nausea Constipation Assistance with feeding	Poor appetite Trouble swallowing Diarrhea Vomiting Cl liquid > 3 days	No appetite Aspiration risk NPO/cl liquid > 3 days

++ *Varies with age group*
Weight loss is not expected in the young pediatric patient (< two years) and may constitute a higher risk factor

Table 3: Nutrition Assessment Data

Clinical	Anthropometric	Laboratory	Dietary
Dental Exam Medical History Physical Exam	Weight, length or height, head circumference, growth percentiles on NCHS growth charts (as appropriate), Triceps skinfold, mid-arm muscle circumference.	Hgb, hct, albumin, total protein, total lymphocyte count, blood urea nitrogen, transferrin, prealbumin, retinol binding protein, specific vitamins and minerals.	Typical intake pattern; vitamin/mineral supplements; calculation of calories, protein and other nutrients as indicated (oral, enteral, parenteral); I/O for assessment of hydration status

Adapted from ASPEN Nutritional Support Guidelines Vol 17 No 4 Supplement July-August 1993

Some of the tests and procedures used for nutrition assessment have not been validated in pediatric patients and may not reflect nutritional status accurately in this population. Laboratory values should be compared to pediatric reference standards. (See Biochemical Assessment section)

ANTHROPOMETRIC ASSESSMENT

In healthy infants and children, growth proceeds at predictable rates. Deviations in rate and pattern of growth of an individual pediatric patient indicates a need for further evaluation.

The National Center for Health Statistics growth curves commonly are used to evaluate growth in infants and children. (See the end of chapter.) Incremental Growth Charts also are available. These charts allow for evaluation of deviations in rate of growth. In the adolescent patient, information about stage of sexual maturation will influence interpretation of growth information. The prepubescent adolescent experiences an acceleration in growth with increased weight gain followed by accelerated gain in stature.

Weight Gain Calculated from 50% of NCHS Growth Grids

Age	Weight Gain
0 - 4 months	20 - 25 g/d
5 - 12 months	15 g/d
12 - 18 months	8 g/d
18 - 24 months	6 g/d
2 - 7 years	38 g/month
7 - 9 years	56 - 62 g/month
9 - 11 years	67 - 77 g/month
11 - 13 years	85 - 110 g/month
13 - 18 years*	6 g/d females; 13 g/d male

* May not reflect growth of prepubescent adolescent

The following growth patterns require further evaluation and may indicate the need for nutrition intervention:
- Weight loss
- Weight and/or stature < 10% or > 90% for age on NCHS growth charts
- Weight/stature < 10% or > 90% on NCHS growth charts
- Rate of weight gain less than expected for age
- Rate of gain in length or height less than expected for age
- Failure to maintain growth in channel (decrease in percentiles over time

Failure to thrive (FTT) is defined as failure to gain in height and/or weight at the expected rate for age and gender. It is identified by evaluation of growth rates rather than absolute size. Weight/stature > 90% indicates overweight. Weight/stature < 10% indicates underweight. The child receiving inadequate energy demonstrates a decline in rate of weight gain before stature is impacted. Under these circumstances, weight/stature declines across channels to < 10%. Chronic undernutrition will result in a decline in rate of growth in stature. Weight/length under these circumstances may fall within normal ranges (stunting).

The presentation of Protein-Energy-Malnutrition (PEM) varies with the degree and duration of protein/energy deficits, age of individual and modifications produced by any associated vitamin/mineral/trace element deficiencies. The most severe presentations include the following:

Kwashiorkor: FTT, edema, irritability and lethargy and changes in skin, hair and mucous membranes. (See Clinical Assessment section)

Marasmus: FTT, irritability, apathy and wasting with significant decrease in subcutaneous fat.

Several classification systems have been used to identify PEM. One is illustrated below.

	> 90% ht for age	< 90% ht for age
> 80% wt for age	NORMAL	SHORT
< 80% wt for age	WASTED	STUNTED

Gomez developed a system for classifying severity based on percent of expected weight for age.

Severity	Standard
Normal	> 90% expected weight for age
Mild or 1st degree	89 - 75% expected weight for age
Moderate or 2nd degree	74 - 60% expected weight for age
Severe or 3rd degree	< 60% expected weight for age

DIETARY ASSESSMENT

A number of tools are available for evaluating an individual patient's dietary intake. The tool used and data collected will be influenced by the identified concerns and the setting. For the hospitalized patient, it is possible to collect intake information during the period of hospitalization. This data may not reflect an individuals usual dietary practices. A diet history, food frequency questionnaire, 3 - 7 day food record, or a 24 hour recall are often used in an outpatient setting to obtain diet history information. The information obtained may be limited by patient/caregiver memory and willingness to share, accuracy of the reporting (particularly portion size) and whether information reflects patient's usual intake. In addition to quantifying intake of individual nutrients, primarily energy and protein, eating patterns that might be problematic can be identified using these tools, (e.g., The absence of dairy products might indicate a concern for calcium intake.)

A quick simple nutrition assessment consists of measurement of weight and height, head circumference and serum albumin. Rate of weight gain is indicative of nutrient intake. After significant failure to gain weight, height velocity is delayed.

NUTRITION SUPPORT OF THE PEDIATRIC PATIENT

To identify the patient in need of nutrition support, some form of nutrition assessment and/or screening must be be performed when the patient is admitted to the hospital and at subsequent intervals.

Nutrition support of the pediatric patient should be designed to correct any identifiable deficits, prevent deviations from expected growth rates of the individual patient and allow resumption of normal growth patterns in individuals where deviations have occurred. Support should take into account the patient's capability for oral feeding and family/patient food preferences. Whenever possible, support established in the hospital that is to continue after hospitalization should allow the patient to resume normal dietary practices and participate in family meals whenever possible. Nutrition support may include any one or a combination of the following:

Stages of Nutrition Support

Voluntary Oral Intake	Continued oral feeding with nutrition counseling and oral supplementation when appropriate.
Enteral Nutrition Support	Supplemental or total tube feeding as indicated by one of several possible routes (NG, OG, gastrostomy, jejunostomy).
Parenteral Support	Partial or total infusion of fat, CHO, protein, vitamins and minerals, centrally or peripherally.

ENTERAL NUTRITION

Enteral nutrition is the preferred method of nutrition support when the gastrointestinal tract can be used and the patient is unable to meet nutrient needs with voluntary oral intake. Enteral nutrition supports GI growth and development and promotes mucosal integrity and GI motility. As with the adult population, there are many indicators for enteral support. Growth failure or malnutrition with an inability to replete by voluntary oral intake may require enteral support. Prematurity and a range of disorders of absorption, digestion, excretion, utilization and storage of nutrients may indicate the need for complete or supplementary enteral support in the patient who is unable to meet his/her needs by voluntary oral intake.

Indication for Enteral Support

Suck-Swallow-Difficulties	Prematurity Respiratory distress Oral-motor or neurologic deficits
Esophageal Anomalies	
Hypermetabolism	
Failure to thrive	Inability or failure to respond to voluntary oral repletion
Cystic Fibrosis	
Renal dysfunction	
Congenital heart disease	
Alteration in gastrointestinal function	Short Gut syndrome IBD Crohns disease
Chronic liver failure	

Formula Selection

To promote optimal growth and development, formula selection should be based on nutritional requirements (calorie, protein, water, vitamins and minerals). Standard infant formulas meet the nutritional needs of infants less than one year of age. Clinical status, disease state and GI function are additional factors to consider. For the hypermetabolic individual modifying the formula to increase caloric density may be necessary to meet energy needs.

Infant formulas are recommended for children less than one year of age. With some modification, these formulas also may meet the needs of some infants beyond one year of age. There are also enteral products designed for the child one to six years of age. These enteral nutrition products should contain less protein (< 18% of calories from protein) and electrolytes than adult formulas thus reducing renal solute load. Higher calcium, phosphorus and vitamin D also are needed to meet the increased needs of this age group. For further information, refer to Barness: *Pediatric Nutrition Handbook for AAP* (American Academy of Pediatrics) Guidelines for Tube Feeding composition for use under 4 years of age).

Route of Delivery

Route selected for tube feeding depends on the anticipated duration of feeding, condition of the gastrointestinal tract, the potential for aspiration and the reason for tube feeding. Feedings may be administered as gastric, duodenal, or jejunal feeds. Gastric feedings are used when the risk for aspiration is minimal and allow utilization of the entire GI tract for absorption and digestion. Nasogastric or oral gastric tubes may be placed. When tube feedings are anticipated to be long term, a gastrostomy tube may be used. Gastric feedings may be administered intermittently or continuously.

Duodenal or jejunal feedings are used when there is an increased risk of aspiration and delayed gastric emptying and/or reflux. Duodenal or jejunal feedings are administered continuously.

Enteral Feeding Site	Comments
Orogastric	May be useful in infants who are obligate nasal breathers. Doesn't require surgery.
Nasogastric	Requires partially functioning GI tract. Doesn't require surgery. May cause nasal necrosis and esophagitis.

Note: Gastric feeding may not be tolerated by patients with delayed gastric emptying, reflux, or risk of aspiration

Nasoduodenal/jejunal	Sometimes indicated in patients with GE refflux and risk of aspiration. Surgery not required. Tube placement may be more difficult than gastric tube placement. Residuals cannot be checked. Complications may include bacterial overgrowth or bowel perforation.
Gastrostomy	Often indicated when need for tube feeding is long term. Surgery and stoma care required. Potential problems include leakage or tube displacement. Easy access and frees oral/nasal cavity from tube placement.

| Jejunostomy | Used when long term feeding is needed in patient at risk for aspiration and delayed gastric emptying. May require surgery. Stoma care required. Potential problems with leakage and tube displacement. |

Administration

Tube feedings are administered either continuously or as intermittent feeding. Decisions regarding administration of tube feedings depend on route of infusion, patient tolerance and functioning of GI tract. Continuous drip feedings may be tolerated better in patients with volume intolerance, malabsorbtion, or alterations in GI motility. In certain disease states, continuous drip feeds may improve growth and nutrient balance. Intermittent feeding allows freedom from the pump to normalize daily activities and is viewed by some as more physiologic.

Isotonic feedings may be initiated and advanced at full strength, at small volumes. The volume of administration and advancement rates depends on the patient's age, size, tolerance, reason for initiating tube feeding and whether the feedings are delivered continuously or intermittently. A number of methods have been used to initiate and advance feeding volume.

When initiating feedings at 10 - 20 cc/kg/d and advancing at 20 - 30 cc/kg/d, the following methods might be used:

Weight		Intermittent q 3 hours	Continuous
4 kg	Initiate	5 - 10 cc/feed	2 - 3 cc/hr
	Advance	Increase 1 - 2 cc/feed	Increase 1 cc/hr every 8 - 12 hours
20 kg	Initiate	25 - 50 cc/feed	8 - 16 cc/hr
	Advance	Increase 3 cc/feed	Increase 2 cc/hr every 8 hours

Individual patients who have no history of intolerance may be advanced more rapidly, with ongoing assessment of tolerance to the increased volumes.

Nutrient Requirements

The 1989 Recommended Dietary Allowances provide an initial estimate of nutrient needs. These recommendations were developed for a healthy population and represent average intakes that maintain good health over time. Individual nutrients may need to be adjusted based on disease states, increased needs or losses, alterations in metabolism or utilization, or drug-nutrient interactions. Disease specific states associated with hypermetabolism may result in significantly increased energy needs for individual patients.

Table 4 demonstrates the RDA for select nutrients by age.

Table 4: RDA for Select Nutrients by Age

Nutrient	0 - 6 months	6 mo - 1 year	1 - 3 years	4 - 6 years	7 - 10 years	11 - 14 years	15 - 18 years
Energy	108 kcal/kg/d	98 kcal/kg/d	102 kcal/kg/d	90 kcal/kg/d	70 kcal/kg/d	47 (F) and 55 (M) kcal/kg/d	40 (F) and 45 (M) kcal/kg/d
Protein	13 g	14 g	16 g	24 g	28 g	45-46g	44 F 59 M
Calcium	400 mg	600 mg	800 mg	800 mg	800 mg	1200 mg	1200 mg
Phosphorus	300 mg	500 mg	800 mg	800 mg	800 mg	1200 mg	1200 mg
Iron	6 mg	10 mg	10 mg	10 mg	10 mg	15 F 12 M	15 F 12 M
Zinc	5 mg	5 mg	10 mg	10 mg	10 mg	12 F 15 M	12 F 15 M
Vitamin A	375 µgRE	375	400	500	700	800 F 1000 M	800 F 1000 M
Vitamin D	7.5 µg	10	10	10	10	10	10

Estimation of energy needs may also be calculated using the following equations in Table 5.

Table 5: Estimation of Energy Needs

Weight	Energy
Up to 10 kg	100 kcal/kg/d
11 - 20 kg	1000 + 50 kcal for each kg > 10
> 20 kg	1500 + 20 kcal for each kg > 20

Behrman RE & Nelson Textbook of Pediatrics 14th edition WB Saunders 1992

These guidelines are for healthy infants and children. The nutrient needs of children with acute and chronic illness are often altered by disease states and medical therapies. Therefore, it is critical to monitor a patient's response to therapy and adjust nutrient recommendations on an individual basis.

Fluid Requirements

Water is needed to replace losses (from skin, lungs, feces and urine) and to provide for growth. Water is needed to handle the solute load presented to the kidneys. The amount of water needed, therefore, is a function of the quantity of solute presented to the kidneys and the renal concentrating abilities. Individual's water needs may vary considerably, particularly in the young infant, secondary to renal immaturity. There are several formulas for estimating fluid requirements for infants and children are demonstrated in **Table 6**.

Table 6: Estimated Water Requirements

Age	Water Requirement (ml/kg/d)
Neonate	80 - 150
Birth - 6 months	130 - 160
6 months - 1 year	120 - 155

1 - 2 years	115 - 135
4 years	100 - 110
6 year	90 - 100
10 years	70 - 85
14 years	50 - 60
18 years	40 - 50

Adapted from Berman RE, Kleigman and RM Nelson. Textbook of Pediatrics

The Food and Nutrition Board recommends 1.5 ml/kcal energy expenditure for infants and children. Fomon recommends basing fluid recommendations for infants on renal solute load (RSL) and renal concentrating ability. Renal concentrating ability in a healthy infant is 900 - 1100 mosm/L. Potential renal solute load (PRSL) refers to solutes that need to be excreted in the urine if none are diverted for synthesis of new tissue and not lost through nonrenal routes. It is assumed that all dietary nitrogen is converted to urea. PRSL can be calculated by the following equation:

$$PRSL = Na + Cl + K + P + (protein/175)$$
with Na, Cl, K and P in mmols and protein in mg.

Prediction of urine concentrating ability may be estimated with the following equation:

$$Urine\ concentration = RSL/\ wf\ L/day - we\ L/day$$
$$(mOs/L) \qquad (mOs/day)$$

Where **wf** is water from food and **we** is extrarenal water.

Attention to water balance is particularly important in patients with altered or immature renal function, patients requiring fluid restriction and patients receiving concentrated formulas.

Electrolyte Requirements for Enteral Nutrition

Estimated sodium, chloride and potassium requirements are given below in **Table 7**.

Table 7: Electrolyte Requirements

Age	Weight (kg)	Sodium	Chloride	Potassium
0 - 5 months	4.5	120 mg	180 mg	500 mg
6 - 12 months	8.9	200	300	700
1 year	11	225	350	1000
2 - 5 years	16	300	500	1400
6 - 9 years	25	400	600	1600
10 - 18 years	50	500	750	2000

Complications and Monitoring

Monitoring of response to therapy, tolerance to feeding and the occurrence of complications is similar to the monitoring of older tube-fed patients, (Refer to section on Enteral Nutrition). Nutrition assessment is the key to monitoring response to therapy. This includes evaluating growth and other anthropometric parameters, biochemical indices and input and output. Adjustments may be made over time when over or underestimates of energy needs occur. Adjustments for growth also are required over time in the pediatric patient.

Enteral feedings complications may be mechanical, gastrointestinal, or metabolic. Gastrointestinal and metabolic problems may be corrected by changing formulas, rates, route, or method or infusion. Mechanical problems include tube occlusion or malposition. Tube position should be checked periodically and the tube should be irrigated properly.

PARENTERAL NUTRITION

Indications

Parenteral nutrition is indicated for pediatric patients who are unable to meet their needs enterally either secondary to inability to utilize the GI tract, poor tolerance, or hypermetabolic states in which increased needs cannot be met enterally. Indications for parenteral nutrition include the following:

Gastrointestinal Disorders
　　Malrotation
　　Meconium ileus
　　Hirschsprung's disease
　　Gastroschisis
　　Intestinal anomalies and atresia
　　Intractable diarrhea
　　Short-bowel syndrome
　　Chronic idiopathic intestinal pseudo-obstruction

Hypermetabolism
　　Severe trauma and burns

Malignancies/bone marrow transplants

Inflammatory bowel disease

Gastrointestinal fistulas

Renal failure

Pancreatitis

Hepatic failure

Chylothorax and chylous ascites

Parenteral solutions may be infused either peripherally or centrally. Peripheral parenteral nutrition is often used when parenteral support is needed short term and there is adequate peripheral access. Infusion of parenteral solutions through a central vein allows for delivery of higher concentrations of nutrients, particularly dextrose concentrations greater than D12.5. It is chosen often when there is limited peripheral access, a need for high concentrations of dextrose or the need for parenteral support is longer than two weeks.

Composition

Parenteral nutrition usually is composed of carbohydrate such as dextrose, protein as amino acids, fat, electrolytes, vitamins, minerals and trace elements. **Carbohydrates** typically provide 60 - 70% of the total calories of parenteral formulas. Excess calories as carbohydrate should be avoided and typical infusions should not exceed 12 - 14 mg/kg/min.

Fat provides EFA and additional calories. Fat is added to a maximum of 3 - 4 g/kg/d as tolerated. Less than 3 gm/g/d for young infants.

Protein is provided as essential and nonessential amino acids. Standard pediatric amino acid solutions are available. Protein needs decrease with age from approximately 3 g/kg/d for preterm infants to 1 - 2 g/kg/d in adults. Sepsis, burns and protein-losing enteropathies may increase need. The patient with renal or hepatic failure may need protein restriction balancing need with tolerance.

Frequent monitoring and adjustment of the content may be necessary.

Table 8: Vitamin Requirements for Parenteral Nutrition.

Vitamin	Dose / Day
A	700 μg
E	7 mg
K	200 μg
D	10 μg
C	80 mg
Thiamin	1.2 mg
Riboflavin	1.4 mg
Pyridoxine	1 mg
Niacin	17 mg
Pantothenate	5 mg
Biotin	20 μg
Folate	140 μg
B_{12}	1 μg

From Greene et al Am J Clin Nutr 48:1324 1988

Table 9: Mineral Requirements for Parenteral Nutrition

Nutrient	
Calcium*	500 - 600 mg/L
Phosphorus*	400 - 450 mg/L
Magnesium*	50 - 70 mg/l
*Assumes average fluid intake of	120 - 150 ml/kg/d
Zinc	250 μg/kg/d < 3 months of age 100 μg/kg/d > 3 months of age Children 50 μg/kg/d (max 5000 μg/d)
If TPN > 4 weeks add the following: Copper Selenium Chromium Manganese Molybdenum Iodide	20 μg/kg/d (max 300 μg/d) 2 μg/kg/d (max 30 μg/d) 0.2 μg/kg/d (max 5 μg/d) 1 μg/kg/d (max 50 μg/d) 0.25 μg/kg/d (max 5 μg/d) 1 μg/kg/d (max 1 μg/d)

From Greene, Am J Clin Nutrition 48:1324, 1988

Note: Manganese and copper should be omitted in patients with obstructive jaundice. Chromium, Selenium and Molybdenum should be omitted in patients with renal dysfunction.

Iron has not been added routinely to parenteral solutions because of concerns regarding adverse reactions and questions regarding appropriate dose.

Iron is recommended for patients on long-term PN, patients not receiving frequent blood transfusions and patients without medical conditions that predispose to iron overload. A patient initially should be evaluated for iron deficiency. 100 ug/kg/d is the recommended dose for term infants.

Electrolytes

Electrolyte requirements vary considerably relative to age, disease states, fluid status, medical therapies and renal function. The following recommendations are guidelines and not absolute requirements.

Sodium	3 - 4 meq/kg/d
Potassium	2 - 3 meq/kg/d
Chloride	2 - 4 meq/kg/d

Frequent monitoring and adjustment of electrolyte content may be necessary.

Complications and Monitoring

Parenteral nutrition complications include mechanical, metabolic and infectious. Mechanical and infectious complications may be reduced by technique and adherence to strict protocols related to care of parenteral lines and sites.

Metabolic complications may occur secondary to infusate composition or rate, or patient utilization or tolerance. Careful monitoring and adjustment of the infusate may reduce the incidence of metabolic complications or correct complications when they occur. See the sections *Complications of Parenteral Nutrition* and *Nutrition Support* in the following section on *Premature and Low Birth Weight Infants*.

A number of monitoring schedules have been proposed for patients on PN. As with the low birth weight infant, care should be taken to minimize the volume of blood routinely drawn in patients and to time laboratory monitors with other labs. The AAP recommends the following monitoring schedule for patients on PN:

Serum electrolytes	2 - 3 times/week
Serum urea nitrogen	2 times/week
Calcium/Magnesium/and Phosphorus	2 times/ week
Glucose	Several times daily until stable then 1 time per week
Acid base status	2 - 3 times/week
Serum ammonia	Weekly
Serum protein (i.e., albumin, prealbumin, transferrin)	Weekly
LFT	Weekly
HgB	2 times/week
Urine glucose	Daily
Clinical assessment	Daily
Blood cell count and	As indicated
differential cultures	As indicated
serum triglycerides	As indicated

Adapted from Barnes, LA: Pediatric Nutrition Handbook

Monitoring more frequently occurs during the initial phase of PN support until the patient is stable.

STAFFING

Pediatrics clinical staffing requirements are determined similarly to the adult population. A productivity study and the identification of the population at risk helps determine the number and type of clinical staff needed. Also, consideration must be given to the methods of clinical coverage for inpatients and outpatients. If the philosophy is to staff by service and provide nutrition care to both the inpatient and outpatient population adjustments will need to be made accordingly.

Acuity should examine the activities required, the time required for each activity and the frequency with which the activities need to occur to provide quality nutrition care.

Clinical staffing needs should be based on levels of care. The following levels of care serve as a guideline for staffing pediatric inpatients:

Level 4 Intensity
RD/patient ratio
Intensive Care Units
Nutrition care need

Complex/In-depth
1 RD/15 pediatric patients
Daily monitoring
Every other day documentation

Level 3 Intensity
RD/patient ratio
Med/Surgical units
Nutrition care needs

Major/Advanced
1 RD/16 - 20 patients
Daily monitoring
Every third day documentation

Dietetic Technician
Nutrition care needs

1 DT/20 - 30 patients
Data collection
Teaching class for general nutrition and formula making
Referral to WIC, as appropriate
Referral to community agencies

Level 2 Intensity
RD/patient ratio
Nutrition care needs

Moderate/Intermediate
1:20 - 25 patients
Monitoring as appropriate
Documentation q 4 - 5 days

Dietetic Technician
Nutrition care given

1 DT/30 - 40 patients
Teaching of general nutrition
Referral to WIC/ community agencies

Level 1 Intensity
RD/patient ratio
Nutrition care given

Basic Care
1 RD/50 patients
Monitoring/documentation q 7 days

Dietetic Technician
Nutrition Care given

1DT/100 patients
Referrals to WIC/community agencies

Staffing Model Example

Inpatient Only

Assumptions:

RD is part of the Health Care Team, therefore does not need a consult
Screening needs to be done first 24 hrs
Assessment of high risk in 48 hours
Daily monitoring
Documentation standards q 3 - 5 days

RVUs

Screening	-	15 min
Assessment	-	60 min
Reassessment	-	30 min

Example Hospital

Bed Size		**500**
% Occupancy	85	425
% At nutrition risk	50	213
% High risk	80	170
% Moderate risk	20	43

Time Needed	**RD**	**DT**	
# New admits per day/screens	50	6.25 hours	6.25 hours
# New high risks	25	25.0 hours	
# New moderate risk	5		2.25 hours
# Reassessments per day	63/12	31.5 hours	4.25 hours
Total Hours Needed Per Day		**62.75**	**12.75**

Assumption -	80% time Nutrition care Number of RDs needed	9.8 FTEs
	70% time in Nutrition Care Number of RDs needed	11.2 FTEs

Same Hospital with Adjoining Clinics

Assumption:

100,000 coverage lives
1 FTE RD/20,000 coverage lives
Need 5 FTEs of RDs in clinic

When determining staffing needs, consideration must be given to the fact that, upon discharge, some patients will be managed in the community and some will be managed in the facility's specialty clinics. Each facility needs to establish medical nutrition care coverage best suiting the patient population of that facility. Consideration may be given to staffing according to medical service. The facility still requires the same number of dietitians, but the responsibilities are divided between inpatient and outpatient.

QUALITY IMPROVEMENT

Quality improvement for the pediatric population can be adapted from the quality improvement in the "Nutrition Support Planning and Management" section. The following form can be used to track QI in the oral, enteral or parenteral pediatric patient.

Nutrition Intervention for the Pediatric Patient

Patient	Admit Date	Feeding Modality	Measurable outcome selected	Goal I = improve M = maintain	Outcome score at discharge I or M N/A = data not available	DC Date	Comments on Ø score

CLINICAL NUTRITION PATHWAYS

Pathways are need for the hospitalized infant and adolescence. The following pathway is designed for the adolescent with Crohns disease. This pathway is intended as a guideline for the creation of others.

Clinical Pathway for the Pediatric Patient

System/ Diagnosis	Potential Problems/ Indicators	Assessment	Intervention/ Monitoring/ Education	Possible Desired Outcome(s)
Gastrointestinal	Malnutrition	Medical goals	**Phase 1 and 2**	Optimal nutrition status
	FTT	Hx: medical, social, dietary, drug	Determine feeding modality – if po, modify fat, fiber, lactose; avoid gas-producing foods	• Preserve/ improve LBM
	Inadequate growth	Weight/growth patterns		• Adequate calorie and protein intake for growth
	Protein losing enteropathy	Biochemical Drug/nutrient interactions, Hydration status	Formulate care plan	
	Diarrhea		Recommend baseline labs	Decrease fecal output
	Acute, severe weight loss secondary to diminished food intake and inflammation	Clinical symptoms/ GI function/vital signs Functional status/ ADLs Feeding modality	Document/ communicate plan **Phase 3** Goal: to achieve desired intake via po or EN/PN	Reduce steatorrhea Normalize electrolytes
	Nutrient deficiencies	Education of parents or care giver		Improve hydration status
	Anemia	Goals of therapy	Review labs, I&Os, medical progress, vital signs, electrolytes, weight Start education process	Comprehension and adherence to dietary recommendations by the parents/ care giver
	Fluid retention	Discharge plans		
	Electrolyte Imbalance	Determine needs: Kcal: per age	Communicate any concerns	If it is determined there is inadequate nutrition knowledge, a plan for continuum of care is implemented
	Intolerance to po	Protein: per age Fluid: per age plus losses	Document progress of care plan and education	
		Electrolytes: standard plus replace losses		
		Vitamins: RDA per age and disease	Adjust care plan as medical condition and/or therapy necessitates	
		Minerals: RDA per age and disease	**Phase 4** Discharge summary and referral	

PREMATURE AND LOW BIRTH WEIGHT INFANT

Premature and low birth weight infants have characteristics that place them at immediate nutritional risk. Born early, with limited nutrient reserve and metabolically and physiologically immature, these infants require immediate and careful consideration of their nutrient needs. The nutrition care of the premie begins once survival chances are determined and metabolic stability is evaluated.

DEFINITION

Premature and low birth weight infants are defined by weight and gestational age. The premature infant is an infant born at 36 weeks gestation. The low birth weight infant weighs less than 2.5 kg. Other definitions are described below.

Premature	< 36 weeks gestation
Low Birth Weight (LBW)	< 2.5 kg (5.5 lbs)
Very Low Birth Weight (VLBW)	< 1.5 kg (3.3 lbs)
Extremely Low Birth Weight (ELBW)	< 1.0 kg (2.2 lbs)

CLASSIFICATION

Infants may be classified based on maturity and intrauterine growth. Using intrauterine growth curves (**Figure 3**), an infant may be classified as large for gestational age (LGA), appropriate for gestational age (AGA), or small for gestational age (SGA). Birthweight greater than the 90th percentile for gestational age are classified as LGA. Infants born of diabetic mothers are often LGA. Birthweights less than the 10th percentile for gestational age are classified as SGA. SGA infants may also be referred to as IUGR or intrauterine growth retarded. An SGA infant may be symmetrically growth retarded; that is, weight, length and/or head circumference at less than the 10th percentile, or asymmetrically growth retarded with weight alone at less than the 10th percentile. Timing and duration of the intrauterine insult may influence the symmetry of the growth retardation. A number of factors may contribute to intrauterine growth retardation, including infectious agents (rubella, CMV, toxoplasmosis, syphilis,

Figure 3: Lubchenco Intrauterine Growth Curves

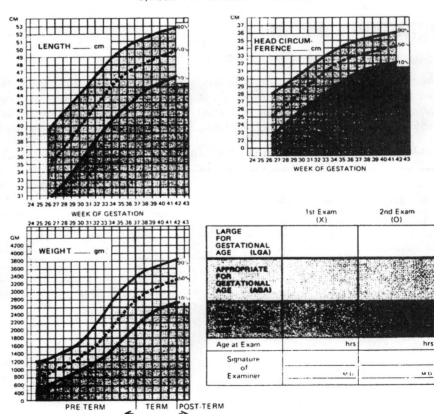

CLASSIFICATION OF NEWBORNS –
BASED ON MATURITY AND INTRAUTERINE GROWTH
Symbols: X - 1st Exam   O - 2nd Exam

Adapted from Lubchenco LC, Hansman C, and Boyd E: Pediatr 37:403, 1966; Battaglia FC, and Lubchenco LC: J Pediatr 71:159, 1967.

herpes), maternal illness (hypertension, renal disease, severe diabetes, malnutrition, toxemia), cigarette smoking and drug abuse, as well as congenital and chromosomal anomalies of the fetus. Classification of a infant as LGA, AGA, or SGA may have implications for early postnatal glucose tolerance, nutritional needs and growth potential.

MEDICAL PROBLEMS

Medical problems frequently seen in the premature infant may impact multiple organ systems and present a major obstacle to providing nutritional support to these infants (**Table 10**).

Table 10: Common Medical Problems of Premature and Low Birth Weight Infants

- Cardiovascular
  Patent ductus arteriosus
- Gastrointestinal
  Hyperbilirubinemia
  Feeding Intolerance
  Necrotizing enterocolitis
- Hematological
  Anemia
- Immunological
  Sepsis
  Pneumonia
  Meningitis

- Metabolic
  Hypoglycemia/hyperglycemia
  Hypocalcemia
  Acidosis
- Neurological
  Intracranial hemorrhage
- Renal
  Fluid and electrolyte imbalance
- Respiratory
  Hyaline membrane disease (Respiratory distress syndrome)
  Bronchopulmonary Dysplasia (BPD)

NUTRITION SUPPORT

Energy and Nutrient Reserves

The premature/low birth weight infant is born prior to accumulating the nutrient reserves of a full term infant. Two thirds of the mineral content of the fetus is accumulated in the last trimester (as shown in **Table 11** for fetal accumulation of calcium and phosphorus). The fat content of the fetus increases from 1 percent to 16 percent of body weight in the last trimester. Estimated energy reserves of an infant by birth weight are shown in **Table 12**.

Table 11: Fetal Calcium, Phosphorus and Magnesium Accretion

| (mg/kg/d) | Gestational Age (weeks) | | | | | | | | | | | |
	25	26	27	28	29	30	31	32	33	34	35	36
Calcium	114	118	121	121	121	120	123	125	130	132	132	130
Phosphorous	65.4	70	72	71	71	71	71	72	74	76	70	80
Magnesium	3.21	3.31	3.37	3.62	3.52	3.2	3.17	3.15	3.14	3.14	3.16	3.18

From: Vitamin and Mineral Requirements in Preterm Infants, Ed: Regina C. Tsang, Marcel Dekker Inc., New York 1985

Table 12: Energy Reserves

Birthweight	Non Protein	Total
500	50	225
800	125	435
1000	165	600
1500	425	1120
2000	1050	1975
3500	4175	5925

With limited nutrient reserves and increased growth rates, the preterm infant has increased requirements for a number of nutrients and a shorter time to depletion when compared to the full term infant. Assuming basal energy needs of approximately 55 - 60 kcal/kg/d, the infant weighing less than 1000 grams may rapidly deplete non-protein energy reserves and begin to catabolize vital tissue protein for energy.

Metabolic and Physiologic Immaturity

Anatomically, the fetal gut by 20 weeks gestation resembles that of a newborn. Functional development, however, is limited prior to 26 weeks gestation, with maturation continuing postnatally. Key developmental issues and their implications for nutritional support are shown in the following table.

Functional Development	Nutritional Implication
Immature suck-swallow-breath coordination appears between 33 and 36 weeks gestation	Impaired nippling ability and increased risk of aspiration and apnea with feeding
Decreased levels of lactase in infants < 34 weeks gestation	Potential for some lactose malabsorption
Decreased lipase and bile acid pool.	Fat intolerance and malabsorption (of long chain fats)
Decreased gastric volume	Volume intolerance
Immature peristaltic and gastricmotility patterns.	Delays in gastric emptying, apparent feeding intolerance (e.g., residuals, regurgitation, abdominal distention) and constipation
Alterations in renal and cardiac function	Fluid and electrolyte imbalance, alteration in protein tolerance – acidosis, azotemia and hyperammonemia

ENTERAL NUTRITION SUPPORT

Advantages

Small amounts of enteral feeding stimulate the production of a number of hormones, including enteroglucagon, gastrin, GIP, motilin and neurotensin, which exert both trophic and motility effects. Enteral feedings also have been associated with improved glucose tolerance and resolution of hyper-bilirubinemia.

Energy Requirements

The preterm infant requires approximately 75 kcal/kg/d to meet maintenance energy needs and 120 - 130 kcal/kg/d for growth approximating intrauterine rates. **Table 13** shows the partitioning of these energy requirements.

Table 13: Energy Requirements of Low Birth Weight Infants

	kcal/kg/d
Basal metabolic rate	50
Activity	15
Cold stress	10
Total Maintenance	75
Specific Dynamic Action	8
Fecal loss	12
Growth	25
Total Additional Requirements	45
Total Energy Needs For Growth	120

Sinclair J., et al Pediatr Clin North Am 17:863 1970

Factors that may alter energy requirements of an individual infant are depicted in **Table 14**.

Table 14: Factors That May Alter Energy Requirements

Trauma/stress

Infection/sepsis

Congenital heart disease/patent ductus arteriosus

Respiratory distress/chronic lung disease

Catch-up growth

Activity

Medications

Increased digestive and absorptive losses

Nutritional Requirements and Advisable Intakes for the Premature Infant

The nutrient requirements of preterm infants are generally higher than those of full term infants. Preterm infants are born with limited body stores, are metabolically and physiologically immature and are expected to grow at increased rates when compared to full term neonates. The exact nutrient requirements for preterm infants (especially the ELBW infant) are still being defined. Recently, a new consensus statement was published accounting for gestational age and weight. Nutrient requirements are defined for three periods (initial, transition and growth). **Table 15** shows the enteral nutritional requirements for the stable, growing, preterm infant.

Table 15: Consensus Recommendations on the Nutritional Needs of the Stable/Growing Enterally Fed Preterm Infant

Energy	120 kcal/kg/d
Protein	3.5 - 4.0 g/kg/d*
Fat Soluble Vitamins	
A	700 - 1500 IU/kg/d
D	150 - 400 IU/kg/d (max 400 IU)
E	6 - 12 IU
K	8 - 10 µg/kg/d
Water Soluble Vitamins	
Vitamin C	18 - 24 mg/d
Thiamin	180 - 240 µg/kg/d
Riboflavin	250 - 360 µg/kg/d
Niacin	3.6 - 4.8 mg/kg/d
Pantothenate	1.2 - 1.7 mg/kg/d
Biotin	3.6 - 6.6 µg/kg/d
Pyridoxin	150 - 210 µg/kg/d
Folate	25 - 50 µg/d
B_{12}	0.3 µg/kg/d
Minerals	
Calcium	120 - 230 mg/kg/d
Phosphorus	60 - 140 mg/kg/d
Magnesium	7.9 - 15 mg/kg/d
Iron	2 mg/kg/d
Zinc	1000 µg/kg/d
Manganese	7.5 µg/kg/d
Copper	120 - 150 µg/kg/d
Iodine	30 - 60 µg/kg/d
Sodium	46 - 69 mg/kg/d
Potassium	78 - 120 mg/kg/d
Chloride	70 - 105 mg/kg/d
Molybdenum	0.3 µg/kg/d
Selenium	1.3 - 3.0 µgkg/d
Chromium	0.1 - 0.5 µg/kg/d

Adapted from Tsang, R: Nutritional Needs of Preterm Infant
*Estimates based on fetal accretion rates. Actual requirements may be influenced by protein quality.

Human Milk versus Formula

The feeding choice for an individual infant should account for desirable growth rate and nutrient accretion as well as metabolic maturity. Human milk offers distinct advantages to the premature infant, providing a feeding that is iso-osmolar and has a low renal solute load. In addition, it provides immunologic and growth factors that may benefit the preterm infant. Certain nutrients, such as fat and iron, are better absorbed from human milk. Preterm infants fed human milk, however, grow at a slower rate than formula fed preterm infants. In addition, the levels of calcium and phosphorus present in human milk do not meet the needs for normal bone mineralization in the preterm infant. Premature formulas have been developed to meet the unique needs of the premature infant, providing increased levels of vitamins and minerals to meet the current guidelines for premature infants at lower volumes than standard formulas. (See **Table 16** for a comparison of: premature and standard formulas). Standard formulas meet the RDA for term infants when an infant consumes approximately one liter of formula, but they do not meet the calcium and phosphorus need of a growing premature infant.

Table 16: Comparison of Premature and Standard Formulas

Premature Formulas	Standard Formulas
24 kcal/oz	20 kcal/oz
Protein: Whey predominant	Protein: whey or casein predominant
CHO: Lactose + glucose polymers	CHO: Lactose
Fat: Medium and long chain triglycerides	Fat: long chain triglycerides
Higher in select vitamins and minerals	Fortified to meet term vitamin and mineral needs
Iso-osmolar	Iso-osmolar

Tables 17/17a shows the nutrient composition of human milk and select standard and premature formulas.

Table 17: Nutrient Composition of Human Milk and Select Standard Formulas per 100 kcal

	Human Milk (term)	Enfamil (20kcal/oz)	Similac (20kcal/oz)
Volume cc	147	148	148
Protein			
Grams	1.54	2.1	2.1
% kcal	6	9	9
Fat			
Source		coconut, soy oil	coconut, soy oil
Grams	5.74	5.3	5.4
% kcal	52	50	48
CHO			
Source	lactose	lactose	lactose
Grams	10.6	10.3	10.7
% kcal	42	41	43

Minerals

Calcium mg	41	78	73
Phosphorus mg	21	53	56
Magnesium mg	5.1	8	6
Iron mg	.04	1.8	1.8
Zinc mg	.18	1.0	0.75
Manganese µg	.9	15	5
Copper µg	37	75	90
Iodine µg	16.2	10	9
Sodium mg	26	27	27
Potassium mg	77	108	105
Chloride mg	62	63	64

Vitamins

A IU	328	300	300
D IU	3	60	60
E IU	.34 (mg)	2	3
K µg	.3	8	8
Thiamin µg	31	80	100
Riboflavin µg	51	140	150
B_6 µg	30	60	60
B_{12} µg	.07	0.3	0.25
Niacin µg	221	1000	1050
Folate µg	7.4	15.6	15
Pantothenate µg	265	500	450
Biotin µg	.6	3	4.4
Vitamin C mg	6	12	9
Choline mg	13.2	12	16
Inositol mg	21.9	17	4.7
Water g	129	134	133
ERSL	11.1	14.2	14.3
Osmolarity (mOsm/liter)	255	270	270

Note: Other formulas are available for standard feeding of full term infants (e.g Gerber, Carnation Good Start, Soy based, Lactofree and Elemental formulas. These formulas, in general, meet the mineral requirements of full term infants. They may vary however in source of CHO, protein and fat.

Table 17a: Nutrient Composition of Select Premature Formulas per 100 kcal (24kcal/oz)

	Similac Special Care	Enfamil Premature Formula
Volume cc	124	124
Protein		
Grams	2.71	3.0
% kcal	11	12
Fat		
Source	MCT, soy and coconut oil	MCT, soy and coconut oil
Grams	5.43	5.1
% kcal	47 4	4
CHO		
Source	Lactose + glucose polymers	Lactose + corn syrup solids
Grams	10.6	11
% kcal	42	44
Minerals		
Calcium mg	180	165
Phosphorus mg	90	83
Magnesium mg	12	7.6
Iron mg	0.37 (1.8)*	0.25 (1.8)*
Zinc mg	1.5	1.56
Manganese μg	12	13
Copper μg	250	130
Iodine μg	6	7.9
Sodium mg	43	39
Potassium mg	129	103
Chloride mg	81	85
Vitamins		
A IU	680	1200
D IU	150	270
E IU	4.0	4.6
K μg	12	13
Thiamin μg	250	250
Riboflavin μg	620	350
B_6 μg	250	250
B_{12} μg	.55	0.3

Niacin μg	5000	4000
Folate μg	37	35
Pantothenate μg	1900	1200
Biotin μg	37	2
Vitamin C mg	37	35
Choline mg	10	7.6
Inositol mg	5.5	4.7
Water g	109	108
ERSL	18.3	18.9
Osmolarity (mOsm/liter)	270	260

Values for iron fortified formula. Tables 17/17a compiled from product information from Ross/Mead Johnson 1989/90

Breast milk does not have a uniform composition. Milk of mothers who deliver preterm differs from milk of mothers delivering at term. The difference appears to be transient and by approximately one month, the milk tends to be similar to term milk. Preterm milk tends to be higher in protein, sodium and possibly other nutrients. **Table 18** shows change in preterm milk over time.

Table 18: Changing Composition of Human Milk: Preterm Versus Term Milk

	Nutrients per 100 cc		
	Preterm < 2 weeks	**Preterm > 3 weeks**	**Term @ 6 weeks**
Protein g	2.4	1.8	1.34
Fat g	3.8	4.0	4.2
CHO g	6.1	7.0	7.0
Sodium mg	50.6	28.9	15
Calcium mg	25	22	35
Phosphorus mg	14	14	15
Copper μg	78	63	39
Zinc μg	475	392	295

Nutrition and Feeding Preterm Infants, Wharton B.A. Blackwell Scientific Publications 1987 pp 8-9

Vitamin and Mineral Supplementation

Vitamin and mineral supplementation depends on the individual infant's nutrient requirements, the formula/milk the infant is fed and the usual volume of formula/milk the infant consumes. (See **Table 19**).

The following exhibit demonstrates how nutrient intake varies based on infant size, volume and type of milk/formula fed.

Nutrient Intake of a 1.5 kg Infant Fed 150 cc/kg/d of Human Milk or a Premature Formula at 24 kcal/oz

Nutrient	Enfamil Premature	Similac Special Care	Human Milk
kcal/kg/d	120	120	105
Protein g/kg/d	3.6	3.3	1.7
A IU	2268	2268	567
D IU	490	272	5
E IU	8	7	0.5 (mg)
C mg	63	67	11.7
Folate µg	63	67	11.7
Calcium mg/kg/d	199	218	50
Phosphorus mg/kg/d	100	109	23

Nutrient Intake of a 2.5 kg Infant Fed 180 cc/kg/d of a Standard Formula at 20 kcal/oz

Nutrient	
kcal/kg/d	120
Protein g/kg/d	2.7
A IU	942
D IU	188
E IU	9.4
C mg	25
Folate µg	47
Calcium mg/kg/d	77 - 91
Phosphorus mg/kg/d	51 - 70
Iron* mg/kg/d	2.3

*Iron fortified formula

Table 19: Vitamin and Mineral Supplementation of Preterm and Low Birth Weight Infants

Human Milk	Enfamil Premature	infant < 1.8 - 2 kg Similac Special Care	Standard
Human Milk fortifier*	Vitamin E	Multiple vitamin supplement which contains Vit E Add A/D for maximum of 1500/400	Usually not fed to infants = 1.8-2.0 kg
Iron**	Iron**	Iron**	Iron**

*Vitamin supplement varies with type of fortifier

Infant > 1.8 - 2 kg	
Standard multivitamin compound Iron**	Usually not fed to infants = 1.8 - 2.0 kg

Adapted from: Nourishing the Premature and Low Birth Weight Infant by Mary O'Leary, in Nutrition in Infancy and Childhood, Peggy Pipes, 4th Ed., Times Mirror/Mosby Publ. 1989
*See Table 20 for composition of currently available human milk fortifiers.
**Preterm infants should receive 2-3 mg/kg/d of iron by 2 months of age. This may be provided as a separate vitamin/ mineral preparation or as iron fortified formula.

Table 20: Nutrient Composition of Human Milk Fortifiers

Natural Care Nutrient	Enfamil Human Milk Fortifier per 4 packets	Similac Human Milk Fortifier per 124 cc
Calories	4	100
Protein g	0.7	2.7
Fat g	< 0.1	5.43
CHO g	2.7	10.6
Vitamins		
A IU	780	680
D IU	210	150
E IU	3.4	4
K µg	9.1	12
Thiamin µg	187	250
Riboflavin µg	250	620
B_6 µg	193	250
B_{12} µg	0.21	0.55
Niacin µg	3100	5000
Folate µg	23	37
Pantothenic acid µg	790	1900
Biotin µg	0.81	37
C mg	24	37
Minerals		
Calcium mg	90	210
Phosphorus mg	45	105
Zinc mg	0.71	1.5
Manganese µg	9	12

Copper µg	80	250
Sodium mg	7	43
Potassium mg	15.6	129
Chloride mg	17.7	81
Osmolarity mOsm/kg H$_2$0	+ 120	300

Note: Enfamil Human Milk Fortifier is a powder added to human milk.
Similac Natural Care Human Milk Fortifier is a liquid added directly to human milk or given as alternate feedings.
Information obtained from product information from Ross Laboratories and Mead Johnson 1990

PARENTERAL NUTRITION

Indications

The need for parenteral nutrition is indicated when the gastrointestinal tract is not functional, when the patient is unable to meet nutrient needs by the enteral route, or when the length of time to achieve adequate intake exceeds infant's nutrient reserves.

Energy and Protein Needs

Premature infants demonstrate adequate growth with parenteral administration of 70 - 90 kcal/kg/d and 2.5 - 3.0 g/kg/d of protein. Provision of 50 - 60 kcal/kg/d and 2 - 2.5 g/kg/d protein is necessary to meet resting metabolic rates and for nitrogen retention to occur. As with enterally fed infants, a number of factors may alter energy expenditure for an individual infant. These estimates assume a relatively inactive infant in a thermoneutral environment.

Maintenance	Growth
50 - 60 kcal/kg/d	70 - 90 kcal/kg/d
2.0 - 2.5 g/kg/d protein	2.5 - 3.0 g/kg/d protein

Vitamin and Mineral Guidelines

The specific requirements for vitamins and minerals in parenteral nutrition are not well known. In addition, difficulty in administering certain nutrients because of solubility (e.g., calcium and phosphorus), adherence of nutrients to tubing or polyvinyl containers (e.g., Vitamin A), environmental losses (e.g., photodegradation) and increased excretion of parenterally administered nutrients (e.g., increased urinary excretion of zinc and copper) must be considered in establishing guidelines for parenteral vitamin and mineral administration. Based on existing data, the Committee on Clinical Practice Issues of the American Society for Clinical Nutrition has established the following guidelines:

Suggested Parenteral Vitamins for Infants and Children

	Term Infants and Children dose/kg/d	Preterm Infants dose/kg/d
A µg RE	700	280
E mg	7	2.8
K µg	200	80
D µg/IU	10/400	4/16

C mg	80	32
Thiamin mg	1.2	0.48
Riboflavin mg	1.4	0.56
Pyridoxin mg	1.0	0.4
Niacin mg	17	6.8
Pantothenate mg	5	2
Biotin µg	20	8
Folate µg	40	56
B12 µg	1	0.4

Greene, Harry L. et al Guidelines for the use of vitamin, traceelements,calcium, magnesium and phosphorus in infants and children receiving total parenteral nutrition: Report of the Subcommittee on Pediatric Parenteral Nutrient Requirements from the Committee on Clinical Practice Issues of the American Society for Clinical Nutrition, Am J Clin Nutr, Vol 48, 1988 pp 1324-1342.

Recommended Parenteral Calcium, Phosphorus and Magnesium

	Preterm Infants (mg/liter)	Term Infants (mg/liter)
Calcium	500 - 600	500 - 600
Phosphorus	400 - 450	400 - 450
Magnesium	50 - 70	50 - 70

Note: To prevent Ca-P precipitation, intakes are described per liter and assume an average fluid intake of 120 - 150 cc/kg/d. Greene et al suggests that these levels be used through a central venous line and not a peripheral line.
From: Greene, Harry L et al, Guidelines for the use of vitamins, trace elements, calcium, magnesium and phosphorus in infants and children receiving total parenteral nutrition.

Recommended Parenteral Trace Elements

	Preterm (µg/kg/d)	Term (µg/kg/d)
Zinc	400	250 < 3 mos 100 > 3 mos
Copper	20	20
Selenium	2	2
Chromium	0.2	0.2
Manganese	1	1
Molybdenum	0.25	0.25
Iodine	1	1

Note: When TPN <4 weeks, only zinc need be added. Copper and manganese should be omitted with obstruction jaundice. Selenium, chromium and molybdenum should be omitted with renal dysfunction.
From: Greene, Harry L et al Guidelines for the use of vitamins, trace elements, calcium, magnesium and phosphorus in infants and children receiving total parenteral nutrition.

Although several parenteral multiple vitamin and trace element preparations are available for use in adult patients, only one multi vitamin preparation is available for use in infants and children (MVI-Pediatric).

Vitamin Content of MVI-Pediatric (per 5 cc)	
A IU	2300
D IU	400
E IU	7
K µg	200
C mg	80
Thiamin mg	1.2
Riboflavin mg	1.4
Pyridoxine mg	1
Niacin mg	17
Pantothenic acid mg	5
Folic Acid µg	140
B_{12} µg	1
Biotin µg	20

It is difficult to provide all the trace elements because of availability and cost. In addition, individual infants may have diffferent needs and tolerance to the addition of trace elements secondary to alteration in organ function. Trace elements for parenteral nutrition are available as multiple trace element preparations (see below for examples) or as individual trace element preparations.

Trace Mineral Composition of Neotrace per 1 cc	
Zn	1.0 mg
Cu	0.1 mg
Mn	25 µg
Chr	1.0 µg

Carbohydrate

Glucose is the major carbohydrate used in parenteral nutrition. The neonate undergoes postnatal metabolic adjustment essential for glucose homeostasis, including utilization of glycogen via gluconeogenesis. The premature infant is particularly susceptible to hypoglycemia and hyperglycemia because of metabolic instability and immaturity. The premature infant has limited glycogen. Immature gluconeogenic mechanisms places them at risk for hypoglycemia in the absence of exogenous glucose. In addition, when presented with a glucose load, hyperglycemia may result secondary to inadequate insulin production or function. To prevent hypoglycemia/ hyperglycemia in the preterm infant, parenteral therapy should begin at 6 mg/kg/min and gradually increase. Advancements in glucose loads greater than 2 mg/kg/min per day are generally not tolerated by the preterm infant < 1500 grams. Glucose loads in excess of 15 mg/kg/min are probably contraindicated.

To Calculate Glucose Load

$$\frac{\text{Dextrose [ ] x 10 x \_\_\_cc/kg/d}}{1440} = \text{mg/kg/min}$$

For example: D7.5 at 148 cc/kg/d provides the following glucose load:

$$\frac{7.5 \text{ x } 10 \text{ x } 148}{1440} = 7.7 \text{ mg/kg/min}$$

Fat

Fat emulsions provide essential fatty acids and concentrated calories with minimal osmolality (e.g., a 10% lipid emulsion provides 1.1 kcal/cc and a 20% provides 2 kcal/cc) The preterm and low birth weight infant is susceptible to essential fatty acid deficiency in the first week of life. Implications of essential fatty acid deficiency may include alteration in skin integrity, decreased immunocompetence, thrombocytopenia, alteration in surfactant production and failure to thrive. Essential fatty acid needs can be met by infusion of .5 - 1.0 g/kg/d of intravenous fat. The potential risks of intravenous fat infusion include hyperlipidemia which may impair pulmonary gas exchange and the potential displacement of bilirubin or albumin in a jaundice infant. To prevent hyperlipidemia, intravenous lipid should be infused slowly and continously over 20 - 24 hours and lipid tolerance should be monitored (e.g., serum triglycerides). In the infant with hyperbilirubinemia, the provision of IV fat may be limited to meeting the individual infant's essential fatty acid needs.

Amino Acids

Amino acid solutions currently available for use in the neonate and preterm infant are listed in **Table 21**. With the exception of Trophamine and Aminosyn PF, these solutions originally were designed for use in adults. Although these solutions are capable of promoting nitrogen balance and appropriate nitrogen accretion in preterm infants, infusion of these solutions results in abnormal plasma amino acid levels when compared to the plasma amino acid levels in breast-fed infants. The implications of these abnormal plasma amino acid levels are not known precisely. Additional complications attributed to infusion of these amino acid solutions include azotemia hyperammonemia, metabolic acidosis and cholestasis. Other factors that might contribute to these complications include excessive protein administration, renal immaturity and alterations in biliary secretion.

Table 21: Concentrations of Amino Acids Adjusted to a 10% Solution

| Amino Acid | Amino Acid Solutions (Mg/100 cc) | | | | |
	Aminosyn	Travasol	Freamine III	Aminosyn P	Trophamine***
Essential					
Isoleucine	720	600	690	760	816
Leucine	940	730	910	1200	1400
Lysine	720	580	730	677	816
Methionine	400	400	530	180	333
Phenylalanine	440	560	560	427	483
Threonine	520	420	400	512	417
Tryptophan	160	180	150	180	200
Valine	800	580	660	673	783
Histidine	300	480	280	312	483

Non Essential

Alanine	1280	2070	710	698	533
Arginine	980	1150	950	1227	1217
Proline	860	680	1120	812	683
Serine	420	500	590	495	383
Taurine*	—	—	—	70	25
Tyrosine*	44	40	—	44	233**
Glycine	1280	1030	1400	385	367
Glutamic Acid	—	—	—	820	500
Aspartic Acid	—	—	—	527	317
Cysteine*	—	—	< 24	—	< 33

Product Information Facts and Comparisons 1988
*May be essential for preterm infants
**As N-acetyl-L-tyrosine
***Amino acids adjusted from a 6% solution for comparison
#Additional Cysteine may be added as Cysteine HCL

Complications of Parenteral Nutrition

A number of complications have been attributed to infusion of parenteral solutions. These complications may be classified as metabolic complications, infectious complications and technical complications.

Metabolic	Abnormal plasma amino acid levels
	Azotemia
	Fluid and electrolyte imbalance
	Hepatic disorders (ie cholestasis)
	Hyperammonemia
	Hyperglycemia
	Hyperlipidemia
	Hypoglycemia
	Metabolic acidosis
	Vitamin and mineral disorders
Infectious	Sepsis
Technical	Catheter malposition
	Pneumothorax
	Hemothorax
	Thrombosis
	Catheter dislodgement
	Perforation of infusion leak

Monitoring

The purpose of monitoring parenteral nutrition is to detect and treat potential or actual complications. Monitoring must take into account the relative probability of a particular complication occurring, the risk of monitoring and the likelihood that the information provided will change clinical actions. Judicious ordering of blood tests is crucial in the preterm infant because of limited blood volume. Although a number of monitoring schedules have been proposed for infants receiving parenteral nutrition, they often represent an "ideal" and compromises must be made for the availability of laboratory tests, the volume of blood a particular test requires and the infant's size and stability. Laboratory monitoring should include the following:

Electrolytes

Acid base studies

Dextrostix/serum glucose

Protein status (e.g., albumin/prealbumin)

Bone mineral status (Ca, Phos and Alkaline phosphatase)

Liver function tests

WBC/culture (as indicated)

Zn/Cu/Iron studies as needed

Lipid tolerance studies (e.g., triglycerides)

Additional tests may be considered as medically and clinically indicated.

ASSESSMENT

The preterm infant often is admitted to the intensive care unit at birth or shortly thereafter with little nutritional history available. Based on size and immaturity, these infants are at high nutritional risk. Nutrition assessment, therefore, becomes an ongoing process of evaluating nutrition intervention in these infants.

Components of nutrition assessment include dietary information, anthropometric data, biochemical data and clinical information. Traditionally, the basis for nutrition evaluation and intervention has been the comparison of an individual with established norms or reference populations. However, it is difficult to establish norms or standards for the preterm or low birth weight infant. Laboratory values initially may reflect placental transfer and be influenced by the infants immaturity and synthetic ability. Body composition of the preterm infant differs from that of the term infant. Postnatal growth initially may reflect body composition differences and necessary changes for adaptation to extrauterine life. Because of these difficulties, it is important to obtain serial measurements and interpret the information with the complete clinical and nutritional history.

Dietary

Dietary history should include an evaluation of calorie and protein intake. For the enterally fed infant, dietary assessment also includes an evaluation of the appropriateness of formula/milk feeding, the appropriateness of vitamin and mineral supplements and tolerance to feeding. Because infant formulas are designed to meet nutrient needs at a particular volume, knowledge of the formula and usual volume taken provides information about overall nutrient intake. More in-depth evaluation of specific nutrient intake may be necessary where there are special concerns such as:

- Infant with frequent feeding changes
- Infant on non standard formula
- Infant who is fluid restricted
- Infant with increased needs and/or increased losses (e.g., medications, short gut)
- Infant with clinical or biochemical evidence of a deficiency or excess

Intolerance to enteral feedings may be assessed by the following information:

Residuals or regurgitation
- Amount (percentage of feed)
- Color
- Consistency
- Frequency

Stools
- Frequency
- Color
- Consistency
- Presence of occult blood
- Presence of reducing substances

Interpretation of these indicators of feeding intolerance should take into account the complete clinical picture. Changes in feeding tolerance, particularly of a previously tolerated feeding may be secondary to changes in medical status, or medical therapies as opposed to feeding composition. Evidence of feeding intolerance with clinical changes in temperature, cardiorespiratory status, glucose intolerance and abdominal distention and/or tenderness may indicate a serious medical complication such as necrotizing enterocolitis. Changes in medication, volume or frequency of feeding, as well as changes in respiratory status may affect feeding tolerance.

For the parenterally fed infant, dietary evaluation includes calorie and protein intake, appropriateness of vitamin and mineral supplements and percentage of calories from carbohydrate, fat and protein.

Careful assessment of hydration status may be indicated in infants with increased losses (short gut syndrome, regurgitation, diarrhea), fluid restricted, or on concentrated formulas.

Growth

Growth measurements include weight, length and OFC. Growth standards have been established for term infants. For the preterm infant, what is ideal or appropriate is controversial. Many individuals rely on intrauterine growth parameters, assuming that continuation of intrauterine rates of growth are the ideal. Postnatal growth patterns may also be used as a basis for comparison. A number of intrauterine and postnatal growth curves are available for use in the preterm infant (see **Figures 1 - 3**). Selection of these curves, however, requires an understanding of the data base and assumptions inherent in their utilization.

Utilization of growth curves depicting intrauterine rates of growth assumes that such growth is the postnatal goal for preterm infants.and does not account for body composition differences and postnatal adaption. The initial period of weight loss is not depicted. The fetus gains approximately 15 g/kg/d. For the infant > 1.2 kg, weight gains of 20-30 g/d duplicates intrauterine rates of growth.

The Dancis curve (**Figure 4**) depicts daily postnatal weight changes in infants from 750 - 2500 grams. These curves reflect initial early postnatal weight loss associated with physiologic redistribution of fluids postnatally and allow for daily measurements. Weight loss in the first one to two weeks of life for the preterm infant may account for 10 - 15% of birthweight, compared to 5 - 10% in term infant. The data base, however, reflects feeding and medical practices and may not reflect optimal standards in todays intensive care settings, particularly for the infant less than 1500 grams. A more recent growth curve developed by Shaffer et al depicts postnatal weigh changes observed in preterm infants cared for under current medical conditions. **Figure 5**.

Available postnatal growth curves (**Figure 6** Babson) reflect birthweight data at various gestational ages and do not reflect longitudinal growth data in preterm infants. They allow for monitoring length, OFC and weight but do not depict the early postnatal weight loss.

Term growth curves such as the NCHS curves also are available. The NCHS curves reflect growth in term infants from birth to 36 months. They require that the preterm infants age be adjusted for prematurity and corrected age > 40 week.

Regardless of which curve is selected, the following patterns are often observed:

- Early postnatal weight loss of 10 - 15% BW for preterm infant. Larger infant may lose 5 - 10%. This weight loss typically occurs in the first 1 - 2 weeks.

- Stable growing infant may duplicate intrauterine rates of growth [20 - 30 g/d weight gain (15 g/kg/d), 0.5 - 1 cm/wk increase in length] and run parallel to postnatal or NCHS curves.

Figure 4: Dancis Curves

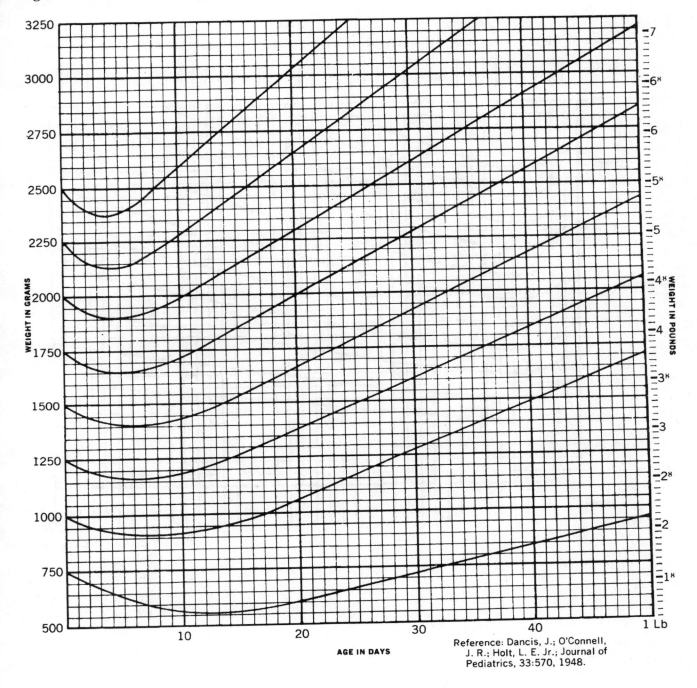

Reference: Dancis, J.; O'Connell, J. R.; Holt, L. E. Jr.; Journal of Pediatrics, 33:570, 1948.

Figure 5: Peds LBW Chart

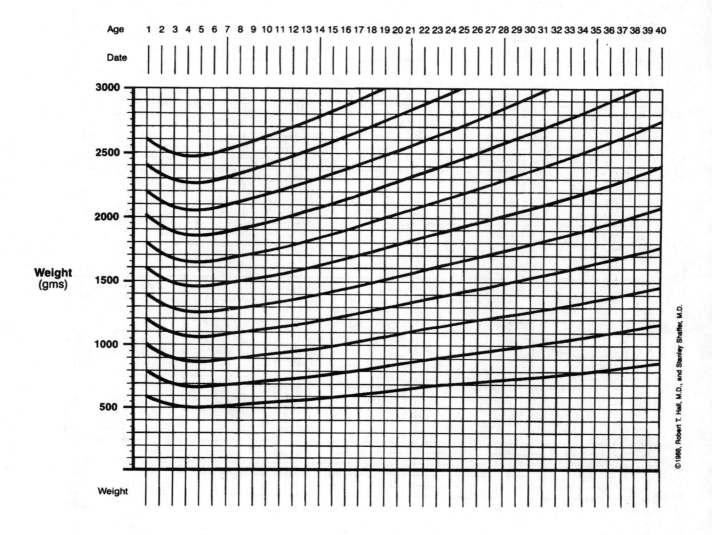

Figure 6: Babson

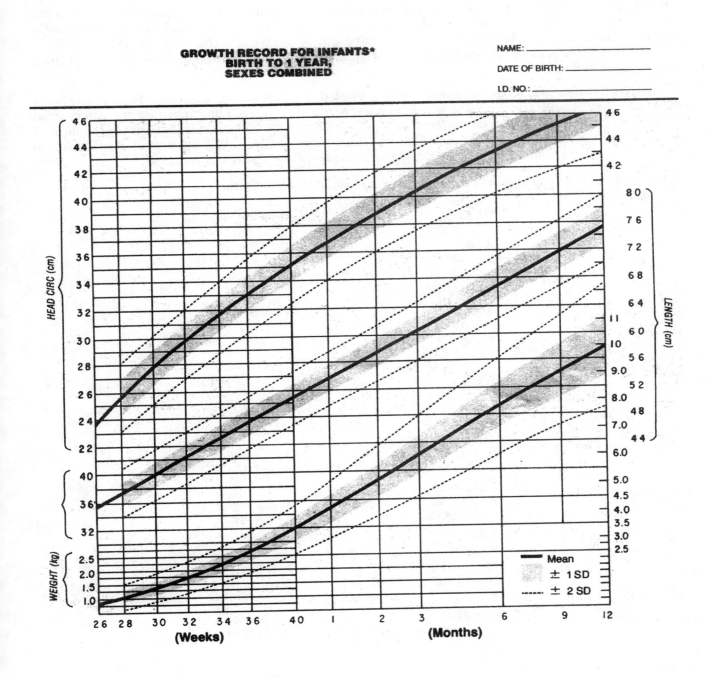

GROWTH RECORD FOR INFANTS*
BIRTH TO 1 YEAR,
SEXES COMBINED

NAME: _____

DATE OF BIRTH: _____

I.D. NO.: _____

Laboratory Assessment

Laboratory indices of nutritional status in adults and children allow for monitoring protein/energy, vitamin and mineral status. Reference values for most of these indices are not available for the preterm infant and interpretation is difficult secondary to immaturity and body composition, as well as medical complications and treatment. In addition, the volume of blood necessary to obtain a single laboratory value may be prohibitive in the small infant with limited blood volume.

In obtaining laboratory indices of nutritional status, it is essential to evaluate the usefulness of a particular test in relation to the risk, evaluate the value in terms of the whole medical and clinical picture and obtain serial measures to ascertain changes in an abnormal value. **Table 22** provides laboratory values for select indices of protein/energy and bone mineral status. Additional laboratory values are available from *Pediatric Clinical Chemistry: Reference (Normal) Values, Samuel Meites (editor in chief), AACC press, 1989.*

Table 22: Laboratory Indices of Protein/Energy and Bone Mineral Status

Albumin	Term 0 - 19 DOL	2.6 - 5.6 g/dl
	Term < 1 year	3.0 - 4.9 g/dl
	Preterm 10 - 55 DOL	2.5 - 4.1 g/dl
Alkaline Phosphatase	Term < 2 years	25 - 500 u/l
	Preterm 10 - 55 DOL	178 - 478
Calcium	Term < 1 year	7.8 - 11.2 mg/dl
	Preterm 10 - 55 DOL	9.4 ± 1.1
Magnesium	Term 0 - 6 DOL 7 - 30 DOL	1.2 - 2.6 mg/dl 1.6 - 2.4 mg/dl
	Preterm 0 - 6 DOL 7 - 30 DOL	1.6 - 2.7 mg/dl 1.8 - 2.4 mg/dl
Phosphorus	Term < 1 year	2.5 - 7.1 mg/dl
	Preterm 10 - 55 DOL	4.7 - 8.5 mg/dl
Prealbumin	Term 0 - 4 DOL 1 mo - 4 years	73 - 144 mg/l 67 - 171 mg/l
	Preterm 10 - 55 DOL	114 ± 36 mg/l

Individual infants may be assessed weekly to summarize progress and provide ongoing monitoring and evaluation of all infants in the intensive care units. (See **Figure 7** for an example of a weekly nutrition assessment).

Figure 7: Neonatal Nutrition Assesssment Form

DATE	TIME

S:

DAY OF LIFE	BIRTHWEIGHT	GESTATION AGE	

CURRENTLY:

☐ NOTHING PER ORAL (NPO)   ☐ VITAMIN SUPPLEMENTS ....

☐ RECEIVING PARENTERAL NUTRITION   ....

☐ ADVANCING FEEDS   ....

☐ ON FULL FEEDS   ....

O:

CURRENT WEIGHT

☐ LOST _____% OF BIRTHWEIGHT   ☐ NO CHANGE IN WEIGHT

☐ REGAINED BIRTHWEIGHT _____ DAY OF LIFE   ☐ INCONSISTENT WEIGHT GAIN PATTERN

CURRENT LENGTH

☐ LOSING WEIGHT   ☐ GAINING _____ gm PER DAY

☐ NO CHANGE IN LENGTH   ☐ INCREASE _____ cm/WEEK   CURRENT INTAKE

DIET HISTORY

☐ STARTED .... DAY OF LIFE   ☐ AVERAGED ....

☐ VITAMIN/SUPPLEMENT ....

A:

☐ ADEQUATE GROWTH   ☐ ADEQUATE CALORIES   ☐ ADEQUATE PROTEIN   ☐ APPROPRIATE VITAMIN/MINERAL SUPPLEMENT

☐ LOSING WEIGHT   ☐ INADEQUATE GROWTH   ☐ INADEQUATE CALORIES   ☐ INADEQUATE PROTEIN

☐ OTHER ....   ☐ NEEDS ....

P:

☐ MONITOR DAILY WEIGHT   ☐ MONITOR WEEKLY LENGTHS   ☐ REEVALUATE ....

☐ INCREASE CALORIES ....   ☐ INCREASE PROTEIN ....

☐ START VITAMIN/MINERAL SUPPLEMENT ....   ☐ OTHER ....

REGISTERED DIETITIAN SIGNATURE   DATE

STAFFING

Clinical staffing requirements are determined similarly to the adult intensive care unit. A productivity or benchmarking study can determine the amount of time and intensity each premie may need. Clinical staffing needs should be based on the identified level of the NICU. A Level Three NICU has a higher acuity level than a Level Two NICU. The following can serve as a guideline for staffing NICUs.

Levels of NICU

Level 3:	Intensity	Complex/In-Depth
	RD/premie ratio Nutrition care needs	1 RD: 15 babies Daily monitoring Every other day documentation
	Dietetic Technician Nutrition care given	1 DT: 20 - 30 babies Data collection Input/output in the computer Plotting growth grids Teaching class for formula making Referrals tp WIC, as appropriate
Level 2:	Intensity	Major/Advanced
	RD/premie ratio Nutrition care needs	1 RD: 16 - 20 patients Daily monitoring Every third day documentation
	Dietetic Technician Nutrition care given	1 DT: 20 - 30 patients Data collection Input/output in the computer Plotting growth grids Teaching class for formula making Referrals to WIC, as appropriate

Staffing Model Example for the NICU Dietitian

Assumptions		Policy is to evaluate survival and metabolic stability after the first 48 hours. Monitoring will be done daily until premie reaches a stable growth pattern. One new admit per day. Percent time in direct care 90% (includes medical rounds).	
	RVU	Assessment Daily monitoring/baby Documentation q 3 day	60 min 15 min 15 min
Bed Size		Level 3	30
% occupancy		90%	27
Time needs per day		1 assessment/day Daily monitoring Documentation Total hrs needed	1.0 hr 6.75 hr 2.25 hr 10 hours
Number of RDs required		(10 hrs/7.2 hrs)	1.4

Staffing needs of the dietitian and dietetic technician are determined by task x time x frequency. Each level of nursery can be evaulated for approrpriate staffing using and/or adapting this model.

QUALITY IMPROVEMENT

Quality improvement provides a means to determine and document that nutritional standards of care are being met. Medical instability and frequent but unpredictable changes in medical status can impact nutritional support. In the VLBW infant's first week of life, it may be difficult to meet basal energy and protein needs secondary to glucose intolerance, metabolic acidosis and fluid and electrolyte imbalances. Exceptions can be built into quality improvement monitoring. **Figure 8** provides an example of Quality Improvement monitoring.

Figure 8: Quality Improvement Monitor for Neonatal Intensive Care

Standard: To minimize tissue catabolism

Goal: By day 5 of life patient will receive ~ 60 kcal/kg/day and 1 gm Pro/kg/day

Hosp. No _____ Patient _____ DOB _____

Patient	DOL	Total kcal/kg Intake	Total protein/kg Intake

Clinical Nutrition Pathway: Neonatal Intensive Care Patient

Objective: to provide optimal nutritional care compatible with medical treatment through planning, implementation and monitoring/evaluating.

CASE STUDY

Patient Data Baby is a 25 week GA 800 gm female

DOL 1 she is receiving D10W at 100 cc/kg/day

How would you develop the nutrition care plan to improve nutritional status? What are your recommendations?

What factors may interfere with the nutrition care plan?

DOL #5 The baby's weight is 720 gms.

What implications must be considered in evaluating this change in weight?

DOL #7 PN is being administered at 150 cc/kg/day.

Solution is D10W; 2.5 gm pro/kg/day; 2.5 gm lipids. Is her nutritional support adequate? Discuss changes that could be made.

Week 3 The baby is medically unstable with worsening lung disease, hyperglycemia, sepsis and, secondary to cardiovascular disease, PDA; she is fluid restricted. PN is D5W at 120 cc/kg/day with 2.5 gm of protein and 2.5 gm lipids. Weight over 5 days has increased from 920 gms to 1120 gms. Assess her growth and intake.

DISCHARGE AND FOLLOW-UP OF THE PRETERM INFANT

Survival rates for preterm infants have dramatically increased over the past ten years. Increasing numbers of ELBW and VLBW infants are surviving and being discharged from the hospital to home. Some infants experienced complicated medical and nutritional courses and are discharged with ongoing medical, nutritional and neurodevelopmental concerns. For some of these infants, transition from hospital to home may be problematic. To ensure continuity of care and continued nutritional rehabilitation the following must be included in discharge planning: identification of nutritional risk, nutritional, educational and support needs; and plans for continued monitoring and communication with health care providers.

Nutrition Risk Factors

Prematurity and LBW	ELBW VLBW Dcd < 37 week CA IUGR/SGA
History of Nutritional Deficits	PN > two weeks Inadequate growth Osteopenia Anemia Other documented deficits
Medical Complications	BPD Heart disease Short gut syndrome Neurologic impairement
Feeding Difficulties	GER History of inadequate intake, choking, ABCs with feeding, respiratory distress with feeding, prolonged feeding times, aversive feeding behavior.

A nutrition discharge summary to community health care providers should include identification of any of the above risk factors, growth and nutritional history, most recent weight/length and pertinent labs as well as feeding plans and instructions. Referal to a clinic dietitian may facilitate management and monitoring of nutrition concerns after discharge.

CLINICAL PATHWAYS FOR NUTRITION INTERVENTION

Following are clinical pathways for preterm infants.

System/ Diagnosis	Potential Problems/ Indicators	Assessment	Intervention/ Monitoring/Education	Possible/Desired Outcome(s)
Prematurity LBW ELBW VLBW	FTT	Medical goals	**Phase 1 and 2**	Optimal nutrition status:
	Inadequate increase in weight and length	Hx: social of parents	Determine feeding modality	• Preserve/ improve LBM
	Protein losing enteropathy	Weight/growth patterns	Formulate care plan	• Adequate calorie and protein intake for growth
	Fluid Balance	Biochemical	Recommend baseline labs	
Arterial Blood gases	Abnormal ABGs	Assessment of respiratory status	Document/ communicate plan	Normalize electrolytes
	Nutrient deficiencies	GI function/vital signs	**Phase 3**	Improve hydration status/ABGs
	Electrolyte Imbalance		Goal: to achieve desired intake	
	Short Gut Syndrome	Hydration status		Administration of adequate nutrients
	Respiratory distress	Feeding modality	Review labs (GGT, SGPT, Bili T/D, Ca, Mg, PO_4, Alk phos, NEFA/Alb, TG, HCT, Cl, CO_2), I&Os, vital signs, ABGs, electrolytes, weight, length	Nutrition education recommendations to the parents/care-giver
	Anemia	Education of parents or care-giver		
	Feeding difficulties	Goals of therapy		If it is determined there is inadequate nutrition knowledge, a plan for continuum of care is implemented
		Discharge plans	Start education process	
		Determine Needs: Kcal: per age If PN 80 - 100 kcal/kg If EN 120 + kcal/kg/d	Communicate any concerns	
			Document progress of care plan and education	
		Protein: per age 2.0 - 2.5 /kg/d	Adjust care plan as medical condition and/or therapy necessitates	
		Fluid: 15 cc/kg plus losses	**Phase 4**	
		Electrolytes: standard per age	Discharge summary and referral	
		Vitamin: RDA per age		
		Minerals: RDA per age		

System/ Diagnosis	Potential Problems/ Indicators	Assessment	Intervention/ Monitoring/ Education	Possible Desired Outcome(s)
Gastrointestinal	Malnutrition	Medical goals	**Phase 1 and 2**	Optimal nutrition status
	FTT	Hx: medical, social, dietary, drug	Determine feeding modality – if po, modify fat, fiber, lactose; avoid gas-producing foods	• Preserve/improve LBM
	Inadequate growth	Weight/growth patterns		
	Protein losing enteropathy			• Adequate calorie and protein intake for growth
		Biochemical	Formulate care plan	
	Diarrhea	Drug/nutrient interactions		Decrease fecal output
	Acute, severe weight loss secondary to diminished food intake and inflammation	Clinical symptoms	Recommend baseline labs	Reduce steatorrhea
		GI function/vital signs	Document/ communicate plan	Normalize electrolytes
	Nutrient deficiencies	Functional status/ ADLs	**Phase 3**	Improve hydration status
	Anemia	Hydration status	Goal: to achieve desired intake via po or EN/PN	Comprehension and adherence to dietary recommendations by the parents/care giver
	Fluid retention	Feeding modality	Review labs, I&Os, medical progress, vital signs, electrolytes, weight	
	Electrolyte Imbalance	Education of parents or care-giver		
	Intolerance to po	Goals of therapy	Start education process	If it is determined there is inadequate nutrition knowledge, a plan for continuum of care is implemented
		Discharge plans	Communicate any concerns	
		Determine Needs:		
		Kcal: per age	Document progress of care plan and education	
		Protein: per age		
		Fluid: per age plus losses	Adjust care plan as medical condition and/or therapy necessitates	
		Electrolytes: standard plus replace losses	**Phase 4**	
		Vitamins: RDA per age and disease	Discharge summary and referral	
		Minerals: RDA per age and disease		

GIRLS: BIRTH TO 36 MONTHS
PHYSICAL GROWTH
NCHS PERCENTILES*

NAME _____   RECORD # _____

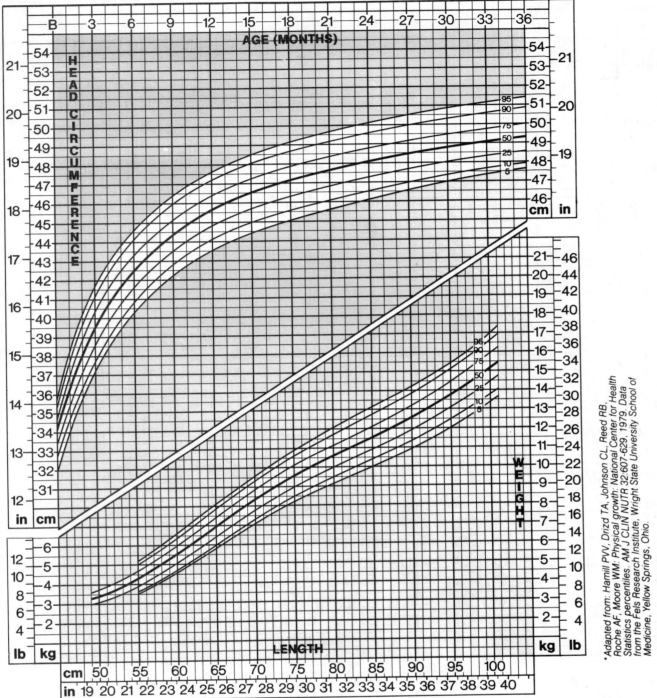

AGE (MONTHS)

HEAD CIRCUMFERENCE

WEIGHT

LENGTH

*Adapted from: Hamill PVV, Drizd TA, Johnson CL, Reed RB, Roche AF, Moore WM: Physical growth: National Center for Health Statistics percentiles. AM J CLIN NUTR 32:607-629, 1979. Data from the Fels Research Institute, Wright State University School of Medicine, Yellow Springs, Ohio.

© 1982 ROSS LABORATORIES

DATE	AGE	LENGTH	WEIGHT	HEAD CIRC.	COMMENT

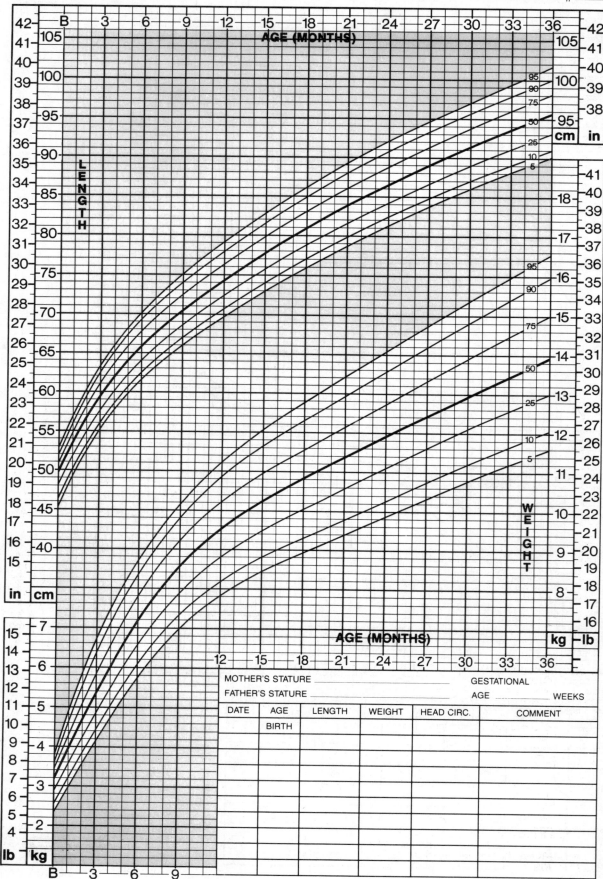

GIRLS: BIRTH TO 36 MONTHS
PHYSICAL GROWTH
NCHS PERCENTILES*

NAME_____ RECORD #_____

Ross
Growth &
Development
Program

AGE (MONTHS)

LENGTH

AGE (MONTHS)

WEIGHT

*Adapted from: Hamill PVV, Drizd TA, Johnson CL, Reed RB,
Roche AF, Moore WM: Physical growth: National Center for Health
Statistics percentiles. AM J CLIN NUTR 32:607-629, 1979. Data
from the Fels Research Institute, Wright State University School of
Medicine, Yellow Springs, Ohio.

MOTHER'S STATURE _____ GESTATIONAL
FATHER'S STATURE _____ AGE _____ WEEKS

DATE	AGE	LENGTH	WEIGHT	HEAD CIRC.	COMMENT
	BIRTH				

GIRLS: PREPUBESCENT
PHYSICAL GROWTH
NCHS PERCENTILES*

NAME_____ RECORD #_____

DATE	AGE	STATURE	WEIGHT	COMMENT

Percentile curves labeled: 95, 90, 75, 50, 25, 10, 5

STATURE

cm 85 90 95 100 105 110 115 120 125 130 135 140 145

in 34 35 36 37 38 39 40 41 42 43 44 45 46 47 48 49 50 51 52 53 54 55 56 57 58

WEIGHT

lb kg (left axis: 25–65 lb / 12–30 kg)

kg lb (right axis)

* Adapted from: Hamill PVV, Drizd TA, Johnson CL, Reed RB, Roche AF, Moore WM: Physical growth: National Center for Health Statistics percentiles. AM J CLIN NUTR 32:607-629, 1979. Data from the National Center for Health Statistics (NCHS) Hyattsville, Maryland.

© 1982 ROSS LABORATORIES

GIRLS: 2 TO 18 YEARS
PHYSICAL GROWTH
NCHS PERCENTILES*

NAME _____ RECORD # _____

MOTHER'S STATURE _____	FATHER'S STATURE _____			
DATE	AGE	STATURE	WEIGHT	COMMENT

AGE (YEARS)

STATURE

WEIGHT

AGE (YEARS)

Ross Growth & Development Program

BOYS: BIRTH TO 36 MONTHS
PHYSICAL GROWTH
NCHS PERCENTILES*

NAME _____   RECORD # _____

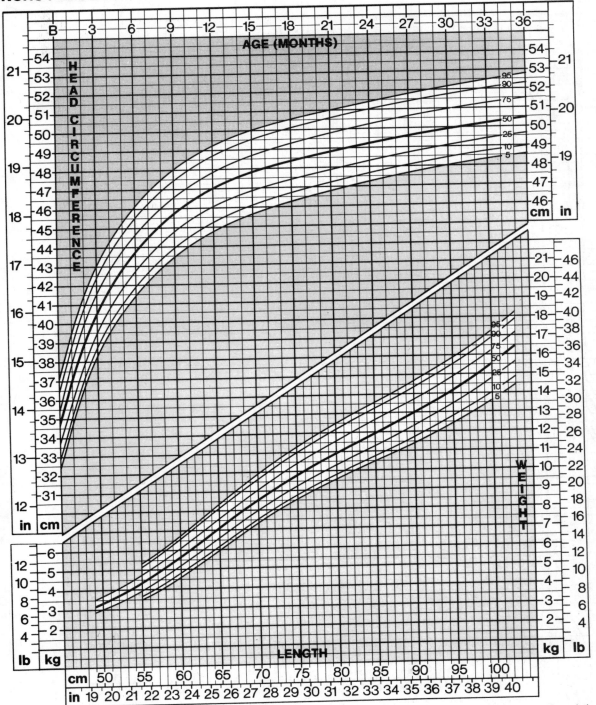

AGE (MONTHS)

HEAD CIRCUMFERENCE

WEIGHT

LENGTH

*Adapted from: Hamill PVV, Drizd TA, Johnson CL, Reed RB, Roche AF, Moore WM: Physical growth: National Center for Health Statistics percentiles. AM J CLIN NUTR 32:607-629, 1979. Data from the Fels Research Institute, Wright State University School of Medicine, Yellow Springs, Ohio.

© 1982 ROSS LABORATORIES

DATE	AGE	LENGTH	WEIGHT	HEAD CIRC.	COMMENT

Recommend the formulation you prefer with the name you trust

SIMILAC®
SIMILAC® WITH IRON
SIMILAC® WITH WHEY
Infant Formulas

The **ISOMIL®** System of
Soy Protein Formulas

ADVANCE®
Nutritional Beverage

ROSS LABORATORIES
COLUMBUS, OHIO 43216
Division of Abbott Laboratories, USA

G105/JUNE 1983   LITHO IN USA

BOYS: BIRTH TO 36 MONTHS
PHYSICAL GROWTH
NCHS PERCENTILES*

NAME＿＿＿＿＿＿＿＿＿＿＿＿＿＿＿＿＿   RECORD #＿＿＿＿＿＿＿＿

Ross
Growth &
Development
Program

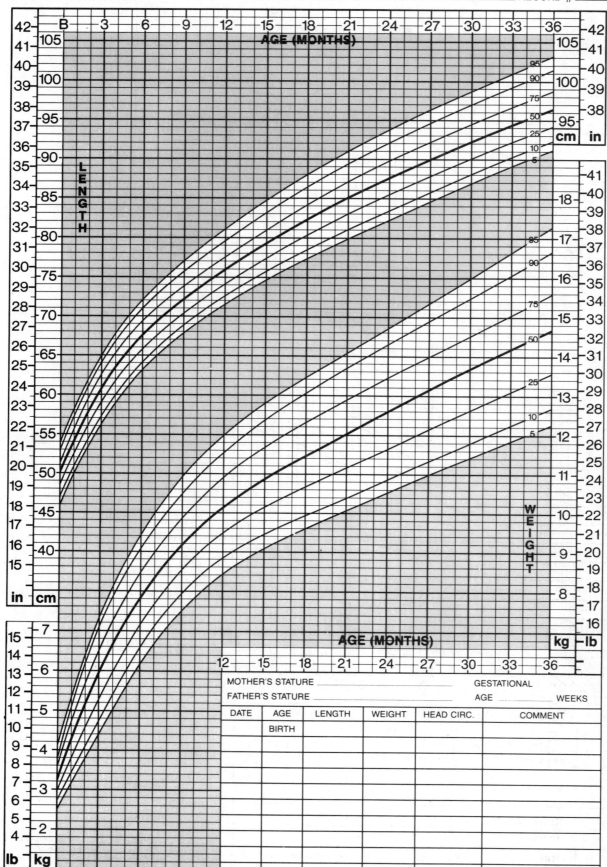

MOTHER'S STATURE ＿＿＿＿＿＿＿＿＿＿＿＿＿   GESTATIONAL
FATHER'S STATURE ＿＿＿＿＿＿＿＿＿＿＿＿＿   AGE ＿＿＿＿ WEEKS

DATE	AGE	LENGTH	WEIGHT	HEAD CIRC.	COMMENT
	BIRTH				

*Adapted from: Hamill PVV, Drizd TA, Johnson CL, Reed RB, Roche AF, Moore WM: Physical growth: National Center for Health Statistics percentiles. AM J CLIN NUTR 32:607-629, 1979. Data from the Fels Research Institute, Wright State University School of Medicine, Yellow Springs, Ohio.

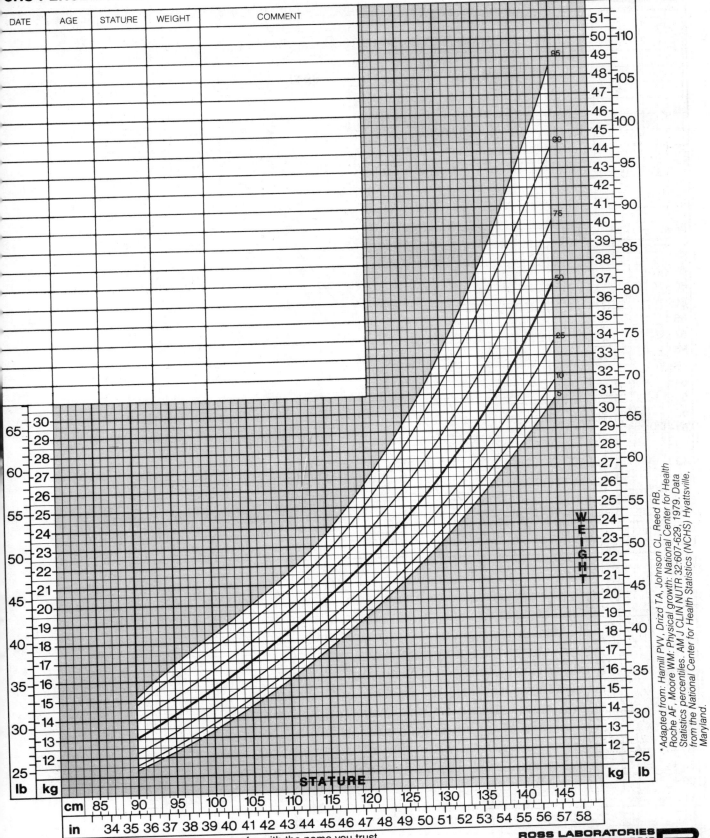

OYS: PREPUBESCENT
HYSICAL GROWTH
CHS PERCENTILES*

NAME_____   RECORD #_____

DATE	AGE	STATURE	WEIGHT	COMMENT

STATURE

cm 85 90 95 100 105 110 115 120 125 130 135 140 145

in 34 35 36 37 38 39 40 41 42 43 44 45 46 47 48 49 50 51 52 53 54 55 56 57 58

WEIGHT

*Adapted from: Hamill PVV, Drizd TA, Johnson CL, Reed RB, Roche AF, Moore WM: Physical growth: National Center for Health Statistics percentiles. AM J CLIN NUTR 32:607-629, 1979. Data from the National Center for Health Statistics (NCHS) Hyattsville, Maryland.

© 1982 ROSS LABORATORIES

Recommend the formulation you prefer with the name you trust

SIMILAC®
SIMILAC® WITH IRON
SIMILAC® WITH WHEY
Infant Formulas

The ISOMIL® System of
Soy Protein Formulas

ADVANCE®
Nutritional Beverage

ROSS LABORATORIES
COLUMBUS, OHIO 43216
Division of Abbott Laboratories, USA ROSS

G107/JUNE 1983   LITHO IN USA

BOYS: 2 TO 18 YEARS
PHYSICAL GROWTH
NCHS PERCENTILES*

NAME_____ RECORD #_____

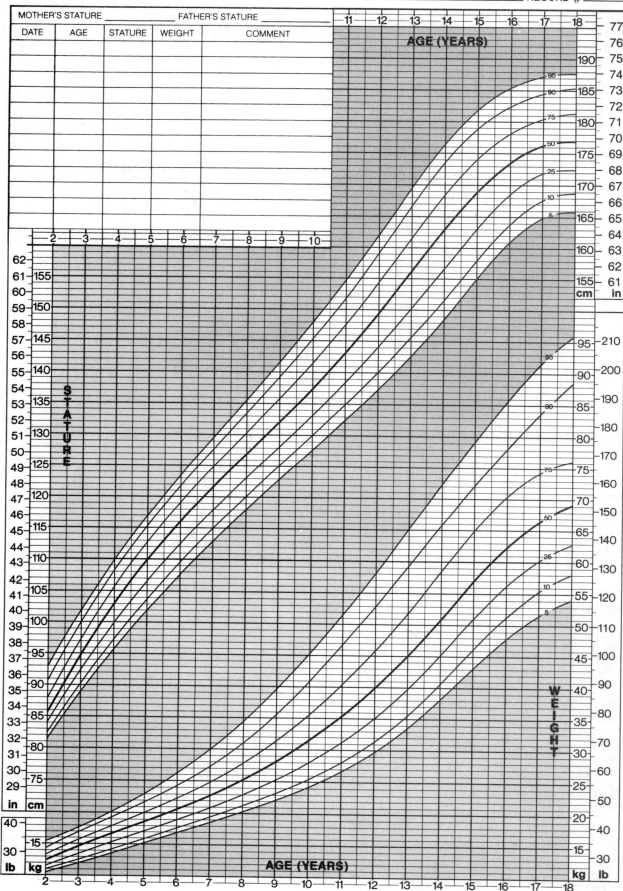

*Adapted from: Hamill PVV, Drizd TA, Johnson CL, Reed RB, Roche AF, Moore WM: Physical growth: National Center for Health Statistics percentiles. AM J CLIN NUTR 32:607-629, 1979. Data from the National Center for Health Statistics (NCHS) Hyattsville, Maryland.

Ross
Growth &
Development
Program

References

- ASPEN Board of Directors. Guidelines for the parenteral and enteral nutrition in adult and pediatric patients. JPEN 1993; 17 (supl): 1993.

- Balistreri, WF and Farrell, MK: Enteral Feeding. Scientific Basis and Clinical Applications. Report of the 94th Ross Conference on Pediatric Research. 1988.

- Barness, LA: Pediatric Nutrition Handbook. Am Academy of Pediatrics, 1993.

- Behrman, RE and Nelson, WE: Textbook of Pediatrics, Philadelphia: WB Saunders, 1992.

- Braunschweig, CL et al: Rationale and guidelines for parenteral and enteral transition feeding of the 3-30 kg child. J Am Diet Assoc 1988; 88:479.

- Cunningham, JJ: Body composition and nutrition support in pediatrics: what to defend and how soon to begin. Nutrit Clin Pract 1995; 10:177.

- Dahlstrom, KA et al: Low blood and plasma carnitine levels in children receiving long-term parenteral support. J Ped Gastro and Nutr 1990; No 3.

- Filer, LJ: Iron needs during rapid growth and mental development. J. Pediatr 1990; 117:143.

- Fomon, SJ: Nutrition of Normal Infants. St Louis: Mosby-Yearbook Inc,1993.

- Greene, HL et al: Guidelines for the use of vitamins, trace elements, calcium, magnesium, and phosphorus in infants and children receiving total parenteral nutrition: report of the subcommittee on pediatric parenteral nutrient requirements. Am J Clin Nutr 1988;48:1324.

- Groh-Wargo, S et al: Nutritional Care for the High Risk Newborn. Chicago: Precept Press, 1994.

- Guo, S et al: Reference data on gains in weight and length during the first two years of life: J Pediatr 1991; 119:355.

- Hallerstein, S et al: Nutritional management of children with chronic renal failure. Ped Nephrol 1987; 1:195.

- Heird, WC et al: Parenteral alimentation of the neonate. Sem in Perinat 1991; 15:493.

- Johnson, CP and Blasco, PA: Infant Growth and Development.

- Kappy, MS: Regulation of growth in children with chronic illness. AJDC 1987; 141:489.

- Marian, M: Pediatric nutition support. Nutrit in Clin Pract 1993; 8:199.

- Merritt, TA et al. Clinical practice guidelines in pediatric and newborn medicine: implications for their use in practice. Pediatr 1997; 99:100.

- Moore, MC and Greene, HL: Tube feeding of infants and children. Ped Clinics of NA 1985; April.

- Pridham, KF. Feeding behavior of 6- to 12-month old infants: assessment and sources of parental information. J Pediatr 1990; 117:S174.

- Preston, PP and Kirby, DF: Short-bowel syndrome: a review of the folw of nutrition support. JPEN 1991; 15:93.

- Ramstack, M and Listernick, R: Safety and efficacy of a new pediatric enteral product in the young child. JPEN 1991; 15:89.

- Schmeling, DJ and Coran, AG: Hormonal and metabolic response to operative stress in the neonate. JPEN 1991; 15:215.

- Schmidt, GL: Review: Parenteral Micronutrition in the Pediatric Patient. In: Baumgartner, TG, ed. Clinical Guide to Parenteral Micronutrition. Fujisawa, USA, Inc, 1991.

•Sutphen, JL: Growth as a measure of nutritional status. J Pediatr Gastro and Nutr 1985; No 2.

• Trahms, CM and Pipes, P: Nutrition in Infancy and Childhood. Boston: McGraw Hill, 1997.

• Tsang, R et al: Nutritional Needs of the Preterm Infant. Pawling, NY: Williams and Wilkins, 1993.

• Waterlow, JC: Classification and definition of protein calorie malnutrition, British Med J 1972; 3:566.

• Wesley, JR: Efficacy and safety of total parenteral nutrition in pediatric patients. Mayo Clin Proc 1992; 67:671.

• American Academy of Pediatrics. Committee on Nutrition. Nutritional needs of low birth weight infants. Pediatrics 1985; 45:976.

• Americn Academy of Pediatrics. Committee on Nutrition. Commentary on Parenteral Nutrition. Pediatrics 1993; 71:547.,

• Pediatric Nutrition Handbook. Elk Grove: American Academy of Pediatrics, 1993.

• Cochran, EB, Phelps, SJ and Helms, R: Parenteral nutrition in pediatric patients. Clin Pharm 1988; 7:351.

• Greene, HL, Hambridge, KF, Schanler, R and Tsang, R: Guidelines for the use of vitamins, trace elements, calcium, magnesium, and phosphorus in infants and children receiving total parenteral nutrition: report of the subcommittee on pediatric parenteral nutrient requirements from the committee on clinical practice issues of the American Society for Clinical Nutrition. Am J Clin Nutr 1988; 48:1324

• Kerner, JA: Parenteral nutrition in the premature infant. Perinat/Neonat 1988. May/June.

• Lebenthal, E, Lee, PC and Heitlinger, L: Impact of development of the gastrointestinal tract on infant feeding. J. Pediatr 1983; 101:1.

• Lebenthal, E: Total Parenteral Nutrition: Indication, Utilization, Complications, and Pathophysiological Considerations. New York: Raven Press, 1986.

• Lindblad, BS: Perinatal Nutrition. Bristol Meyers Nutrition Symposium. Vol. 6. Academic Press, 1988.

• Lucas, A, Bloom, SR, Aynsley-Green, A. Gut hormones and 'minimal enteral feeding'. Acta Paediatr Scand 1986; 75:719.

• Meites, S: Pediatric Clinical Chemistry: Reference (Normal) Values Washington DC: AACC Press, 1989.

• National Research Council. Recommended Dietary Allowances. Washington DC: National Academy Press, 1989.

• O'Leary, M: Nourishing the premature and low birth weight infant. In: Pipies, PL, ed. Nutrition in Infancy and Childhood. Times Mirror/Mosby College Publishing, 1989.

• Tsang, RC: Vitamin and Mineral Requirements in Preterm Infants. New York: Marcel Dekker Inc, 1985.

• Tsang, RC: Nichols, BL. Nutrition During Infancy. Philadelphia: Hanley and Belfus Inc, 1988.

• Wharton, BA: Nutrition and Feeding of Preterm Infants. Boston: Blackwell Scientific Publications, 1987.

• Ziegler, E, Biga, RL and Fomon, SJ Nutritional Requirements of the Premature Infant. In: Suskind, RM, ed. Textbook of Pediatric Nutrition. New York: Raven Press, 1981.

Figures

Tables:

APPENDIX

CASE STUDIES

Tube Feeding in the Elderly

Patient Data	80 year old male diagnosed to have squamous cell carcinoma of the lip. Was admitted to the surgical service for a radical lip and neck dissection. An N.G. tube was put in place during surgery.
Medical History	Following the administration of the tube feeding, the patient developed diarrhea (with an estimated output of 800 ml per day) and a post-op wound infection with a temperature ranging up to 40° C. After three weeks the patient often complained of thirst and became increasingly lethargic. The infection was controlled but his temperature once again rose. Lethargy increased to stupor. Skin and mucous membranes were dry. Average urinary output was 1200 ml in 24 hours.

Physical Exam

Respirations	26/min
B.P.	110/75 (lying)
	90/55 (sitting)
Pulse	96/min

Anthropometry

Ht.	182 cm
IBW	75 kg
Usual wt	80 kg
Current wt	65 kg

Laboratory

Na	158.0 mEq/L
K	5.0 mEq/L
Cl	116.0 mEq/L
Creatinine	1.6 mg/dl
BUN	96.0 mg/dl
HCT	52.0 %
Albumin	3.6 gm/dl
Prealbumin	20 mg/ml
Glucose	240.0 mg

Specific Gravity	1.010
Nutrition	Current tube feeding provides 3000 calories, 2100 cc and support 140 gm Protein, 110 mEq sodium, 93 mEq potassium, and 41 mEq chloride.

Implications of Findings

Elevated Serum Lytes	Indicative of water depletion due to excessive solute loading by administration of hyperosmolar tube feeding (800 mOsm/L) without adequate free water.
Elevated BUN	Dehydration as a result of hemoconcentration.
Albumin	Lab value reflects a low normal range whereas the true value is actually lower because albumin is elevated in dehydration.
Elevated HCT	Reflects hemoconcentration.
Glucose	Elevated in dehydration.
Specific Gravity	Dehydration; inability to concentrate urine.
Postural Hypotension	Indicative of hypovolemia.
Thirst	Primary response to maintain hydration status. Major symptom of hypernatremia.
Stupor	Symptomatic cerebral dysfunction resulting from osmotic shift of water out of the brain and cerebrospinal fluid in response to rising serum sodium.
Dry Skin/Membranes	Due to dehydration.
Urinary Output	Decreases with dehydration due to compensation attempts to reduce urinary water losses.
Temperature	Increased due to dehydration.
Diarrhea	Due to high osmolar load not dehydration.

Nutrient Needs

Total Calories	2200 - 2400
Protein	75 - 80 gms. Increased needs due to catabolism associated with surgery.
Fluid	Assuming a commercial isotonic tube feeding is used, 2400 cc yields approximately 1965 cc. Will need extra water: 500 - 600 cc.
Assessment	Abnormal fluid losses through diarrhea and increased temperature. Patient dehydrated secondary to fluid loses and by receiving a hyperosmolar tube, high protein feeding without adequate additional water. Goal is to rehydrate the patient and support protein repletion and a minor weight gain. Suggest discontinuing the tube feeding and correct hydration status with IV's. Restart tube feeding, check residuals, monitor labs for hydration and the patient should be weighed bi-weekly.

Crohns Disease

Patient Data	37 year old male with a ten year history of progressive Crohn's disease. Has continued severe, frothy diarrhea, pain and weight loss.
Medical History	Past medical and surgical treatment includes multiple resections of the small bowel and steroid therapy.
Physical Exam	Thin, poorly nourished male in some distress. Stool is quaiac positive. An upper GI series showed marked narrowing of the lumen of several areas in the remaining bowel with some fistulas evident.
Medical Treatment	Resection of the small bowel, leaving only the proximal duodenum, anastomosed to the mid-transverse colon. A central line for parenteral nutrition was established.

Anthropometry		
	Ht	178 cm
	Usual Wt	77 kg
	Current Wt	64 kg
	IBW	75 kg

Laboratory		
	Na	142.0 mEq/L
	K	3.1 mEq/L
	Albumin	2.8 gm/dl
	Calcium	8.2 gm/dl
	HCT	32.0 %
	Glucose	90.0 mg %
	Mg	1.3 mEq/L
	PO_4	1.8 mEq/L
	Prealbumin	5.2 mg/ml

Drugs	Prednisone	30 mg

Implications of Findings

Albumin	Depressed due to recent surgery and malnutrition.
Calcium	Depressed due to the low albumin and steatorrhea.
Potassium	Low secondary to diarrhea.
HCT	Low value indicates poor nutritional status and recent surgery.
Steroids	Increased protein catabolism, loss of muscle mass, increased potassium excretion and decreased calcium absorption.
Mg	Reduced values occur with malabsorption and diarrhea.
PO_4	Decreased secondary to none to little in the TPN solution and malnutrition.

Nutrient Needs

Total Calories	3000 - 3300
Protein	100 - 120 gms (1.5 gm/kg IBW)
Fat Lipids	10% - 500 cc 3 times per week
Assessment	Parenteral nutrition should be administered until remaining small bowel has hypertrophied. Need some p.o. intake for stimulus. 10% AA's; D50W; plus lipids three times per week at 125 ccs per hour should yield adequate calories for weight gain and protein repletion. May need to add more PO4 secondary to starvation.
Oral Nutrition	When appropriate. Six small, modified fiber, low lactose, low LCT feedings as tolerated. Limit liquids to reduce transit time.

Alcoholism

Medical History	Forty year old female presenting with vague abdominal pain and bright red hematemesis following heavy alcohol consumption. Two years of intermittent ascites.
Social History	Divorced and lives alone. Currently has no cooking facilities. Unemployed, receives monthly compensation and food stamps. Average alcohol consumption is 10 (12 oz) beer per day.
Physical Exam	Thin, poorly nourished female with epigastric tenderness; hepatomegaly, splenomegaly, spider angiomas of the neck and chest and palmar erythema.

Anthropometry

Height	168 cm
IBW	58 kg
Usual weight	60 kg
Current weight	68 kg

Laboratory

Na	148 mEq/L
K	3.1 mEq/L
Ca	8.1 mg
Mg	1.1 mEq/L
HCT	35%
MCV	Elevated
Albumin	2.9 gm/dL
AlkPhos	223 U/dl
SGOT	40 IU
SGPT	19 IU
Stool	Guiac positive

Drugs	Lasix, Aldactone, Pitressin, Vit. K, Lomotil, Folic Acid

Problem List

1. Mild Laennec's Cirrhosis
2. Ascites secondary to # 1
3. Peripheral Edema secondary to #1
4. Portal hypertensicn secondary to #1
5. L. Hydrothorax secondary to #4
6. Esophagitis secondary to ETOH intake
7. Esophageal Varices secondary to #4
8. Macrocytic Anemia
9. Possibility of portal systemic shunt

Implications of Findings:

Serum Albumin	Values decrease with hepatocyte damage and poor intake.
Alkaline Phosphatase	Intracellular enzymes found in the liver, small intestines, kidney, bones. Plasma concentration rises with hepatic injury and/or biliary obstruction.
Magnesium	Low secondary to alcoholism, vomiting, poor intake and malabsorption.
SGOT, SGPT	Intracellular enzymes involved in transamination reactions; released from damaged hepatocytes.
Prothrombin Time	Sole site for synthesis of prothrombin clotting factors. Clotting time prolonged in liver disease.
Total Bilirubin	Indicative of liver's ability to conjugate and excrete bilirubin. Normally rapidly removed from plasma by hepatocytes and excreted in bile. Abnormal in liver disease causing jaundice.

Nutrient Needs

Total Calories	1600 minimum per day is sufficient for maintenance and prevention of further nutritional deterioration and catabolism of endogenous nitrogen. Introduce additional calories after food intake increases and is stable.
Protein	Unrestricted. Most cirrhotic patients are in nitrogen equilibrium at about 0.7 gm/kg. Since there are no clinical signs of encephalopathy, 50 - 60 gms can probably be tolerated.
Sodium	500 - 1000 mgs/day. With use of diuretics, further restriction is seldom necessary. Once edema and ascites are no longer evident, there should be a liberalization of intake. Possibly 2 - 3 gms/day.
Fluid Restriction	Not necessary since there are no clinical signs of impaired renal function and/or hyponatremia. If the disease was advanced, water loads would not be handled normally. Need sufficient fluid to ensure reasonable urine flow.
Potassium	Patient is hypokalemic. Cirrhotic patients may have limited K stores and additional losses often result from diuretic therapy. KCl is needed since oral intake may be inconsistent.
Folic Acid	Increased MCV diagnostic of macrocytic anemia attributable to folic acid deficiency.
Vitamin K	Needed for hypoprothrombinemia.
Oral Iron	Iron deficiency anemia secondary to inadequate intake and/or blood loss. Dosage must be carefully calculated and serum monitored.
B Complex & Vit C	Alterations in intermediary metabolism and/or intestinal absorption of thiamine, niacin, and folate are indicative of undernourished alcoholics.

Pancreatitis

Medical History	Forty-five year old female with a chief complaint of severe pain, nausea, vomiting, and weight loss. Five year existing history of recurring abdominal pain and a six month history of bulky, foul smelling stools and continued weight loss.
Physical Exam	Thin female in obvious distress with icteric sclera and jaundice abdominal tenderness and hypoactive bowel sounds.

Anthropometry

Height	168 cm
IBW	59 ± 3kg
Usual weight	63 kg
Current weight	44 kg
Wrist	6 in
TSF	10 mm
AMC	18 cm

Laboratory

Na	138 mEq/L
K	3.5 mEq/L
Albumin	3.7 gm/dL
Calcium	8.0 mg/dL
Amylase	632 units
Lipase	3.5 cc
Bilirubin	3.5 mg%
Carotene	5.0 mg%
FBS	250 mg%
3 day fecal fat	50 gms/24 hours

Secretin stimulation and duodenal aspiration revealed decreased bicarbonate and total volume and content of pancreatic enzymes.
X-ray revealed calcifications of the pancreas.

Problem List

1. Chronic pancreatitis
2. Jaundice
3. Malabsorption
4. Steatorrhea
5. Diabetes Mellitus 2° to #1

Implications of Findings

Carotene	Elevated due to impaired fat digestion and absorption.
Calcium	Decreased. Fatty acids, released by lipolysis in the abdomen, combine with calcium to form soaps, thus depleting plasma levels of the ion.
FBS	Elevated due to impaired secretion of insulin in response to glucose and inflammatory destruction of islets of Langerhans. It has been suggested that glucagon released from alpha cells may contribute to the elevation of blood glucose.
Fecal Fat	Elevated as a result of impaired digestion of fat due to impaired secretion of pancreatic enzyme. Normal stool fat is 5 - 6 gm/100 gm stool.
Amylase	Elevated due to the liberation of digestive enzymes from the pancreas into neighboring tissues and the blood stream.
Lipase	Elevated due to liberation of lipase from the pancreas into the blood stream.
Bilirubin	Elevated possibly secondary to compression of the distal common duct within the pancreas, calculous biliary stones, or inflammation of the liver and bile ducts.
Decreased Bicarbonate Total Volume, and Enzymes	Due to recurrent attacks of pancreatic inflammation.

Nutrient Needs

Total Calories	Approximately 3000 enteral. Caloric intake should be as high as possible to replace losses from malabsorption.
Protein	Approximately 120 gms per day. Protein is necessary for optimal pancreatic function and to combat the loss of protein.
Fat	50 - 70 gms per day. 20% maximum should be long chain to prevent increased diarrhea. MCT oil may relieve steatorrhea.
CHO	Fifty percent of total calories. Dietary restriction of CHO is generally considered unwarranted in pancreatic diabetes. Concentrated CHO may be restricted because of the associated hyperglycemic peaks.
Pancreatic Enzymes	A replacement of pancreatic enzymes through the administration of pancreatic extracts.
Fluids	Fluid replacement is essential.

Respiratory Management

G.L. is an 87 year old white female, tachypneic, cyanotic, and somewhat delirious, admitted to the hospital where initial exam showed unremarkable auscultation, chest x-ray with some congestion thought to be pulmonary edema. ABG's were 7.25 pH, 55 PO_2 and 55 CO_2. Her respiratory rate was 40. In a state of near exhaustion, an endotracheal tube was placed and she was connected to the respirator.

Initially the patient was thought to have congestive heart failure, but failed to improve with diuresis, and EKG and enzyme confirmation of heart problems was not found. Sputum cultures could not document pneumonia. This patient has "idiopathic pneumonitis," or lung inflammation of unknown origin.

Implications of Findings

ABG's	These numbers indicate she was acidotic, hypoxic and hypercarbic.
Respiratory Rate	Indicates the diagnosis of respiratory failure.

To correct her blood gas abnormalities, she was placed on an IMV of 14, a Vt of 700 and an FiO_2 of 0.6. Her CO_2 was high, so at least 14 breaths per minute at 700 cc were necessary to ventilate her; oxygen was low so 60% (vs 20% room air) was used. At that time, her gases were pH 7.32, pCO_2 44 and pO_2 60. Her ventilation improved, but oxygenation remained poor. Since 70% oxygen and higher is toxic to the lungs and brain, PEEP was added. Her gases were then pH 7.30, pCO_2 50 and pO_2 70. PEEP makes CO_2 worse but O_2 better, a necessary tradeoff.

Nutrient Needs

Total Calories	~1800
Protein	70 gms

Nutrition Care: A decision was made to use tube feedings but she became distended and had diarrhea. Implication: distention adversely affects mechanical respiration by preventing lung expansion. TPN was begun with D50W and 8.5% AAs. Her pCO_2 increased. Implication: oxidation of glucose yields CO_2. In a normal person this is not a problem but in a patient with respiratory compromise, oxidation of even normal calories can dangerously increase pCO_2 and aggravate acidosis. Dextrose was decreased and fat calories increased.

Summary

- Patients with severe respiratory distress require careful evaluation.
- Tachypnea greatly increases caloric requirements.
- Tachypnea increases insensible water loss.
- Oxidation of TPN glucose yields CO_2 and in some cases aggravate acidosis.
- Need to decrease carbohydrate calories and add fat calories.
- IV fats cause fewer problems with CO_2 retention.
- Patients on PEEP may retain CO_2.
- If a respirator patient gets markedly distended, tube feeding is inappropriate secondary to poor lung expansion.

Bone Cancer

Medical History	Twenty eight year old male with a five month history of progressive nausea, vomiting, ascities, constipation and weight loss of 12 kg.
Physical Exam	Emaciated but in no acute distress. Skin pale, with few bruises. Sclerae were icteric due to biliary tract obstruction. Lungs clear; no gallop rhythm or heart mumur; protuberant abdomen is dull to percussion and has a fluid wave; liver measures 15 cm; spleen tip palpable; ankes 1 - 2+ pitting edema; mouth with multiple yellow ulcers of 3 - 6 mm over the gingival, buccal, and palatal mucosa resulting from chemotherapy.

Anthropometry		
	Height	175 cm
	IBW	72 kg
	Usual weight	70 kg
	Current weight	44 kg

Laboratory		
	Na	143 mEq/L
	K	3.54 mEq/L
	Albumin	2.8 gm/dL
	Calcium	11.2 mg/dL
	Cl	100 mEq/L
	CO_2	27 mEq/L
	Creatinine	0.8 mg/dL
	BUN	14 mg/dL
	Prealbumin	7 mg/dL
	FBS	130 mg%
	Mg	2.0 mg
	Phos	5.0 mg/dL
	Hg	10 gm/dL
	HCT	31%
	SGOT	42 U/dL
	Bili	4 mg/dL
	Alkphos	160 IU

Vital Signs		
	BP	100/76
	Temp	37°
	Pulse	100/min
	Respirations	20/min

Drugs	Vincristine sulfate, cyclophosphamide, doxorubicin, methotrexate.
Social History	Lives with supportive parents; is a student at the local university.

Implications of Findings

Albumin	Low; suggests poor nutritional status; decrease in albumin and globulin results from decrease in both protein and synthesis of plasma proteins.
Prealbumin	Indicates inadequate po intake.
Hg	Low; reflects bone marrow depression and poor intake.
SGOT	Elevated. Indicates malfunction of liver cells, a result of chemotherapy.
Bilirubin	Elevated. Suggests obstruction of the bilary tract, probably caused by metastasis.
Alk. Phos.	Elevated. Indicates inflammation of the biliary tract and metastatic bone cancer.
Phos	Increased secondary to bone tumors.
Ca	Increased. Bone metastasis; malignant tumors.

Nutrient Needs: Parenteral Nutrition

Total Calories	Approximately 2200 - 2500 (30 - 35 kcal/kg) to stop weight loss and catabolism.
Protein	Approximately 90 gms per day. Protein is necessary for anabolism.
Fat	Lipids 3 - 4 times per week.
CHO	Fifty percent of total calories. Not to exceed the maximum oxidation rate.
Vitamins	Standard/RDAs.
Fluids	Fluid replacement is essential.

Renal Disease

Medical History	Fifty one year old male with a ten year history of hypertension. Unknown treatment with probable noncompliance.
Physical Exam	Nausea and vomiting, dizziness, lethargy, pallor, stomach cramps, diarrhea, itching, joint and bone pains, oliguria, confused and disoriented. Cardiomegaly with marked edema. Both kidneys are small.

Anthropometry		
	Height	168 cm
	IBW	69 kg
	Usual weight	66 kg (dry)
	Current weight	69 kg

Laboratory		
	Na	129 mEq/L
	K	6.2 mEq/L
	Albumin	2.5 gm/dL
	Calcium	7.5 mg/dL
	Cl	113 mEq/L
	Bicarb	20 mEq/L
	Creatinine	13 mg/dL
	Creatinine clearance	25ml/min
	BUN	160 mg/dL
	Hg	11 gm
	HCT	35.5
	WBC	8000
	Phos	12.4
	Alkphos	250 IU

Vital Signs		
	BP	170/130
	Temp	37°

Drugs	Vincristine sulfate, cyclophosphamide, doxorubicin, methotrexate.
Social History	Lives with supportive wife. Father (deceased) had a twenty year history of HTN. Brother and sister have been treated for nehprolithiasis.

Implications of Findings

Albumin & Prealbumin	Low secondary to renal disease and possible poor intake.
K+	Elevated; indicates impaired renal function and possible tissue destruction.
Na+	Decreased. Indicates dilutional fluid; edema.
BUN	Increased in renal disease. Waste product of protein metabolism; dialysis removes urea nitrogen.
Hg and HCT	Decreased. Excessive fluid. Water overload.
Alkphos & Creatinine	Elevated with impaired renal function.
Phos	Increased secondary to uremia and impaired renal function.
Ca	Decreased secondary to a low albumin.
Edema	Impaired renal function; need to control Na and fluid intake; some may be caused from a decreased albumin.

Nutrient Needs: Patient Placed on Peritoneal Dialysis

Total Calories	Approximately 2200 - 2500 (30 - 35 kcal/kg) to stop weight loss and catabolism.
Protein	Approximately 1.5 gm/kg/day. Higher needs secondary to greater protein losses.
Na	130 mEq (2 - 3 gm/day).
K	40 - 65 mEq/day (2 - 3 gm/day).
Vitamins	Nephrocaps plus Vit E
Fluids	750 ccs plus urine output

Depression and Malnutrition

Medical History	Sixty five year old female admitted to psych unit with depression secondary to a DUI.
Problem List	Depression; malnutrition; 40 - 45# weight loss past two months; severe anorexia; nausea; diarrhea; dehydration; dizziness; lack of self care; ETOH abuse?; pellegra?; scurvy?
Physical Exam	Depressed; malnourished; poor state of hygiene; sores all over hands; rash on chest; sores on elbows; dry skin; skin yellow and sallow; scaly eczemoid rash about upper arms.

Anthropometry		
	Height	157 cm
	IBW	56 kg
	Usual weight	82 - 84 kg
	Current weight	66 kg

Laboratory		
	Na	145 mEq/L
	K	4.2 mEq/L
	Albumin	2.5 gm/dL
	Prealbumin	7.2 mg/dL
	Calcium	8.2 mg/dL
	Glucose	95 mg%
	Creatinine	13 mg/dL
	BUN	19 mg/dL
	Cholesterol	89 mg/dL
	TGs	122 mg/dL
	LDH	370 units/L
	Phos	3.0 mg/dL
	Alk. Phos.	258 IU
	SGOT	203 units/L
	SGPT	96 units/L

Vital Signs		
	BP	110/80
	Temp	37°

Drugs	Antidepressants; Librium; Theragran; Vit B$_6$; Folate.
Social History	Lives alone. College graduate; was selling real estate; is on Medicare; three grown children who are college graduates.

Implications of Findings

Albumin & Prealbumin	Low secondary to poor intake and possible alcoholism.
Ca	Decreased secondary to a low albumin.
Na$^+$	Increased. Dehydration; insufficient intake of fluids.
Cholesterol	Decreased. Low in malnutrition.
SGOT	Increased with liver disease.
SGPT	Increased with liver disease.
Alk. Phos.	Elevated. Indicates liver disease.
Drugs	Medications may contribute to nausea and diarrhea.

Nutrient Needs

Total Calories	Approximately 1600 - 1800 (30 - 35 kcal/kg) to stop weight loss and catabolism.
Protein	70 - 80 gms. Approximately 1.5 gm/kg/day.
Vitamins	Thergran; B_6 and Folate.
Fluids	35 cc/kg plus fluid losses.

AIDS

Medical History	Thirty eight year old male admitted with AIDS.
Physical Exam	Three day history of 101° fever, chills, odynophagia, 9 kg weight loss past two months; 5 - 8 diarrheal stools per day past 2 weeks; nausea and vomiting past 3 days; GI consult reveals CMV in the esophagus; stool culture + for Cryptosporidum.

Anthropometry		
	Height	184 cm
	IBW	76 kg
	Usual weight	73 kg
	Current weight	62 kg

Laboratory		
	Na	142 mEq/L
	K	4.2 mEq/L
	Albumin	2.9 gm/dL
	Prealbumin	15 mg/dL
	Calcium	8.2 mg/dL
	Glucose	95 mg%
	Creatinine	130 mg/dL
	BUN	7 mg/dL
	Creatinine	0.6 mg/dL
	Hg	14 gm/dL
	HCT	38%
	CD_4	200

Vital Signs		
	BP	130/80
	HR	85/min
	Temp	38°

Drugs	ATZ
Social History	Lives with supportive wife and 3 children. College graduate; worked as an engineer.

Implications of Findings

Albumin & Prealbumin	Low secondary to poor intake.
Ca	Decreased secondary to a low albumin.
CD_4	Low; indicative of AIDS.
Drugs	Medications may contribute to nausea and diarrhea.

Nutrient Needs: TPN

Total Calories	Approximately 2100 - 2400 (30 - 35 kcal/kg) to stop weight loss and catabolism.
Protein	Approximately 100 gm (1.5 gm/kg/day)
Fluids	35 cc/kg plus fluid losses.

ABBREVIATIONS

A	Assessment
AA	Amino acid
aa	Amount to be taken
ac	Before meals
AB	Abortion
abd	Abdomen
ABW	Actual/average body weight
ABG	Arterial blood gases
ACH	Adrenocortical hormone
ACLS	Advanced coronary life support
ACTH	Adrenocorticotropic hormone
ad lib	As desired
ADH	Antidiuretic hormone
ADL	Activities of daily life
adm	Admission
AGA	Appropriate for gestational age
AI	Aortic insufficiency
AIDS	Acquired immune deficiency syndrome
AKA	Above knee amputation
alb	Albumin
alk phos	Alkaline phosphatase
ALL	Acute lymphocytic leukemia
AM	Morning
AMA	Against medical advice
amb	Ambulate
AML	Acute (myeloid) (monocytic) leukemia
AMML	Acute monyelocytic leukemia
Amp	Ampicillin
Amt	Amount
ANLL	Acute nonlymphocytic leukemia
Ao	Aortic
AOB	Alcohol on breath
AODM	Adult onset diabetes mellitus
AP	Anterior-posterior
Aq	Aqueous
ARC	AIDS-related complex
ARDS	Adult respiratory distress syndrome
ARF	Acute renal failure
Art	Arterial
AS	Aortic stenosis
As tol	As tolerated
ASAP	As soon as possible
ASCVD	Arteriosclerotic cardiovascular disease
ASHD	Arterosclerotic heart disease
ASD	Arterial septal defect
ASHD	Ateriosclerotic heart disease
ASMI	Anteroseptal myocardial infarct
ATG	Antithymocyte globulin
AUL	Acute undifferentiated leukemia
AV shunt	Ateriovenous shunt
AV block	Atrioventricular block
AVN	Avascular necrosis
BBT	Basal body temperature
BCAAs	Branch chain amino acids
BEC	Before exam completed
BE	Barium enema
BEE	Basal energy expenditure
BF	Breast feeding

BID	Twice a day	CHI	Closed head injury
BJM	Bones, joints and muscles	CHO	Carbohydrate
BK	Below the knee	Chol	Cholesterol
BKA	Below the knee amputation	CLL	Chronic lymphocytic leukemia
BM	Bowel movement	Cm	Centimeter
BMI	Body mass index	CME	Cystoid macular edema
BMR	Basal metabolic rate	CML	Chronic myelocytic leukemia
BMT	Bone marrow transplant	CNS	Central nervous system
BNO	Bladder neck obstruction	CO2	Carbon dioxide
BP	Blood pressure	Comp	Compound
BPH	Benign prostatic hypertrophy	Cont	Continuously
BR	Bedrest	COPD	Chronic obstructive pulmonary disease
BRP	Bath room priviledges	CPAP	Continuous positive airway pressure
BS	Blood sugar	CPK	Creatinine phosphokinase
BSA	Body surface area	Cpm	Counts per minute
BSS	Balanced salt solution	CPM	Continuous passive motion
BTL	Bilateral tubal ligation	CrCl	Creatinine clearance
BUN	Blood urea nitrogen	CRP	C-reactive protein
BW	Body weight	CT	Computed tomography
BX	Biospy	CTA	Clear to ausculation
CA	Cancer	CTR	Cadaver renal transplant
CABG	Coronary artery bypass graft	CVA	Cerebrovascular accident
CAD	Coronary artery disease	CVP	Central venous pressure
Cal	Calorie	CXR	Chest xray
CAPD	Chronic ambulatory peritoneal dialysis	D	Day
Cath	Catherization	D/c	Discontinue
CBC	Complete blood count	DB	Decibel
CC	Chief complaint	DC	Discharge
CCC	Critical care center	D&C	Dilatation and curettage
CCE	Clubbing, cyanosis or edema	Decub	Decubitus
CCU	Coronary care unit	Def	Deficiency
CF	Cystic fibrosis	DJD	Degenerative joint disease
CHD	Congential heart disease	Dl	Deciliter
CHF	Congestive heart failure	DKA	Diabetic ketoacidosis

DM	Diabetes mellitus		F/U	Follow-up
Dm	Decimeter		FB	Foreign body
DMI	Diaphragmatic myocardial infarction		FBS	Fasting blood sugar
DNA	Deoxyribonucleic acid		FS	Full strength
DOA	Dead on arrival		FSH	Follicle-stimulating hormone
DOB	Date of birth		FTT	Failure to thrive
DOE	Dyspnea on exertion		FUO	Fever of undetermined origin
DOL	Day of life		GA	Gestational age
DR	Diabetic retinopathy		GBD	Gallbladder disease
DS	Discharge summary		GC	Gonorrhea
DTR	Deep tendon reflex		GDM	Gestational diabetes mellitus
DTs	Delirium tremens		G-tube	Gastrostomy tube
DVT	Deep venous thrombosis		Gent	Gentamicin
Dx	Diagnosis		GFR	Glomerular filtration rate
E	Energy		GI	Gastrointestinal tract
ECG	Electrocardiogram		GN	Glomerular nephritis
Echo	Echocardiogram		GSW	Gunshot wound
ECT	Electroconvulsive therapy		GTT	Glucose tolerance test
EDV	End-diastolic volume		GVHD	Graft-versus-host disease
EEG	Electroencephalogram		Gyn	Gynecology
EENT	Eyes, ears, nose, throat		HA	Headache
EFA	Essential fatty acid		HAA	Hepatitis antigen
ELBW	Extremely low birth weight < 1 kg		HBV	High biologic value
EN	Enteral nutrition		Hct	Hematocrit
ESP	End systolic pressure		HD	Hemodialysis, hospital day
ESRD	End stage renal disease		HDL	High-density lipoprotein
ERCP	Endoscopic retrograde cholangiopancreatography		HEENT	Head, eyes, ears, nose and throat
			HEP	Hepatitis
ESR	Erythocyte sedimentation rate		HepB	Hepatitis B
ETA	Estimated time of arrival		HIV	Human immunodeficiency virus
ETOH	Ethanol, ethyl alcohol		HgbA1C	Hemoglobin A1C test (glucose)
EUA	Examination under anesthesia		HHNK	Hyperosmolar hyperglycemic nonketotic syndrome
Fib	Fibrillation			
FiO$_2$	Fractional inspired oxygen concentration		HJR	Hepatojugular reflex
			HM	Hand motion

HR	Heart rate		L	Liter
Hr	Hour		LA	Left atrium
Ht	Height		Lab	Laboratory
HTN	Hypertension		Lac	Laceration
HUS	Hemolytic uremic syndrome		LAD	Left anterior descending
Hx	History		Lap	Laparotomy
Hypo	Hypodermic		LAP	Left atrial pressure
I-CA	Ionized calcium		Lat	Lateral
I&D	Incision and drainage		LBM	Lean body mass
I&O	Intake and output		LBP	Lower back pain
IPD	Intermittent peritoneal dialysis		LBV	Low biologic value
IBW	Ideal body weight		LBW	Low birth weight < 2.5 kg
ICU	Intensive care unit		LCT	Long chain triglycerides
IDDM	Insulin dependent diabetes mellitus		LDH	Lactic acid dehydrogenase
IIC	Intermediate intensive care		LDL	Low-density lipoproteins
IGT	Impaired glucose tolerance		L.E.	Lupus erythematosus
IM	Intramuscular		LES	Lower esophageal sphincter
IMV	Intermittent mandatory ventilation		LFT	Liver function test
Inj	Injection		LGA	Large for gestational age
IPPB	Intermediate positive pressure breathing		LH	Luteinizing hormone
I.U.	International units		LLQ	Left lower quadrant
IUGR	Intrauterine growth retarded		LMP	Last menstrual period
IUP	Intrauterine pregnancy		LRDT	Living related donor transplant
IV	Intravenous(ly)		LS	Lumbosacral
IVF	Intravenous fluids		Lt	Left
IVDA	Intravenous drug abuse		LUQ	Left upper quadrant
J-tube	Jejunostomy tube		LV	Left ventricular
JODM	Juvenile onset diabetes mellitus		Lytes	Electrolytes
JVD	Jugular venous distention		M	Murmur
JVP	Jugular venous pulse		MA	Milliampere
K/P	Kidney/pancreas transplant		MAO	Monoamine oxidase
Kcal	Food kilocalories		MAP	Mean arterial pressure
Kg	Kilogram		MAT	Multifocal atrial tachycardia
KUB	Kidney, ureter, bladder		MCA	Middle cerebral artery

MCL	Midclavicular line	NROM	Normal range of motion
MCP	Metacarpophalangeal (joint)	NS	Normal saline
MD	Muscular dystrophy	NSR	Normal sinus rhythm
Meds	Medications	NSVD	Normal spontaneous vaginal delivery
MG	Myasthenia gravis	N&V	Nausea and vomiting
MI	Myocardial infarction	O	Objective
MN	Midnight	Ocs	Oral contraceptives
MODM	Maturity onset diabetes mellitus	OD	Overdose
MOF	Multiple organ failure	OFC	Head circumference
MR	Mitral regurgitation	OHD	Organic heart disease
MRI	Magnetic resonance imaging	OLT	Orthotopic liver transplant
MS	Multiple sclerosis, mental status	OOB	Out of bed
Msec	Millisecond	OP	Operation
MVA	Motor vehicle accident	OR	Operating room
MVI	Multiple vitamins intravenously	Osm	Osmolality
MVR	Mitral valve replacement	OTC	Over-the-counter
N	Noon	P	Pulse
NAD	No acute distress	P2	Pulmonary second sound
NC	Noncontributory	PA	Postero-anterior
NEC	Necrotizing entercolitis	PAC	Premature atrial contraction
NED	No evidence of disease	Pc	After meals
Neg	Negative	PAP	Pulmonary artery pressure
NG	Nasogastric	Pap smear	Papanicolaou smear
NH	Nursing home	Para	Paraplegic
Ni	No improvement	PAT	Paroxysmal atrial tachycardia
NIA	Nutrient intake analysis	PCM	Protein calorie malnutrition
NIDDM	Non-insulin dependent diabetes mellitus	PCO_2	Partial pressure of carbon dioxide
		PCR	Protein catabolic rate
NINK	No information/not keeping	PD	Peritoneal dialysis
Nl	Normal	PDR	Proliferative diabetic retinopathy
Noc	Night	PE	Pulmonary embolus
NPC	Nodal premature contraction	PEEP	Positive end-expiratory pressure
NPDR	Nonproliferative diabetic retinopathy	PEM	Protein energy malnutrition
NPN	Non-protein nitrogen	PERRLA	Pupils equal, round, reactive to light & accommodation
NPO	Nil per os (nothing by mouth)		

PID	Pelvic inflammatory disease		PTA	Prior to admission
PIH	Pregnancy-induced hypertension		PFT	Pulmonary function test
PIP	Peak inspiratory pressure		PUD	Peptic ulcer disease
PKU	Phenylketonuria		PVC	Premature ventricular contraction
PM	Afternoon		PVD	Peripheral vascular disease
PN	Parenteral nutrition		R	Respiration
PPN	Peripheral parenteral nutrition		R/O	Rule out
PND	Paroxysmal nocturnal dyspnea		RA	Right atrium, room air
PNS	Peripheral nerve stimulator		RBC	Red blood cell count
PNV	Prenatal vitamins		RDS	Respiratory distress syndrome
PO	Per os (by mouth)		REE	Resting energy expenditure
Post-op	Postoperative		Ref	Reference
POD	Post operative day		REM	Rapid eye movement
PP	Post partum		RI	Renal insufficiency
PML	Premature labor		RLQ	Right lower quadrant
PTL	Preterm labor		RQ	Respiratory quotient
Q	Every		RR	Respiratory rate
QAM	Every morning		RRR	Regular rate and rhythm
Qd	Every day		RS	Reducing substances
Qhr	Every hour		Rt	Right
Qid	Four times a day		RUQ	Right upper quadrant
Qnoc	Every night		RV	Right ventricle
Qhs	Every bedtime		Rx	Prescription
Qod	Every other day		Rxn	Reaction
Qs	Every shift		S	Subjective
Q(number)hr	Every (number) hours		S/P	Status post
Quad	Quadriplegic		SAB	Spontaneous abortion
PRBC	Packed red blood cells		SBE	Subacute bacterial endocarditis
Premie	Premature < 36 weeks		SBO	Small bowel obstruction
PRN	Pro re nata (as needed)		SCI	Spinal cord injury
Pre-op	Preoperative		SGA	Small for gestational age
Prep	Prepare		SI	Small intestines
Psi	Pounds per square inch		SIADH	Syndrome of inappropriate antidiuretic hormone
Pt	Patient		SIDS	Sudden infant death syndrome

SLE	Systemic lupus erythematosus		URI	Upper respiratory infection
SOB	Shortness of breath		U/S	Ultrasound
STAT	Immediately		UTI	Urinary tract infection
STD	Sexually transmitted disease		UUN	Urine urea nitrogen
Strep	Streptococcus		Vag	Vaginal
Subq	Subcutaneous		VC	Vital capacity
Surg	Surgery		Ve	Minute ventilation
Sx	Symptoms		VE	Vaginal examination
Synd	Syndrome		VD	Veneral disease
SZ	Seizure		VLBW	Very low birth weight < 1.5 kg
T, temp	Temperature		VMA	Vanillymandelic acid
T,C,DB	Turn, cough, deep breath		VO_2 max	Maximum oxygen uptake
TAH	Total abdominal hysterectomy		VOD	Venous occlusive disease
T & C	Type and crossmatch		VSD	Ventricular septal defect
TIA	Transient ischemic attack		VT	Tidal volume
TID	Three times a day		VZV	Varicella zoster virus
TF	Tube feeding		W/O	Without
TKO	To keep open		W/U	Workup
TM	Tympanum membrani (eardrum)		WAIS	Wechsler Adult Intelligence Scale
TJM	Temporomandibular joint		WB	Whole blood
TLC	Total lung capacity		WBC	White blood cell count
TNM	Tumor, node, metastases		WNL	Within normal limits
TOP	Termination of pregnancy		WS	Watt seconds
TPE	Total pelvic exenteration		Wt	Weight
TPN	Total parenteral nutrition		Wx	Wound
TPR	Temperature, pulse, respiration		X	Times
Trach	Tracheostomy		XRT	Xray therapy/treatment
TUN	Total urine nitrogen			
TUR(P)	Transurethral resection (of prostrate)			
TX	Transplant			
U	Unit			
UA	Urinalysis			
UBW	Usual body weight			
UGI	Upper gastrointestinal			

MISCELLANEOUS INFORMATION

Milliequivalent / milligram Terms

Milligrams (mg):	Describes mass or weight of an element. Limited usage because atoms react on the basis of equivalent numbers and charges; i.e., NaCl is not 50% Na^+ and 50% Cl^-.
Equivalent (mEq):	Amount of a particular element that can react completely with an equivalent amount of another element. Takes into account molecular weight and charge of a substance.
Mole (mol):	Weight in grams equal to numerical molecular weight of element divided by valence; i.e., molecular weight of Na^+ is 23, therefore, 1 mole of Na^+ = 23 grams.
Milliosmol (mOsm):	Total number of milliequivalents dissolved in solution.

Milliequivalent/milligram Conversions

To determine milliequivalents of an electrolyte, divide milligrams by the atomic weight of the element. Multiply the result by the valence.

$$mEq = (\text{mg of an element} / \text{atomic weight}) \times (\text{valance})$$

To determine milligrams of an electrolyte multiply the equivalents by the atomic weight. Divide the results by the valence.

$$mg = (mEq \times \text{atomic weight}) / (\text{valence})$$

Table 1: Atomic Weight and Valence

Electrolyte	Atomic Weight	Valence
Sodium	23.0	1
Potassium	39.0	1
Magnesium	24.3	2
Calcium	40.0	2
Chloride	35.5	1
Phosphorus	31.0	2
Zinc	65.37	2

Table 2: Weights and Measures

Unit	Abbreviation	Equivalents
Ounce	oz	28.35 gm, 8 dr
Pound	lb	453.6 gm
Grain	gr	.0666 gm
Gram	gm	1000 mg, 5 gr, .0353 oz
Kilogram	kg	1000 gm, 2.205 lb
Milligram	mg	1000 mcg, .001 gm
Microgram	mcg/µg	1000 ng, 10^{-6} gm
Nanogram	ng	1000 pg, .001 mcg, 10^{-9} gm
Picogram	pg	.001 ng, 10^{-12} gm
Dram	dr	60 gr
Minim	M	0.166 fl dr
Cubic centimeter	cc	1000 mm³, 1 ml
Milliliter	ml	.001 L, .0352 fl oz
Liter	L	1.05 qt, 33.8 oz
Deciliter	dl	.1 L, 100 ml
Cubic millimeter	mm	3 .001 cc
Microliter	uL	.000001 L, .001 ml
Milligram percent	mg%	mg/1000 ml
Tablespoon	TB	15 ml, 15 gm, 0.5 oz
Teaspoon	tsp	5 ml, 5 gm, 0.16 oz
Fluid ounce	fl oz	30 cc, .03 L, 8 dr
Pint	pt	473 cc, .473 L, 16 fl oz
Quart	qt	946 cc, .946 L, 32 fl oz
Inch	in	2.54 cm, .025 m
Foot	ft	30.48 cm, .305 m
Yard	yd	.914 m
Mile	mi	1.609 km
Meter	m	1000 mm, 3.25 ft
Centimeter	cm	10 mm, .39 in
Millimeter	mm	.1 cm, .001 m, .039 in
Cubic centimeter	cm³	.001 cc

Centi	c	10^{-2}	
Milli	m	10^{-3}	
Micro	u/µ	10^{-6}	
Nano	n	10^{-9}	
Pico	p	10^{-12}	
Femto	f	10^{-15}	
Atto	a	10^{-18}	

Table 3: Approximate pH of Certain Beverages

Beverage	pH	Beverage	pH
Carbonated			
Club soda	4.7	Cider	2.9 to 3.3
Cream soda	3.9	Cranberry	2.5 to 2.7
Cherry soda	3.0	Currant	3.0
Cola	2.4	Grapefruit	2.9 to 3.4
Ginger ale (dry)	2.7	Grape	3.5 to 4.5
Grape	3.0	Lemon	2.2 to 2.6
Grapefruit	3.0	Lime	2.2 to 2.4
Lemon	2.9	Pineapple	3.4 to 3.7
Lemon-lime	3.1	Prune	3.7 to 4.3
Orange	3.2	Tomato	3.9 to 4.4
Quinine	2.5		
Other Beverages			
Raspberry	3.1	Milk (cow's)	6.4 to 6.8
Root beer	4.0	Milk (evaporated)	5.9 to 6.3
Sarsaparilla	4.0	Milk (acidophilus)	4.0
Canned Juices		Buttermilk	4.5
Cherry	3.4 to 3.6	Beer	4.0 to 5.0
Wines	2.3 to 3.8		

ARM ANTHROPOMETRY NOMOGRAM FOR ADULTS AND CHILDREN

To obtain Arm Muscle Area: Lay a ruler between the values for arm circumference and triceps skinfold. Read arm muscle area where the ruler crosses the center line. *Note:* Values in the nomogram have not been adjusted for bone area. (Subtract 10 cm² for men and 6.5 cm² for women).

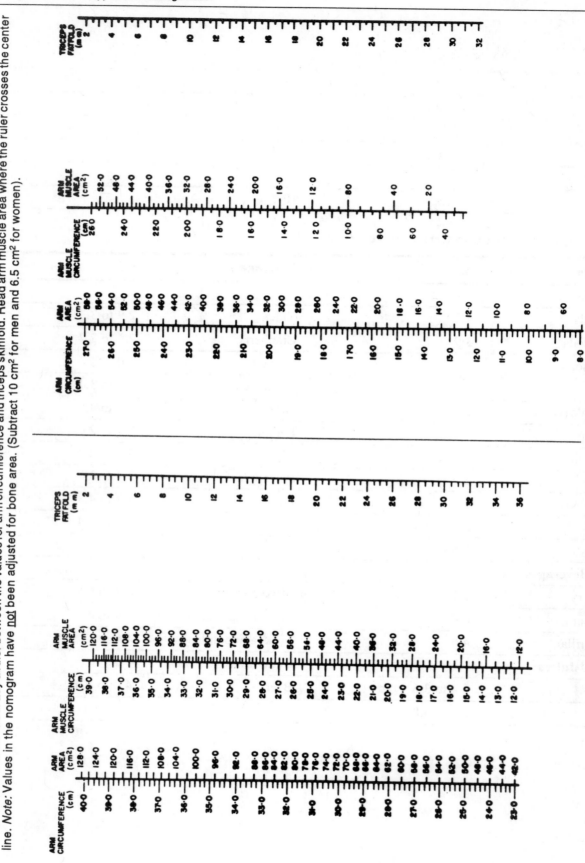

Reproduced with permission from: Gurney, J. and Jelliffe, D.: Arm anthropometry in nutritional assessment: nomogram for rapid calculation of muscle circumference and cross-sectional muscle and fat areas. Amer. J. Clin. Nutr. 26:912, 1973.

INDEX

Please send me ———— copies of **Nutrition Assessment, Support and Management**

Name _____

Address _____

City _____ State/Province _____

County _____ Zip _____

Daytime Telephone (   ) _____ _____ Copies at $40.00 each $_____

Send check or money order to:
Anne Grant/Susan DeHoog
  P.O. Box 75057
    Northgate Station
    Seattle, WA 98125
(206) 362-9323 or (425) 885-2849

Please allow 3-4 weeks for delivery

Make Check or money order payable to
Anne Grant or Susan DeHoog

Washington residents add state $ _____
and local sales tax

Postage and handling $4.00 $_____
Each additional book add $2.00
Canada $6.00
Other $10.00

Payable in U.S. Funds Only

Total Enclosed $_____

▶▶▶◀◀◀◀

Please send me ———— copies of **Nutrition Assessment, Support and Management**

Name _____

Address _____

City _____ State/Province _____

County _____ Zip _____

Daytime Telephone (   ) _____ _____ Copies at $40.00 each $_____

Send check or money order to:
Anne Grant/Susan DeHoog
  P.O. Box 75057
    Northgate Station
    Seattle, WA 98125
(206) 362-9323 or (425) 885-2849

Please allow 3-4 weeks for delivery

Make Check or money order payable to
Anne Grant or Susan DeHoog

Washington residents add state $ _____
and local sales tax

Postage and handling $4.00 $_____
Each additional book add $2.00
Canada $6.00
Other $10.00

Payable in U.S. Funds Only

Total Enclosed $_____